AF700430

Tech, Sex and Health

This book presents recent sociological research investigating the intersection of technology, human sexuality, and health.

Rapid advances within biomedical, biomechanical, and biodigital domains have prompted scholarly exploration into the ways these technologies are being integrated into, or are reshaping, human sexual and intimate practices and the resulting health implications. Scholarship has also focused on the potential for new technologies to extend the imagined, and real, possibilities for enhancing human sexual experiences. The chapters in this book delve into the interconnected themes of sex, health, bodies, and risk in relation to emerging technologies. They illuminate the intricate interplay between human bodies, sexual practices and technologies, spotlight how novel technologies and human practices collaboratively shape or remodel cultures of sex and intimacy, and critically interrogate the discourses of risk and pleasure that frame our understanding of technology and sex.

Researchers within the fields of sociology, technology studies, human sexuality, and health, as well as educators and professionals seeking a comprehensive understanding of how people engage with technologies in their intimate relationships and sex lives, will find this collection engaging and informative. Additionally, individuals interested in the cultural, societal, and ethical implications of emerging technologies in relation to sexual experiences and health will also benefit from the insights presented in this volume. The chapters in this book were originally published in several journals, including *Health Sociology Review*, *Journal of Gender Studies*, and *Information & Communications Technology Law*.

Jennifer Power is a Principal Research Fellow based at the Australian Research Centre in Sex, Health and Society at La Trobe University, Melbourne, Australia. Her work focuses on sexuality and sexual health, including sexual health among young people, LGBTQA+ health and wellbeing and quality of life among people living with HIV.

Andrea Waling is Senior Lecturer in the School of Psychology and Public Health, and a Senior Research Fellow at the Australian Research Centre in Sex, Health and Society at La Trobe University, Melbourne, Australia. Her research examines men, bodies, technologies, sex, and sexuality, and LGBTIQ+ health and well-being. Her most recent book is *Exploring the Cultural Phenomenon of the Dick Pic* (2023).

Tech, Sex and Health

The Place of New Technologies in Sex, Sexual Health, and Human Intimacy

Edited by
Jennifer Power and Andrea Waling

Routledge
Taylor & Francis Group
LONDON AND NEW YORK

First published 2024
by Routledge
4 Park Square, Milton Park, Abingdon, Oxon OX14 4RN

and by Routledge
605 Third Avenue, New York, NY 10158

Routledge is an imprint of the Taylor & Francis Group, an informa business

Introduction © 2024 Jennifer Power and Andrea Waling
Chapters 4–11 © 2024 Taylor & Francis
Chapter 1 © 2022 Jennifer Power, Lily Moor, Joel Anderson, Andrea Waling, Alexandra James, Nicole Shackleton, Anne-Maree Farrell, Elizabeth Agnew and Gary W. Dowsett. Originally published as Open Access.
Chapter 2 © 2022 Anne-Maree Farrell, Nicole Shackleton, Elizabeth Agnew, Samantha Hopkins and Jennifer Power. Originally published as Open Access.
Chapter 3 © 2023 Jennifer Power, Gary W. Dowsett, Andrea Waling, Alexandra James, Lily Moor, Nicole Shackleton and Anne-Maree Farrell. Originally published as Open Access.

With the exception of Chapters 1, 2 and 3, no part of this book may be reprinted or reproduced or utilised in any form or by any electronic, mechanical, or other means, now known or hereafter invented, including photocopying and recording, or in any information storage or retrieval system, without permission in writing from the publishers. For details on the rights for Chapters 1, 2 and 3, please see the chapters' Open Access footnotes.

Trademark notice: Product or corporate names may be trademarks or registered trademarks, and are used only for identification and explanation without intent to infringe.

British Library Cataloguing in Publication Data
A catalogue record for this book is available from the British Library

ISBN13: 978-1-032-71681-7 (hbk)
ISBN13: 978-1-032-71684-8 (pbk)
ISBN13: 978-1-032-71685-5 (ebk)

DOI: 10.4324/9781032716855

Typeset in Minion Pro
by Newgen Publishing UK

Publisher's Note
The publisher accepts responsibility for any inconsistencies that may have arisen during the conversion of this book from journal articles to book chapters, namely the inclusion of journal terminology.

Disclaimer
Every effort has been made to contact copyright holders for their permission to reprint material in this book. The publishers would be grateful to hear from any copyright holder who is not here acknowledged and will undertake to rectify any errors or omissions in future editions of this book.

Contents

Citation Information

The following chapters were originally published in various volumes and issues of the journals *Sexual Health*; *Information & Communications Technology Law*; *Sexuality Research and Social Policy*; *Health Sociology Review*; and *Journal of Gender Studies*. When citing this material, please use the original page numbering for each article, as follows:

Chapter 1

Traversing TechSex: benefits and risks in digitally mediated sex and relationships
Jennifer Power, Lily Moor, Joel Anderson, Andrea Waling, Alexandra James, Nicole Shackleton, Anne-Maree Farrell, Elizabeth Agnew and Gary W. Dowsett
Sexual Health, volume 19, issue 1 (2022), pp. 55–69

Chapter 2

Regulating tech-sex and managing image-based sexual abuse: an Australian perspective
Anne-Maree Farrell, Nicole Shackleton, Elizabeth Agnew, Samantha Hopkins and Jennifer Power
Information & Communications Technology Law, volume 32, issue 2 (2023), pp. 189–206

Chapter 3

Rethinking Risk in Adults' Engagement with Sexual Digital Imagery
Jennifer Power, Gary W. Dowsett, Andrea Waling, Alexandra James, Lily Moor, Nicole Shackleton and Anne-Maree Farrell
Sexuality Research and Social Policy (2023), DOI: 10.1007/s13178-023-00844-w

Chapter 4

Dating apps as public health 'problems': cautionary tales and vernacular pedagogies in news media
Kath Albury, Anthony McCosker, Tinonee Pym and Paul Byron
Health Sociology Review, volume 29, issue 3 (2020), pp. 232–248

Chapter 5

'I don't think my torso is anything to write home about': men's reflexive production of 'authentic' photos for online dating platforms
Andrea Waling, Michael Kehler, Jennifer Power, Lucille Kerr and Adam Bourne
Journal of Gender Studies, volume 32, issue 5 (2023), pp. 471–485

Chapter 6

Building community, one swipe at a time: hook-up apps and the production of intimate publics between women
Jonathan Petrychyn, Diana C. Parry and Corey W. Johnson
Health Sociology Review, volume 29, issue 3 (2020), pp. 249–263

Chapter 7

'It's like getting an Uber for sex': social networking apps as spaces of risk and opportunity in the Philippines among men who have sex with men
Brooke Maria Hollingshead, Gary W. Dowsett and Adam Bourne
Health Sociology Review, volume 29, issue 3 (2020), pp. 264–278

Chapter 8

Data-driven intimacy: emerging technologies in the (re)making of sexual subjects and 'healthy' sexuality
Jacinthe Flore and Kiran Pienaar
Health Sociology Review, volume 29, issue 3 (2020), pp. 279–293

Chapter 9

Conceptualising the continuum of female genital fashioning practices
Alexandra James, Jennifer Power and Andrea Waling
Health Sociology Review, volume 29, issue 3 (2020), pp. 294–311

Chapter 10

The age of LARC: making sexual citizens on the frontiers of technoscientific healthism
Jenny Dyck Brian, Patrick R. Grzanka and Emily S. Mann
Health Sociology Review, volume 29, issue 3 (2020), pp. 312–328

Chapter 11

Producing bodies at risk in sexual health – an ethnographic comparative analysis between the combined oral contraceptive pill and pre-exposure prophylaxis in Switzerland
Marlyse Debergh
Health Sociology Review, volume 29, issue 3 (2020), pp. 329–343

For any permission-related enquiries please visit:
www.tandfonline.com/page/help/permissions

Notes on Contributors

Elizabeth Agnew, School of Law, Queens University, Ireland.

Kath Albury, Swinburne University of Technology, Hawthorn, Australia.

Joel Anderson, Australian Research Centre in Sex, Health and Society, La Trobe University; School of Psychology, Australian Catholic University, Melbourne, Australia.

Adam Bourne, Australian Research Centre in Sex, Health and Society, La Trobe University, Bundoora, Australia.

Jenny Dyck Brian, The Honors College, Arizona State University, Tempe, AZ, USA.

Paul Byron, University of Technology, Sydney, Australia.

Marlyse Debergh, Faculty of Social and Behavioural Sciences, University of Amsterdam, Netherlands.

Gary W. Dowsett, Australian Research Centre in Sex, Health and Society, La Trobe University, Melbourne; Centre for Social Research in Health, UNSW, Sydney, Australia.

Anne-Maree Farrell, Edinburgh Law School, University of Edinburgh, Edinburgh, United Kingdom.

Jacinthe Flore, University of Melbourne, Melbourne, Victoria, Australia.

Patrick R. Grzanka, Department of Psychology, The University of Tennessee, Knoxville, TN, USA.

Brooke Maria Hollingshead, Australian Research Centre in Sex, Health and Society, La Trobe University, Melbourne, Australia.

Samantha Hopkins, School of Law, Queen's University Belfast, Belfast, UK.

Alexandra James, Australian Research Centre in Sex, Health and Society, La Trobe University, Melbourne, Australia.

Corey W. Johnson, Department of Parks, Recreation and Tourism Management, College of Natural Resources, NC State University, USA.

Michael Kehler, Werklund School of Education, University of Calgary, Calgary, Canada.

Lucille Kerr, Australian Research Centre in Sex, Health and Society, La Trobe University, Bundoora, Australia.

Emily S. Mann, Department of Health Promotion, Education, and Behavior, University of South Carolina, Columbia, SC, USA.

Anthony McCosker, Swinburne University of Technology, Hawthorn, Australia.

Lily Moor, Australian Research Centre in Sex, Health and Society, La Trobe University, Melbourne, Australia.

Diana C. Parry, Department of Recreation and Leisure Studies, University of Waterloo, Waterloo, Canada.

Jonathan Petrychyn, Ryerson University, Ontario, Canada.

Kiran Pienaar, School of Humanities and Social Sciences, Deakin University, Melbourne, Australia.

Jennifer Power, Australian Research Centre in Sex, Health and Society, La Trobe University, Melbourne, Australia.

Tinonee Pym, Swinburne University of Technology, Hawthorn, Australia.

Nicole Shackleton, Australian Research Centre in Sex, Health and Society, La Trobe University, Melbourne, Australia.

Andrea Waling, School of Psychology and Public Health, Australian Research Centre in Sex, Health and Society, La Trobe University, Melbourne, Australia.

Introduction

Jennifer Power and Andrea Waling

This updated special edition brings together new sociological work exploring the nexus between technology, human sexuality and health. In recent decades, rapid advances in biomedical, biomechanical and biodigital technologies have inspired scholarship that seeks to understand the ways in which practices of sex and intimacy are being transformed by such technologies and the implications this has for health. For example, scholars have tracked the biomedicalisation of sexuality, charting the rising prominence of pharmaceuticals such as Viagra and Flibanserin ('female Viagra') that have redefined cultural perceptions of 'normal' sexual desire and function (Flore, 2018). Meanwhile, new biomechanical products for sex have filtered into public imagination via sensationalised media reports of lifelike sex robots (Sparrow, 2017), sex via virtual reality, or haptic technologies to communicate using simulated touch (Elsey, van Andel, Kater, Reints, & Spiering, 2019). These technologies produce unprecedented possibilities for imagining the augmentation of human sexual bodies. This is occurring in the context of advances in biodigitally enabled apps and global communication networks that facilitate intimate human connection over vast distances (Attwood, Hakim, & Winch, 2017; Renold & Ringrose, 2017). The papers in this collection explore themes of sex, health, bodies and risk in relation to new technologies. They reveal the complex ways in which these themes are intertwined, focusing on how new technologies and human action collaboratively produce or transform sexual and intimate cultures and sexual subjectivities.

We open with Power and colleagues (2022) who collected survey data on adult digital sexual practices during COVID-19 social lockdown periods. COVID-19 marked a significant time in the uptake of technology for social connection (Duguay, Dietzel, & Myles, 2022). The findings from this survey show the commonplace role that technologies play in people's intimate lives and relationships, mostly in the form of dating apps, pornography and sexual image sharing. Many participants acknowledged that digital connectivity could support emotional or sexual connection with their partners or potential partners although there were concerns, particularly among women, about non-consensual exposure of intimate images.

Building on the theme of risk, Farrell et al., (2023) utilise a case study focused on the management of image-based sexual abuse (ISBA) within Australia's recently reformed online safety laws. The response to ISBA has largely focused on criminal law. In this paper, the authors advocate a regulatory approach that recognises the increasing role digital technologies play in people's intimate lives and respects adult sexual agency, while seeking to prevent and respond to harms. In part this involves mobilising sufficient political will to engender and, where possible, enforce commitment to appropriate standards across the technology industry.

Continuing the theme of risk and benefits of new technologies, Power et al., (2023) present findings from a qualitative study about Australian adult's use of digital imagery in their sex lives. Study participants described the creation and sharing of sexual images as a practice which fostered intimacy, sexual tension, and eroticism within their relationships. While some participants were wary of non-consensual exposure, the sense of risk and vulnerability often contributed to an enhanced sense of trust, intimacy or eroticism.

Each of the above papers critiques and reframes narratives of risk in research on sex and new technologies. Building on this, Albury and colleagues (2020) interrogate the production of media discourses that uncritically position dating apps as a social problem through analysis of the relationship between media reporting and research. Albury et al. (2020) identify a strand of media reporting that educates people about enjoyable and safe use of dating apps in a way that does not entrench risk narratives.

Waling et al., (2022) explore men's engagement with dating apps, specifically delving into the emerging emphasis on body image among cisgender, heterosexual men and their sentiments regarding dating app profile pictures. Drawing insights from interviews with cisgender, heterosexual men in Australia, this study investigates men's construction of dating app profile pictures, specifically the decisions they make about the content of these images. The authors argue that the men in the study strived to portray their authentic selves online while grappling with concerns about body image and conflicting desires to convey a muscular, athletic image while not appearing vain or narcissistic.

Petrychyn et al. (2020) similarly focus their discussion away from hook-up apps as a social problem to explore their role in developing 'intimate publics'. This paper draws attention to unexpected outcomes of dating app technology, focusing on intimacy that is created through common use of these apps in everyday life, not just between people who meet potential sexual partners via the apps. A sense of intimacy and sociability develops between women who use the apps based on shared experiences, familiarity and conversations about their app use.

Hollingshead et al. (2020) also look beyond the prescribed function of hook-up and social networking apps to make sense of how they are transforming sexual cultures among men who have sex with men (MSM) in the Philippines. The authors argue that networking apps have agentic capacity to transform sexual networks and subjectivities among MSM, and that this has implications for how we may approach HIV prevention. Flore and Pienaar (2020) draw on similar themes to explore the agentic capacity of technologies in their study of marketing discourse and the function of wireless-enabled sex toys (teledildonics). Flore and Piennar utilise the concept of 'sexuotechnical-assemblages' to encourage us to think about wireless sex toys not as objects that reflect cultural or gendered norms, but as objects that have potential to bring into being new sexual cultures and subjectivities. This is produced through an assemblage of human sexual desire, gendered cultural scripts and teledildonic products.

Three papers engage with the relationship between new technologies and women's bodies. James et al. (2020) explore young women's perceptions of genital modification using old and new technologies for hair removal (razors, wax), adornment (tattooing, vajazzling), or cosmetic surgery (labiaplasty). The authors argue that the high public profile of new surgical technologies reduces the extent to which young women perceive 'old' technologies and everyday practices, such as pubic hair-removal, to be product of gendered beauty standards. Brian et al. (2020) present a critical reading of reproductive health policy in relation to Long Acting Reversible Contraception (LARC). Discourses of freedom, choice and empowerment for women have long been associated with the contraceptive pill. However, the authors argue that these discourses of health and empowerment obscure the ways reproductive health policy relating to LARC limits reproductive choice for women who are culturally positioned as irresponsible or 'risky', something often determined along lines of race and class. Debergh's (2020) paper examines clinical encounters in which the bodies of women seeking access to The Pill, or men seeking pre-exposure prophylaxis (PreP), are assessed as 'safe' or 'risky'. Bodies that are unable to tolerate medical contraception or PrEP, usually due to medical conditions such as high blood pressure, are deemed 'risky' sexual bodies, expanding the reach of biomedicine in shaping human sexuality.

This special issue provides a backdrop for exploring the relationships between technology and practices of human intimacy and sexual connection. Our aim is to look broadly at processes through which technologies materialise sexual practices and intimacies and the ways in which commercial markets, policy and health promotion form part of this. Technologies are not simply neutral objects that we use to fulfil our needs. Nor do they determine how we live our lives. Rather, technologies are part of human intimacies and part of human sexual practices. Our aim with this collection of papers is to explore how technologies and human practices are shaping each other in, often, unpredictable ways.

References

Albury, K., McCosker, A., Pym, T., & Byron, P. (2020). Dating apps as public health 'problems': Cautionary tales and vernacular pedagogies in news media. *Health Sociology Review*. https://doi.org/10.1080/14461242.2020.1777885

Attwood, F., Hakim, J., & Winch, A. (2017). Mediated intimacies: Bodies, technologies and relationships. *Journal of Gender Studies*, *26*(3), 249–253. https://doi.org/10.1080/09589236.2017.1297888

Brian, J., Grzanka, P. R., & Mann, E. S. (2020). The age of LARC: Making sexual citizens on the frontiers of technoscientific healthism. *Health Sociology Review*. https://doi.org/10.1080/14461242.2020.1784018

Debergh, M. (2020). Producing bodies at risk in sexual health – An ethnographic comparative analysis between the combined oral contraceptive pill and pre-exposure prophylaxis in Switzerland. *Health Sociology Review*. https://doi.org/10.1080/14461242.2020.1823870

Duguay, S., Dietzel, C., & Myles, D. (2022). The year of the 'virtual date': Reimagining dating app affordances during the COVID-19 pandemic. *New Media & Society*, 14614448211072257. https://doi.org/10.1177/14614448211072257

Elsey, J. W., van Andel, K., Kater, R. B., Reints, I. M., & Spiering, M. (2019). The impact of virtual reality versus 2D pornography on sexual arousal and presence. *Computers in Human Behavior*, *97*, 35–43.

Farrell, A.-M., Shackleton, N., Agnew, E., Hopkins, S., & Power, J. (2023). Regulating tech-sex and managing image-based sexual abuse: An Australian perspective. *Information & Communications Technology Law*, *32*(2), 189–206. https://doi.org/10.1080/13600834.2022.2119208

Flore, J. (2018). Pharmaceutical intimacy: Managing female sexuality through Addyi. *Sexualities*, *21*(4), 569–586.

Flore, J., & Pienaar, J. (2020). Data-driven intimacy: Emerging technologies in the (re)making of sexual subjects and 'healthy' sexuality. *Health Sociology Review*. https://doi.org/10.1080/14461242.2020.1803101

Hollingshead, B., Dowsett, G. W., & Bourne, A. (2020). 'It's like getting an Uber for sex': Social networking apps as spaces of risk and opportunity in the Philippines among men who have sex with men. *Health Sociology Review*. https://doi.org/10.1080/14461242.2020.1820366

James, A., Power, J., & Waling, A. (2020). Conceptualising the continuum of female genital fashioning practices. *Health Sociology Review*. https://doi.org/10.1080/14461242.2020.1811749

Petrychyn, J., Parry, D. C., & Johnson, C. W. (2020). Building community, one swipe at a time: Hook-up apps and the production of intimate publics between women. *Health Sociology Review*. https://doi.org/10.1080/14461242.2020.1779106

Power, J., Dowsett, G. W., Waling, A., James, A., Moor, L., Shackleton, N., & Farrell, A.-M. (2023). Rethinking risk in adults' engagement with sexual digital imagery. *Sexuality Research and Social Policy*. https://doi.org/10.1007/s13178-023-00844-w

Power, J., Moor, L., Anderson, J., Waling, A., James, A., Shackleton, N., Farrell, A.-M., Agnew, E., & Dowsett, G. W. (2022). Traversing TechSex: Benefits and risks in digitally mediated sex and relationships. *Sexual Health*, 19(1), 55–69.

Renold, E., & Ringrose, J. (2017). Selfies, relfies and phallic tagging: Posthuman part-icipations in teen digital sexuality assemblages. *Educational Philosophy and Theory*, *49*(11), 1066–1079.

Sparrow, R. (2017). Robots, rape, and representation. *International Journal of Social Robotics*, *9*(4), 465–477.

Waling, A., Kehler, M., Power, J., Kerr, L., & Bourne, A. (2022). 'I don't think my torso is anything to write home about': Men's reflexive production of 'authentic' photos for online dating platforms. *Journal of Gender Studies*, *32* (4), 1–15. https://doi.org/10.1080/09589236.2022.2027236

Open Access

Traversing TechSex: benefits and risks in digitally mediated sex and relationships

Jennifer Power, Lily Moor, Joel Anderson, Andrea Waling, Alexandra James, Nicole Shackleton, Anne-Maree Farrell, Elizabeth Agnew and Gary W. Dowsett

ABSTRACT

Background Digital technologies play a significant role in people's sexual and intimate lives via smart phones, cameras, dating apps and social media. Although there is a large body of research on the potential risks posed by these technologies, research on benefits and pleasures is limited. **Methods** This study explored digital sexual practices, including perceptions of risks and benefits among a sample of Australian adults ($n = 445$). Data were collected in 2020 via an online survey. Descriptive and bivariate analyses were undertaken to identify significant relationships between demographic variables and the use of technologies in relation to perceived risks and benefits. The mean age of participants was 42 years, over half were women (58.5%) and identified as heterosexual (61.1%). **Results** Findings reveal that use of digital media was common in participants' sex lives and relationships; 60.3% of participants had viewed pornography online, 34.9% had used dating apps, and 33.9% had sent sexual or naked self-images to another person. Over one in three reported positive outcomes from this: 38.2% felt emotionally connected to their partners due to online communication; 38.0% agreed that digital technologies facilitated closer connections; however, the majority of participants were aware of potential risks associated with online sexual engagement, particularly non-consensual exposure of their sexual or naked images, with women expressing greater concern. **Conclusions** Policy, legal and educational responses should be based on holistic understanding of digital sexual engagement, acknowledging the ways in which technologies can support sexual relationships while also building people's knowledge and capacity to manage risks.

Introduction

Digital technologies increasingly play a part in people's sex lives and relationships via dating apps, social media and internet-enabled communication.[1–3] Smartphones and other devices equipped with cameras mean digitally mediated sex is highly accessible

This is an Open Access article distributed under the terms of the Creative Commons Attribution-NonCommercial-NoDerivatives License (http://creativecommons.org/licenses/by-nc-nd/4.0/), which permits non-commercial re-use, distribution, and reproduction in any medium, provided the original work is properly cited, and is not altered, transformed, or built upon in any way.

and phones/devices are commonly used for meeting potential lovers, sending messages, 'chatting', sharing sexualised images ('sexting'), communicating via video, and accessing pornography.[2–4]

There is now a large body of research dedicated to understanding the social, health, legal and emotional impact of sex-related uses of digital technologies. Much of this work has focused on risks and dangers, such as concerns about public health implications, including increased rates of sexually transmissible infections (STIs), resulting from popularity of dating and hook-up apps,[5–7] and safety implications, such as sexual violence linked to image-based abuse[8] and non-consensual exposure of sexual images ('revenge porn').[9] In recent decades, there has also been high-profile public debates in Australia, and internationally, centred on mental health, legal and safety concerns about young people sending sexual self-images ('sexting', naked or sexual 'selfies').[10–13] More recently, law reform, including the recent Australian *Online Safety Act 2021*, has been enacted in response to harms arising from non-consensual dissemination of sexual images, cyber-stalking, digital harassment and online sexual violence.[14–17] Although such laws are important to address serious harms, their introduction has raised concern that the dominant focus on risk and danger in both policy and research could lead to censorship or curtailment of consensual online sexual activity or content.[18] Further, digital sexual literacy education is likely to be more effective if education about risk is balanced with recognition of reasons why people use digital technologies in their sex and intimate lives, and that pleasure or sexual connection gained via technologies is important for many people.[19–21]

Partially in response to these concerns, there is an emerging body of literature exploring the unique role that digital technologies play in facilitating sexual intimacy.[4,10,20,22,23] This research has shown how smartphones enable people to communicate spontaneously and intimately with longdistance lovers,[1] or to share images or words that express sexual desire, pleasure or affection.[1,2,24] Conversations via email or text messages can also facilitate an open exchange of emotion or explicit conversations in ways that build sexual and emotional intimacy.[1,25] Further, the internet enables people to explore new sexual practices or fantasies in safe ways[2,26] and has been an important space in which lesbian, gay, bisexual, transgender and queer and other genderdiverse people have sought community and connection.[22,27,28]

This paper presents findings from an Australian survey that explored people's engagement with a range of online sexual practices and their perceptions of the benefits and pleasures, as well as the risks, associated with those practices. The paper has two aims:

1. To identify a range of ways in which people engage with digital technologies in their sex lives and relationships and explore which practices are more common.
2. To explore what is perceived to be the most important benefits and most relevant risks or concerns associated with use of digital technologies in sex lives or relationships and whether these are associated with particular demographic characteristics or experiences using technologies.

Guiding these aims is an overarching interest in the ways people engage with digital technologies to establish, support or enhance sex and intimacy. The literature cited above suggests that the benefits of digital technologies can best be understood in the context of human relationships and intimacy, the pursuit of sexual pleasure, or to explore sexual identity and seek information and support for this.[1,4,22,29,30] The form and function of the technology is significant in that the internet enables affordable, accessible connection and the small, portable nature of smart devices enables constant and spontaneous communication, often involving visual communication via photos or video.[4,24,25] However, the functionality of devices or platforms does not wholly determine people's use or experiences of technology within their sex or intimate lives. Rather, this is produced though the interaction between technologies, human action and human relationships. Online pornography, online dating, messaging and use of webcams are all part of an infrastructure that increasingly forms part of people's sex lives and intimate relationships, producing unique forms of sexual communication, intimacy and experiences.[4,23] Drawing from this sociomaterial approach to understanding human interaction with technologies,[24] in this study, we explored the ways people engage with technologies in their sex lives, with a focus on sexual relationships, intimacies, experiences and pleasures.

The study is intended to lay groundwork for holistic digital sexual literacy education and effective legal, policy and educational responses that recognise the complexity and breadth of people's online sexual experiences. This study is also intended to support further quantitative research into the use and impact of digital technologies in people's sex and intimate lives by trialling previously untested measures regarding perceived benefits and risks in the context of human sexual relationships, intimacy and pleasure.

Data were collected when Australia and many parts of the world experienced an extended period of social lockdown due to the SARS-CoV-2 virus (i.e. the COVID-19 pandemic).[31] Although one part of this study, to be published elsewhere, looked at the impact of lockdowns on people's use of digital technologies, the broad aim was to explore use of digital technology in sex lives over people's lifetimes, and that is what is reported here. That said, the pandemic and associated lockdowns provided a unique context for this study in that digital technologies were part of many people's social and intimate lives in likely unprecedented ways.[24,32]

Materials and methods

Ethics approval was granted by the La Trobe University Human Research Ethics Committee (HEC20130). A cross-sectional survey of adults (aged ≥18 years) currently living in Australia was used to collect data via an online questionnaire. The survey was widely advertised on Facebook as a study about digital sex and intimacy, including use of technology to establish or maintain relationships. Participants could opt-in to the study by clicking a link that directed them to the questionnaire. Participants were advised that the survey was anonymous and that responses to all items were optional. Data were collected between May and July 2020. There were 445 valid responses. Although this is a relatively small sample drawn using convenience sampling, the aim of the study was to explore use of new digital technologies in sexual relationships rather than draw conclusions on the pattern of digital technology use across the population. Hence, the sample size and sampling strategy was appropriate.

Measures

Demographic characteristics

Standard measures were used to gather information on: age; gender; sex assigned at birth; sexual orientation; country of birth; cultural identity; place of residence; Australian citizenship/residency status; religious affiliation; current household income; employment status; and highest level of education. Participants were also asked their current relationship status, whether they cohabited with their partner(s), and living arrangements at the time of the survey (e.g. live alone, live with others).

Use of digital technologies for sexual purposes

Participants were asked about the use of digital technologies in their sex lives and relationships, including: use of dating apps to arrange in-person hooks-ups, dates and/or to meet potential sexual or romantic partners; use of digital devices for sexual communication via texting or talking; production and/or dissemination of home-made pornography or sexual/naked self-images (sexting) or videos; and sending sexual self-images to someone met online or offline. Participants were also asked about perceived benefits of such practices, including sexual gratification or emotional closeness. Participants were also asked about whether they use technologies to view pornography online or to seek information about sex or sexual health.

Perceived benefits

Participants were asked about perceived benefits of digital technologies in three areas: access to information and sexual cultures; developing or enhancing sexual intimacy/connection; and whether technology facilitates sexual gratification. The items used were a combination of novel items developed for this survey as well as items adapted with permission from Lehmiller *et al.*,[3] who reported on US adults' use of digital technologies to facilitate sex and intimacy. Three benefits scales were created: (1) 'access to information about sexual cultures' (four items: e.g. 'The internet has enabled me to explore sexual cultures I did not have access to previously'); (2) 'sexual connection online' (five items: e.g. 'I feel more sexually connected to my partner(s) because of our online communication'); and (3) 'sexual gratification from online sexual contact' (four items: e.g. 'I find it sexually gratifying or exciting to have sex online via a webcam with another person or persons'). All responses were measured on a five-point Likert scale, ranging from 1 (*strongly agree*) to 5 (*strongly disagree*). All three benefits scales yielded good estimates of internal consistency in this sample ($\alpha > 0.78$).

Perceived risks

To measure risks associated with the use of digital technologies for sex and intimacy, participants were asked to indicate the extent to which they were concerned about a defined set of circumstances and outcomes and the extent to which they worried about exposure associated with the use of digital technology related to sexual activity. Two risks scales were created to capture concerns about consequences: (1) 'concerns about potential problems or consequences of online sexual engagement' (four items: e.g. 'sharing explicit or naked images or videos risks criminal prosecution'); and (2) 'worries about unwanted exposure' (five items: e.g. 'I worry that if I search for pornography online, my search history will be seen by others'). Responses were measured on a four-point Likert scale, ranging from 1 (*not at all concerned*) to 4 (*very concerned*). Both scales yielded good estimates of internal consistency in this sample ($\alpha > 0.75$).

Analysis

Descriptive analysis was used to explore demographic characteristics and responses to the perceived risks and benefits statements. Bivariate analysis was undertaken to identify significant relationships between demographic variables and the use of technologies in relation to the risks and benefits scales. For continuous variables, correlation analyses using a Pearson's product-moment test were conducted. For categorical variables, chi-squared tests of independence and *t*-tests were used. Multivariate analysis was not undertaken as bivariate findings pointed to a range of issues relevant to perceived risks and benefits of digital technologies and sex, as per the study aims.

Participants

Participant characteristics are described in Table 1. Some data were missing (range: 26.5–40.2%). Little's missing completely at random (MCAR) test revealed all data were missing at random, $P > 0.133$, possibly reflecting fatigue or boredom effects as non-response rates increased toward the end of the questionnaire. Participant ages ranged from 18 to 80 years ($M = 42.00$, s.d. = 16.24). Most participants were female (58.5%) (inclusive of cisgender and transgender women) and identified as heterosexual (61.1%). Over half the participants were partnered (56.4%) and 36.2% were cohabiting with their partner. Most participants were born in Australia (71.7%) and identified as Caucasian/Anglo Saxon/White (67.4%). The majority indicated they did not hold religious views or affiliations (56%). The sample was well educated, with 65.3% holding a university qualification, and 60.0% were currently employed.

Results

Digital technology in participants' sex lives and relationships

Viewing pornography online was the most common means by which participants used technology in their sex lives, with 60.3% reporting 'ever' having viewed pornography online, whereas 34.9% had used dating or hook-up apps 'ever' and 33.9% had sent sexual images (sexts) to a lover or partner whom they knew offline (Table 2). Participants were less likely to have sent sexual images to someone they did not know offline, with 13.6% reporting they had done so, and 20% had received an unsolicited sexualised message or image.

Those aged under 30 years were more likely than other age groups to have sent sexual images to partners ($\chi^2[3455] = 32.95$, $P < 0.001$), used the internet to seek information on sexual health ($\chi^2[3275] = 26.06$, $P < 0.001$), or have received unsolicited sexual images

Table 1. Characteristics of participants.

	n (%)
Age range (mean)	18–80 (42 years)
Gender identity	
Female (includes cisgender and transgender, *n* = 2 women identify as transgender)	252 (58.5)
Male (includes cisgender and transgender, *n* = 3 men identify as transgender)	146 (33.9)
Nonbinary or gender fluid	28 (6.3)
Other	5 (1.2)
Sex assigned at birth	
Female	267 (62.7)
Male	148 (34.7)
Other/prefer not to say	11 (2.5)
Identify as transgender	13 (3.1)
Born with intersex characteristics	3 (<1%)
Sexual identity	
Heterosexual or straight	256 (61.1)
Bisexual	60 (14.3)
Gay/homosexual/lesbian	39 (9.3)
Queer	25 (6.0)
Pansexual	13 (3.1)
Other or prefer not to specify	26 (6.2)
Relationship status (multiple responses permitted)	
Partner/s who lives with me	161 (36.2)
Partner/s who does not live me	90 (20.2)
No partner/single	131 (29.4)
Other	15 (3.4%)
Current living arrangement (household makeup) (multiple responses permitted)	
Live alone	64 (14.4)
Live with partner/spouse	161 (36.2)
Live with dependent children	54 (12.1)
Live with other family members	52 (11.7)
Live with friends/flatmates	60 (13.5)
Live with pets	57 (12.8)
Aboriginal or Torres Strait Islander	6 (1.4)
Country of birth	
Australia	292 (71.7)
Other	115 (28.3)
Cultural or ethnic identity	
Caucasian/Anglo/white/Australian	300 (67.4)
South East Asian	21 (4.7)
South Asian	10 (2.2)
Greek	8 (1.8)
Aboriginal or Māori	6 (1.4)

(*Continued*)

Table 1. Continued.

	n (%)
Eastern European	5 (1.1)
Other	16 (3.6)
Religiosity	
None/atheist	225 (56.0)
Christian	82 (20.4)
Agnostic	39 (9.7)
Buddhist	11 (2.7)
Jewish	9 (2.2)
Muslim	8 (2.0)
Hindu	2 (<1)
New age	2 (<1)
Other/prefer not to say	23 (5.7)
Importance of religion	
Not at all or a little important	236 (67.6)
Important, very or extremely important	113 (32.4)
Have a disability that affects ability to engage in everyday activities or work	61 (15.5)
Highest level of education completed	
Primary school only	1 (<1)
Up to 4-years high school (year 10)	15 (3.8)
Leaving certificate/HSC/Year 12	56 (14.1)
Tertiary diploma/trade certificate/TAFE	61 (15.3)
Undergraduate university degree	100 (25.1)
Postgraduate university degree	160 (40.2)
Prefer not to say	5 (1.3)
Annual household income in 2019 (Australian dollars)	
<AUD50 000	94 (23.8)
AUD50 000–AUD99 999 per year	113 (28.5)
AUD100 000–AUD199 999 per year	110 (27.8)
≥AUD200 000 per year	30 (7.6)
Don't know or prefer not to say	49 (12.4)
Current employment status (multiple responses permitted)	
Employed full time	138 (31.0)
Employed part time or casual	129 (29.0)
Unemployed	47 (10.6)
Retired	32 (7.2)
Home duties	13 (12.9)
Student	74 (16.6)
Other	23 (5.2)
Currently working from home (at time of survey)	
Working from home entirely	147 (42.4)
Working from home part of the time	51 (14.7)
Not working at home	149 (42.9)

Table 2. Use of online technology in participants' sex lives.

Dating and hook up apps	Occasional or regular use, *n* (%)[A]
Dating apps/websites to meet people for casual dates	108 (30.1)
Dating apps/websites to meet people for long-term relationships	79 (22.3)
Dating apps/websites to meet people for casual sex	79 (22.0)
Ever used dating apps for casual dates, long-term relationships or casual sex	128 (34.9)
Production or consumption of pornography and erotic imagery	**Occasional or regular use, *n* (%)[A]**
Viewed pornography online	207 (60.3)
Sent erotic images (sexts) to a lover or partner you were also seeing in real life	117 (33.9)
Received sexually explicit messages or images without asking for them	68 (20.0)
Sent erotic images (sexts) to someone you knew online but not in real life	47 (13.6)
Information-seeking related to sex and sexual health (ever in lifetime)	Frequently or occasionally, n (%)[B]
I have used the internet to find information about sex	146 (32.8)
I have used the internet to find information about sexual health	151 (33.9)

[A]People reporting regular or occasional use compared to those who have never used technologies for these purposes. Valid percentages, missing data excluded.
[B]Percentage of total dataset reported as it was not possible to differentiate between 'no' and missing data for these items.

from another person ($\chi^2[3455] = 12.86$, $P = 0.005$; Table 3). Participants who had a sexual partner with whom they were not cohabiting were most likely to have used dating apps ($\chi^2[2375] = 19.00$, $P < 0.001$), sent sexual images to partners ($\chi^2[2375] = 26.78$, $P < 0.001$), or used the internet to find information on sexual health ($\chi^2[2268] = 15.99$, $P < 0.001$; Table 3).

Men and gender non-binary people were more likely than women to have viewed pornography online ($\chi^2[2426] = 23.29$, $P < 0.001$); however, women and non-binary people were more likely than men to have sent sexual images to partners ($\chi^2[2426] = 6.73$, $P = 0.035$). With respect to sexual identity, participants who identified as lesbian, gay, bisexual/pansexual or queer were more likely than heterosexual participants to have used dating apps ($\chi^2[1419] = 25.49$, $P < 0.001$), sent sexual images to partners ($\chi^2[1419] = 10.47$, $P = 0.002$), sent images to someone met online ($\chi^2[1419] = 16.30$, $P < 0.001$), sought information about sexual health online ($\chi^2[1275] = 13.32$, $P < 0.001$), or to have received unsolicited sexual images ($\chi^2[1419] = 28.22$, $P < 0.001$; Table 3).

Access to information and new sexual cultures

When asked whether information found online had helped them feel more comfortable about sex, 54.4% agreed, whereas 49.1% agreed that the internet had enabled them to explore sexual cultures to which they did not previously have access (Table 4). Participant characteristics associated with a greater likelihood of perceving benefits associated with accessing sexual information and cultures online included: being younger ($r = -0.173$, $P = 0.006$); identifying as lesbian, gay, bisexual/pansexual or queer ($t[245] = -2.94$, $P = 0.004$); past use of digital technology to view pornography ($t[245] = 4.55$, $P = < 0.001$); and having sent erotic/sexual images to partners ($t[245] = 3.45$, $P < 0.001$; Table 5).

Table 3. Regular or occasional use of digital technology × characteristics of participants.

	Used dating apps ever	Viewed pornography online	Sent erotic images (sexts) to a lover/ partner you were also seeing in real life	Sent erotic images (sexts) to someone you knew online but not in real life	Received sexually explicit messages or images without asking for them	Used the internet to find information about sex	Used the internet to find information about sexual health
Age (years)							
<30	38 (29.2)	66 (50.8)	54 (41.5)	16 (12.3)	29 (22.3)	55 (67.9)	58 (71.6)
30–39	33 (34.4)	54 (56.3)	28 (29.2)	11 (11.5)	19 (19.8)	38 (60.3)	40 (63.5)
40–49	19 (29.2)	27 (41.5)	17 (26.2)	10 (15.4)	6 (9.2)	19 (48.7)	21 (53.8)
50+	38 (24.7)	60 (39.0)	18 (11.7)	10 (6.5)	14 (9.1)	34 (37.0)	32 (34.8)
	χ^2 (3455) = 2.75	χ^2 (3455) = 8.78*	χ^2 (3455) = 32.95***	χ^2 (355) = 4.80	χ^2 (3455) = 12.86**	χ^2 (3275) = 18.37***	χ^2 (3275) = 26.06***
Gender[A]							
Male	46 (31.5)	91 (62.3)	29 (19.9)	21 (14.4)	24 (16.9)	42 (49.4)	40 (47.1)
Female	70 (27.8)	98 (38.9)	78 (31.0)	21 (8.3)	38 (15.1)	89 (52.7)	97 (57.4)
Non-Binary	12 (42.9)	18 (64.3)	10 (35.7)	5 (17.9)	6 (21.4)	6 (21.4)	14 (70.0)
	χ^2 (2426) = 2.95	χ^2 (2426) = 23.29***	χ^2 (2426) = 6.73*	χ^2 (2426) = 4.87	χ^2 (2426) = 0.80	χ^2 (2274) = 4.33	χ^2 (2274) = 4.37
Sexuality							
LGBQ[A]	73 (44.8)	88 (54.0)	60 (36.8)	31 (19.0)	46 (28.2)	76 (66.1)	78 (67.8)
Heterosexual	55 (21.5)	119 (46.5)	57 (22.3)	16 (6.3)	22 (8.6)	70 (43.8)	73 (45.6)
	χ^2 (1419) = 25.49**	χ^2 (1419) = 2.24	χ^2 (1419) = 10.47**	χ^2 (1419) = 16.30***	χ^2 (1419) = 28.22***	χ^2 (1275) = 13.41***	χ^2 (1275) = 13.32***
Disability status							
No reported disability	106 (31.9)	178 (53.6)	101 (30.4)	39 (11.7)	53 (16.0)	118 (51.1)	125 (54.1)
Disability	22 (36.1)	29 (47.5)	16 (26.2)	8 (13.1)	15 (24.6)	28 (63.6)	26 (59.1)
	χ^2 (1393) = 0.40	χ^2 (1393) = 0.76	χ^2 (1393) = 0.43	χ^2 (1393) = 0.09	χ^2 (1393) = 2.68	χ^2 (1275) = 2.34	χ^2 (1275) = 0.37
Relationship status							
Cohabiting r/ship	32 (20.4)	80 (51.0)	30 (19.1)	14 (8.9)	24 (15.3)	50 (46.7)	46 (43.0)
Non-cohabiting r/ship	39 (44.8)	54 (62.1)	44 (50.6)	16 (18.4)	18 (20.7)	43 (66.7)	47 (74.6)

(Continued)

Table 3. Continued.

	Used dating apps ever	Viewed pornography online	Sent erotic images (sexts) to a lover/partner you were also seeing in real life	Sent erotic images (sexts) to someone you knew online but not in real life	Received sexually explicit messages or images without asking for them	Used the internet to find information about sex	Used the internet to find information about sexual health
Single	51 (38.9)	68 (51.9)	37 (28.2)	14 (10.7)	24 (18.3)	49 (50.0)	53 (54.1)
	χ^2 (2375) = 19.00***	χ^2 (2375) = 3.09	χ^2 (2375) = 26.78***	χ^2 (2375) = 5.06	χ^2 (2375) = 1.20	χ^2 (2268) = 6.75*	χ^2 (2268) = 15.99***
Living arrangements							
Live alone	32 (50.0)	37 (57.8)	19 (29.7)	8 (12.5)	10 (15.6)	25 (54.3)	29 (63.0)
Live with other adults	96 (25.2)	170 (44.6)	98 (25.7)	39 (10.2)	58 (15.2)	121 (52.8)	122 (53.3)
	χ^2 (1455) = 16.45***	χ^2 (1455) = 3.83	χ^2 (1455) = 0.45	χ^2 (1455) = 0.30	χ^2 (1455) = 0.01	χ^2 (1275) = 0.06	χ^2 (1275) = 1.48
Annual household income (AUD)							
<50 000	35 (37.2)	50 (53.2)	32 (34.0)	10 (10.6)	20 (21.3)	36 (61.0)	37 (62.7)
50 000–99 000	40 (35.4)	55 (48.7)	35 (31.0)	16 (14.2)	20 (17.7)	44 (52.4)	42 (50.0)
100 000–199 000	39 (35.5)	64 (58.2)	33 (30.0)	14 (12.7)	21 (19.1)	38 (50.7)	46 (61.3)
≥200 000	8 (26.7)	19 (63.3)	9 (30.0)	6 (20.0)	3 (10.0)	12 (48.0)	10 (40.0)
	χ^2 (3347) = 1.13	χ^2 (3347) = 3.14	χ^2 (3347) = 0.44	χ^2 (3347) = 1.85	χ^2 (3347) = 2.00	χ^2 (3243) = 1.93	χ^2 (3243) = 5.74
Importance of religion							
Not/a little important	83 (35.2)	132 (55.9)	82 (34.7)	29 (12.3)	43 (18.2)	91 (54.8)	96 (57.8)
Important[B]	35 (31.0)	56 (49.6)	25 (22.1)	16 (14.2)	22 (19.5)	41 (53.2)	44 (57.1)
	χ^2 (1349) = 0.60	χ^2 (1349) = 1.25	χ^2 (1349) = 5.73	χ^2 (1349) = 0.24	χ^2 (1349) = 0.79	χ^2 (1243) = 0.52	χ^2 (1243) = 0.01
Country of birth							
Australian born	93 (31.8)	131 (44.9)	82 (28.1)	32 (11.0)	51 (17.5)	104 (51.5)	107 (53.0)
Born overseas	35 (30.4)	76 (66.1)	35 (30.4)	15 (13.0)	17 (14.8)	42 (57.5)	44 (60.3)
	χ^2 (1407) = 0.08	χ^2 (1407) = 14.87***	χ^2 (1407) = 0.22	χ^2 (1407) = 0.35	χ^2 (1407) = 0.43	χ^2 (1275) = 0.79	χ^2 (1275) = 1.15

[A]Includes lesbian, gay, bisexual, pansexual and queer-identified participants.
[B]Religion important, very important or extremely important.
$^*P < 0.05$, $^{**}P < 0.01$, $^{***}P < 0.001$.

Developing intimacy and sexual connection

When asked about intimacy and sexual connection, 38.2% reported that they felt more emotionally connected to their partners due to online communication, 38.0% agreed that connecting with people online helped them develop closer connections, and 27.4% felt more sexually connected with partners due to online communication (Table 4). Participant characteristics associated with a greater sense of connection included: being younger ($r = -0.131$, $P = 0.004$); not cohabiting with partners ($t[154] = -2.81$, $P = 0.005$); experience in using digital technology to view pornography ($t[247] = 2.63$, $P = 0.009$); having sent sexual or naked images to someone met online ($t[247] = 3.33$, $P = 0.001$); or having sought information online about sexual health ($t[237] = 3.67$, $P < 0.001$; Table 5).

Sexually gratifying connection

There were 30.9% who indicated they found it sexually gratifying to share sexual text messages with someone they met online, whereas 30.6% indicated they found it sexually gratifying to receive erotic or sexual images from someone they had met online (Table 4). Participant characteristics associated with a greater sense of gratification included: being

Table 4. Perceived benefits of sex online, n(%).

	Agree	Unsure or disagree	Not applicable
Access to information and sexual cultures[A] (*perceived benefits scale 1*)			
Information I have found online has helped me feel more comfortable about sex	149 (54.4)	78 (28.5)	47 (17.2)
The internet has enabled me to explore sexual cultures I did not have access to previously	134 (49.1)	73 (26.7)	66 (24.2)
Thanks to the internet, I have tried new things in my sex life	132 (48.5)	82 (30.1)	58 (21.3)
I have used the internet to find information about sex that has improved my sexual experiences	122 (44.5)	95 (34.7)	57 (20.8)
Intimacy and sexual connection[B] (*perceived benefits scale 2*)			
I feel emotionally connected to my partner(s) because of our online communication	110 (38.2)	81 (28.1)	97 (33.7)
Connecting with someone online helps me to develop a closer connection with them	108 (38.0)	127 (44.7)	49 (17.3)
I feel more sexually connected to my partner(s) because of our online communication	79 (27.4)	103 (35.8)	106 (36.8)
I feel that I can be more honest with someone online than in person	79 (27.4)	160 (55.6)	49 (17.0)
I feel as emotionally connected with someone when communicating online as I do in real life	61 (21.3)	183 (63.8)	43 (15.0)
Sexually gratifying connection[C] (*perceived benefits scale 3*)			
I find it sexually gratifying or exciting to share explicit text messages with someone I have met online	101 (30.9)	124 (37.9)	102 (31.2)
I find it sexually gratifying or exciting to receive erotic or sexual images from someone I have met online	100 (30.6)	149 (45.6)	110 (33.6)
I find it sexually gratifying or exciting to share erotic or sexual images of myself with someone I have met online	68 (20.8)	149 (45.6)	110 (33.6)
I find it sexually gratifying or exciting to have sex online via a webcam with another person or persons	49 (15.0)	159 (48.6)	119 (36.4)

[A]Missing responses: $n = 170$.
[B]Missing responses: $n = 157$.
[C]Missing responses: $n = 118$.

Table 5. Perceived benefits (bivariate) of technology use according to participant characteristics and use of technologies in sex life, *n* (%)

	Access to information and culture	Intimacy and sexual connection	Sexually gratifying connection
Age	$r = -0.173^{**}$	$r = -0.131^{*}$	$r = -0.111$
Gender[A]			
Male	3.47 (0.98)	3.10 (0.95)	3.20 (1.08)
Female	3.36 (0.94)	2.84 (0.91)	2.51 (1.17)
	$t(226) = 0.78$	$t(227) = 1.98$	$t(220) = 4.30^{***}$
Sexuality			
LGBQ[B]	3.64 (0.86)	3.63 (0.79)	2.92 (1.16)
Heterosexual	3.29 (0.97)	2.84 (0.94)	2.64 (1.19)
	$t(245) = -2.94^{**}$	$t(247) = 0.22$	$t(241) = 0.41$
Disability status			
No reported disability	3.43 (0.93)	2.90 (0.91)	2.78 (1.17)
Disability	3.52 (1.01)	3.10 (0.90)	2.65 (1.29)
	$t(245) = -0.57$	$t(247) = -1.10$	$t(241) = 0.62$
Relationship status			
In relationship	3.45 (0.99)	2.93 (0.93)	2.79 (1.24)
Single	3.40 (0.86)	2.92 (0.87)	2.66 (1.10)
	$t(239) = 0.33$	$t(241) = 0.29$	$t(234) = 0.79$
Cohabiting with partner			
Cohabiting	3.39 (1.02)	2.75 (0.97)	2.44 (1.16)
Not cohabiting	3.56 (0.94)	3.16 (0.83)	3.26 (1.18)
	$t(152) = -1.03$	$t(154) = -2.81^{**}$	$t(140) = -4.14^{***}$
Living arrangements			
Live alone	3.42 (0.92)	2.99 (0.92)	2.88 (1.22)
Live with other adults	3.44 (0.95)	2.91 (0.91)	2.75 (1.18)
	$t(245) = -0.13$	$t(247) = 0.49$	$t(241) = 0.67$
Household income (AUD)[C]			
<50 000 p/a	3.46 (0.99)	2.90 (0.99)	2.76 (1.18)
≥50 000 p/a	3.43 (0.92)	2.93 (0.89)	2.77 (1.18)
	$t(245) = 0.23$	$t(247) = -0.24$	$t(241) = -0.09$
≥100 000 p/a	3.37 (0.9)	2.93 (0.89)	2.65 (1.21)
	$t(245) = 1.02$	$t(247) = 0.02$	$t(241) = 1.41$
Importance of religion			
Not important or a little important	3.40 (0.94)	2.94 (0.94)	2.73 (1.20)
Important, very or extremely	3.60 (0.90)	2.89 (0.92)	2.83 (1.20)
	$t(216) = -1.45$	$t(184) = -0.78$	$t(186) = 0.42$
Country of birth			
Australian born	3.42 (1.00)	2.94 (0.88)	2.62 (1.19)
Born overseas	3.48 (0.76)	2.90 (1.00)	3.12 (1.09)
	$t(245) = -0.43$	$t(247) = 0.33$	$t(241) = -2.97^{**}$
Viewed pornography online			
Never or once or twice	3.08 (1.03)	2.73 (0.91)	2.08 (1.08)
Occasionally or regularly	3.63 (0.83)	3.04 (0.89)	3.15 (1.07)
	$t(245) = 4.55^{***}$	$t(247) = 2.63^{**}$	$t(241) = 7.43^{***}$

(*Continued*)

Table 5. Continued.

	Access to information and culture	Intimacy and sexual connection	Sexually gratifying connection
Sent erotic images (sexts) to a lover or partner you were also seeing in real life			
Never or once or twice	3.29 (0.96)	2.85 (0.93)	2.37 (1.15)
Occasionally or regularly	3.71 (0.96)	3.04 (0.87)	3.38 (0.97)
	$t(245) = 3.45$***	$t(247) = 1.96$	$t(241) = 7.15$***
Received sexually explicit messages or images without asking for them			
Never or once or twice	3.32 (0.91)	2.87 (0.92)	2.62 (1.19)
Occasionally or regularly	3.86 (0.93)	3.13 (0.84)	3.17 (1.07)
	$t(245) = 3.83$***	$t(247) = 1.96$*	$t(241) = 3.22$**
Sent sexual or erotic images (sexts) to someone you knew online but not in real life			
Never or once or twice	3.32 (0.93)	2.84 (0.91)	2.54 (3.75)
Occasionally or regularly	4.03 (0.72)	3.35 (0.79)	3.75 (0.84)
	$t(245) = 4.50$***	$t(247) = 3.33$**	$t(241) = 6.78$***
I have used the internet to find information about sex			
Never or once or twice	2.99 (0.92)	2.65 (0.91)	2.36 (1.23)
Occasionally or frequently	3.77 (0.81)	3.12 (0.87)	3.08 (1.06)
	$t(245) = 6.97$***	$t(237) = 4.06$***	$t(210) = 4.61$***
I have used the internet to find information about sexual health			
Never or once or twice	3.05 (0.97)	2.66 (0.93)	2.43 (1.20)
Occasionally or frequently	3.70 (0.83)	3.10 (0.86)	3.00 (1.13)
	$t(245) = 5.51$***	$t(237) = 3.67$***	$t(210) = 3.53$**

[A]Non-binary gender identity excluded from this analysis due to low numbers.
[B]Includes lesbian, gay, bisexual, pansexual, queer.
[C]Income categories: <AUD50 000 vs ≥AUD50 000 and <AUD100 000 vs ≥AUD100 000.
*$P < 0.05$, **$P < 0.01$, ***$P < 0.001$.

male ($t[220] = 4.30$, $P < 0.001$); not cohabiting with a partner ($t[140] = -4.14$, $P < 0.001$); being born overseas ($t[241] = -2.97$, $P = 0.002$); experience in using digital technology to view pornography ($t[241] = 7.43$, $P < 0.001$); having sent sexual images to a partner ($t[241] = 7.15$, $P < 0.001$); having sent images to someone they met online ($t[241] = 8.19$, $P < 0.001$); or having sought information about sexual health online ($t[210] = 3.53$, $P < 0.001$; Table 5).

Perceived risks or negative consequences

When asked about their level of concern with potentially negative consequences of online sexual engagements, participants were most likely to agree that sharing naked or explicit images or videos could cause them embarrassment (58.7%), or that online sexual engagement could cause them problems in the workplace (51.3%; Table 6). Participant characteristics associated with a greater sense of concern about potential consequences or problems included: identifying as heterosexual ($t[246] = 4.52$, $P < 0.001$); never having sent sexual images to a partner ($t[246] = -3.47$, $P = 0.001$); and having less experience in using the internet to search for information on sexual health ($t[246] = -1.98$, $P = 0.049$; Table 7).

In relation to the potential exposure of their digital sexual histories, 50.8% indicated that they worried their search history could be seen by others if they searched for pornography, and 26.0% indicated they worried that their data might be hacked if they shopped for sex products online. A similar number (24.0%) worried about providing personal contact details when shopping for sex products online (Table 6). Participant

Table 6. Concerns and perceived problems and knowledge of law, *n* (%).

Concerns about potential problems or consequences of online sexual engagement (*perceived risks scale 1*)			**Concerned**	**Not concerned**
Sharing sexually explicit or naked images or videos with someone could cause me *embarrassment*			158 (58.7)	111 (41.3)
Sharing sexually explicit or naked images or videos with someone could cause me *problems in the workplace*			138 (51.3)	131 (29.4)
Sharing sexually explicit or naked images or videos with someone could cause me *problems with friends or family*			123 (45.7)	146 (54.3)
Sharing sexually explicit or naked images or videos with someone could cause me *legal problems*			112 (41.6)	157 (58.4)
Worries about unwanted exposure (*perceived risks scale 2*)	**Agree**	**Disagree**	**Not applicable**	**Don't know**
I worry that if I search for pornography online my search history will be seen by others	135 (50.8)	83 (31.2)	35 (13.2)	13 (4.9)
I worry that my data will be hacked if I purchase sex products online	68 (26.0)	125 (47.7)	31 (11.8)	38 (14.5)
I worry about giving my personal contact details to companies if I purchase sex toys online	63 (24.0)	143 (54.4)	45 (17.1)	12 (4.6)
I worry that my friends or family will find out if I purchase sex toys online	58 (22.1)	154 (58.6)	40 (15.2)	11 (4.2)
Knowledge of rights and ownership	**Agree**	**Disagree**	**Not applicable**	**Don't know**
Sharing explicit or naked images or videos of myself online or via text means I no longer have control over where that image(s) or video appear(s)	231 (85.9)	13 (4.9)	17 (6.3)	8 (3.0)
Sharing explicit or naked images or videos of other people risks criminal prosecution	208 (77.3)	23 (8.5)	17 (6.3)	21 (7.8)
Sharing explicit or naked images or videos could potentially lead me to lose my job	159 (59.1)	43 (16.0)	35 (13.0)	32 (11.9)
Uploading sexually explicit or naked images or videos to a website means that website owns that image/video	151 (56.1)	34 (12.6)	27 (10.0)	57 (21.2)
Sharing explicit or naked images or videos of myself to a website means I have no right to ask for that image/video to be removed	76 (28.3)	113 (42.1)	28 (10.4)	51 (19.0)

Missing responses excluded (~n = 176).

characteristics associated with greater concerns about potential exposure were: being female ($t[247] = -2.33$, $P = 0.021$); not cohabiting with a partner ($t[165] = 2.14$, $P = 0.034$); earning >AUD50 000 per annum (household income; $t[267] = -2.82$, $P = 0.005$); and never having sent sexual messages to a partner ($t[267] = -3.45$, $P = 0.001$) or to a person known only online ($t[267] = -3.49$, $P = 0.001$; Table 7).

Knowledge of rights and data ownership

When asked about knowledge of copyright and ownership of digital content, 85.9% were confident that sending or uploading an image meant that they lost control of where those images appeared, and 77.3% agreed that sharing explicit images of other people risked criminal prosecution in some circumstances. Participants reported uncertainty about whether uploading a sexual image to a website meant the website then owned the image; 56.1% agreed that the website would own those images, but 21.2% did not know. In addition, 19.0% indicated they did not know if they had a legal right to ask for their images to be removed from a website (Table 6).

Table 7. Risk and concerns (bivariate) about technology according to characteristics of participants and use of technologies in their sex life, *n* (%).

	Worries about exposure	Concerns about problems
Age	$r = 0.083$	$r = -0.004$
Gender[A]		
Male	2.25 (0.71)	2.39 (0.88)
Female	2.42 (0.68)	2.69 (0.99)
	$t(227) = 1.70$	$t(247) = -2.33$*
Sexuality		
LGBQ[B]	2.10 (0.68)	2.58 (0.97)
Heterosexual	2.49 (0.67)	2.66 (0.98)
	$t(246) = 4.52$***	$t(267) = 1.70$
Disability status		
No reported disability	2.33 (0.67)	2.59 (0.95)
Disability	2.23 (0.86)	2.52 (1.08)
	$t(246) = 0.32$	$t(267) = 0.46$
Relationship status		
In a relationship	2.33 (0.68)	2.68 (0.96)
Single	2.36 (0.75)	2.44 (0.96)
	$t(240) = -0.34$	$t(261) = 1.96$
Cohabiting with partner		
Cohabiting	2.37 (0.70)	2.80 (0.96)
Not cohabiting	2.27 (0.64)	2.47 (0.93)
	$t(155) = 0.83$	$t(165) = 2.14$*
Living arrangements		
Live alone	2.41 (0.69)	2.64 (0.95)
Live with other adults	2.32 (0.70)	2.56 (0.97)
	$t(246) = 0.76$	$t(267) = 0.50$
Household income (AUD)[C]		
<50 000 p/a	2.22 (0.81)	2.26 (1.01)
≥50 000 p/a	2.36 (0.67)	2.66 (0.94)
	$t(246) = -1.72$	$t(267) = -2.82$**
≥100 000 p/a	2.41 (0.70)	2.71 (1.0)
	$t(246) = -1.72$	$t(267) = -2.31$*
Importance of religion		
Not important or a title important	2.28 (0.66)	2.58 (0.94)
Important/very/extremely	2.44 (0.79)	2.52 (1.04)
	$t(181) = -1.52$	$t(195) = 0.51$
Country of birth		
Australian born	2.36 (0.72)	2.59 (0.95)
Born overseas	2.25 (0.65)	2.53 (1.02)
	$t(246) = 1.04$	$t(267) = 0.45$
Viewed pornography online		
Never or once or twice	2.43 (0.72)	2.58 (1.05)
Occasionally or regularly	2.28 (0.68)	2.57 (0.91)
	$t(246) = -1.69$	$t(267) = -0.03$
Sent erotic images (sexts) to a lover or partner you were also seeing in real life		
Never or once or twice	2.45 (0.71)	2.71 (1.00)
Occasionally or regularly	2.13 (0.63)	2.31 (0.85)
	$t(246) = -3.47$**	$t(267) = -3.45$**

(*Continued*)

Table 7. Continued.

	Worries about exposure	Concerns about problems
Received sexually explicit messages or images without asking for them		
Never or once or twice	2.37 (0.68)	2.62 (1.01)
Occasionally or regularly	2.20 (0.77)	2.40 (0.76)
	$t(246) = -1.55$	$t(267) = -1.60$
Sent sexual or erotic images (sexts) to someone you knew online but not in real life		
Never or once or twice	2.40 (0.70)	2.64 (0.97)
Occasionally or regularly	1.98 (0.68)	2.16 (0.80)
	$t(246) = -3.48$**	$t(267) = -3.49$**
I have used the internet to find information about sex		
Never or once or twice	2.40 (0.73)	2.63 (1.05)
Occasionally or frequently	2.25 (0.67)	2.53 (0.89)
	$t(246) = -2.10$*	$t(267) = -0.79$
I have used the internet to find information about sexual health		
Never or once or twice	2.43 (0.76)	2.64 (1.03)
Occasionally or frequently	2.25 (0.66)*	2.52 (0.91)
	$t(246) = -1.98$	$t(267) = -1.05$

[A]Non-binary gender identity excluded from this analysis due to low numbers.
[B]Includes lesbian, gay, bisexual, pansexual, queer.
[C]Income categories: <AUD50 000 vs ≥AUD50 000 and <AUD100 000 vs ≥AUD100 000.
*$P < 0.05$, **$P < 0.01$, ***$P < 0.001$.

Discussion

This paper contributes to a body of research striving to understand how new digital technologies enhance and facilitate face-to-face and digitally mediated sex and intimacy, while also exploring how people perceive associated risks and problems. The purpose is to build a nuanced understanding of the ways people engage with technologies in their sex lives and relationships to inform educational, health promotion, legal and policy responses to potential risks. People rarely take risks with their health or safety outside a context in which they are seeking some form of benefit or human connection. A better understanding of this context will lead to more appropriately targeted responses.

The findings from this study align with previous research that has shown the use of the internet to view pornography and to seek casual partners via dating apps or websites is not uncommon.[33,34] Indeed, nearly half the participants had viewed pornography online, and almost one in three had used dating apps at some point in their lives. However, these findings also suggest that digital technology plays an ongoing part in people's relationships, and is not simply a medium through which people meet sexual or romantic partners. The use of technology to seek sexual intimacy or gratification was common among participants who were in non-cohabiting relationships, and these participants were more likely to report that online communication facilitated a sense of sexual or emotional connection with partners and that online sexual communication was sexually gratifying.

Interestingly, people who were born overseas were more likely to report receiving sexual gratification from digitally mediated sex. Although these findings cannot explain why this is so, previous research has indicated that migrants often connect with people from their home countries via dating apps or stay in touch with lovers/partners via digital technologies (phones, text, webcams). Dating apps may also provide a way for newly arrived or temporary migrants to engage in social or dating cultures in their 'new' country.[35–37]

There is a tendency for digital communication to be viewed as superficial or inferior to face-to-face contact or physical intimacy, or as something that people do only when physical contact is not an option.[24,38,39] Although digital communication may not replicate the experience of physical intimacy, the perception of it being inferior ignores the possibility that digital technologies offer a unique medium for facilitating sexual or emotional connections between people.[22,38,40–42] Technology may also provide opportunities for people to explore or understand their sexuality or sexual connections in ways not available offline or elsewhere in daily life.[43–46] The findings from this study confirm technologies provided both these experiences for participants. More than half reported that information they found online helped them to feel more comfortable with sex, and just under half agreed that the internet had enabled them to explore sexual cultures to which they had no previous access. In addition, more than one in three agreed that connecting with someone online helped them achieve a greater sense of sexual or emotional intimacy with that person.

Lesbian, gay, bisexual or queer participants in this study were more likely than heterosexual participants to have used dating apps, met someone online, sent sexualised images to another person, or sought sexual health information online. These findings reflect gay and bisexual men's early adoption of mobile phone hook-up technologies[47] and the part that online spaces play in connecting people of diverse sexualities.[48] For these reasons, technology may be more integrated into the sex and social lives of lesbian, gay, bisexual or queer people than it is for heterosexual people. This is important given the internet is a key site through which specific lesbian, gay, bisexual or queer sexuality education can be made available to young people and school-leavers who have not had access to such content in school-based sexuality education.[49,50]

There were distinctly gendered patterns in these findings. Women were less likely than people of other genders to report accessing pornography online but were more likely, along with non-binary people, to have sent sexualised or naked images of themselves to people met online. Men were more likely than people of other genders to report that they received sexual gratification from the use of digital technologies in their sex lives. These findings are not surprising given men are generally afforded greater freedom than women to express sexual desire or gratification,[51,52] and sexualised images and pornography are more commonly created for a heterosexual male gaze.[53,54] Women, particularly young women, may feel more pressure than men to send naked images to sexual partners.[55]

Participants in this study, particularly women, were also aware of a range of personal, reputational and employment harms that could result from non-consensual use of data and audio-visual materials derived from digital technologies. Given well-publicised media reports and research on such harms,[9,56–59] there is good reason to be aware of such risks.[15,60] Participants were, however, less certain about their rights regarding ownership or control of digital content. Legislative reforms may need to be supported by initiatives that aim to educate users on legal consent, ownership and privacy associated with digital sexual data and audio-visual materials, and what legal or other redress is available to those who suffer harm arising from nonconsensual sharing of digital images (A Farrell, N Shackleton, E Agnew, unpubl. data).[15,61]

Limitations

Revealing information on personal sexual and intimate practice can be uncomfortable for some, particularly concerning practices that might be considered harmful or shameful. Hence, responses may have been influenced by some social desirability bias.

Conclusions

Findings from this study build on existing work[22] to show that people's digital sexual experiences are often about engaging sexual intimacies, and that pleasure and connection are part of many people's online sexual experiences, even where risks are present.[1,10,29] As we know from decades of research on sexual health education,[62–64] people's choices and actions in sex and relationships rarely stem from simple, rational choices about risk and safety. Rather, choices and actions sit within a context of social, cultural and sexual practices and pleasures, as well as gendered relationships and patterns of inequality.[27,65] Understanding what people perceive to be the benefits of online sexual engagements, as well as the risks people take and how these are perceived in relation to – and in balance with – pleasure and intimacy, is necessary for developing comprehensive educational and legal responses that build people's confidence and capacity to engage safely with digital technologies and online environments.

Acknowledgements

Professor Jayne Lucke assisted with the development of the project, funding acquisition and development of the survey. We are grateful to all survey participants.

Data availability

Data are available on request subject to appropriate ethics/institutional review board approval. Please contact the corresponding author.

Conflicts of interest

The authors have no conflicts of interest to declare.

Declaration of funding

This project was funded by an Australian Research Council Discovery Grant (DP190102027).

ORCID

Jennifer Power https://orcid.org/0000-0002-6566-3214
Andrea Waling https://orcid.org/0000-0003-1370-5600

References

1 Murray CE, Campbell EC. The pleasures and perils of technology in intimate relationships. *J Couple Relatsh Ther* 2015; 14(2): 116–40. doi:10.1080/15332691.2014.953651
2 Gesselman AN, Druet A, Vitzthum VJ. Mobile sex-tech apps: how use differs across global areas of high and low gender equality. *PloS ONE* 2020; 15(9): e0238501. doi:10.1371/journal.pone.0238501
3 Lehmiller JJ, Garcia JR, Gesselman AN, *et al.* Less sex, but more sexual diversity: changes in sexual behavior during the COVID-19 coronavirus pandemic. *Leis Sci* 2021; 43(1–2): 295–304. doi:10.1080/01490400.2020.1774016

4 Paasonen S. Infrastructures of intimacy. In: Andreassen R, Petersen MN, Harrison K, Raun T, editors. Mediated intimacies: connectivities, relationalities and proximities. New York: Routledge; 2017. pp. 103–16.
5 Cabecinha M, Mercer CH, Gravningen K, *et al.* Finding sexual partners online: prevalence and associations with sexual behaviour, STI diagnoses and other sexual health outcomes in the British population. *Sex Transm Infect* 2017; 93(8): 572–82. doi:10.1136/sextrans-2016-052994
6 Heijman T, Stolte I, Geskus R, *et al.* Does online dating lead to higher sexual risk behaviour? A cross-sectional study among MSM in Amsterdam, the Netherlands. *BMC Infect Dis* 2016; 16(1): 1–13. doi:10.1186/s12879-016-1637-5
7 Knox J, Chen Y-N, He Q, *et al.* Use of geosocial networking apps and HIV risk behavior among men who have sex with men: casecrossover study. *JMIR Public Health Surveill* 2021; 7(1): e17173. doi:10.2196/17173
8 Drouin M, Ross J, Tobin E. Sexting: a new, digital vehicle for intimate partner aggression? *Comput Human Behav* 2015; 50: 197–204. doi:10.1016/j.chb.2015.04.001
9 Henry N, Powell A, Flynn A. Not just 'revenge pornography': Australians' experiences of image-based abuse. A summary report. Melbourne: RMIT University; 2017.
10 Albury K, Hasinoff AA, Senft T. From media abstinence to media production: sexting, young people and education. In: Allen L, Ramussen M, editors. The Palgrave handbook of sexuality education. London: Springer; 2017. pp. 527–45.
11 Albury K, Crawford K. Sexting, consent and young people's ethics: beyond Megan's story. *Continuum* 2012; 26(3): 463–73. doi:10.1080/10304312.2012.665840
12 Angelides S. 'Technology, hormones, and stupidity': the affective politics of teenage sexting. *Sexualities* 2013; 16(5–6): 665–89. doi:10.1177/1363460713487289
13 Döring N. Consensual sexting among adolescents: risk prevention through abstinence education or safer sexting? *Cyberpsychol J Psychosoc Res Cybersp* 2014; 8(1): 1–9. doi:10.5817/CP2014-1-9
14 Evans M. Regulating the non-consensual sharing of intimate images (revenge pornography) via a civil penalty regime: a sex equality analysis. *Monash UL Rev* 2018; 44: 602. doi:10.26180/5dc678820944f
15 Henry N, McGlynn C, Flynn A, *et al.* Image-based sexual abuse: a study on the causes and consequences of non-consensual nude or sexual imagery. Routledge; 2020.
16 Sentencing Advisory Council. Sentencing image-based sexual abuse offences in Victoria. Melbourne: Sentencing Advisory Council; 2020.
17 Australian Government. Online safety bill – reading guide. Canberra: Australian Department of Infrastructure, Transport, Regional Development and Communications; 2020.
18 Stardust Z. A new online safety bill could allow censorship of anyone who engages with sexual content on the internet. *Conversation* 2021. February 18. Available at https://theconversation.com/a-new- online-safety-bill-could-allow-censorship-of-anyone-who-engages- with-sexual-content-on-the-internet-154739
19 Dobson A. Sexting, intimate and sexual media practices, and social justice. In: Dobson A, Robards B, Carah N, editors. Digital intimate publics and social media. Cham, Switzerland: Springer; 2018. pp. 93–110.
20 Albury K, Byron P. Taking off the risk goggles: exploring the intersection of young people's sexual and digital citizenship in sexual health promotion. In: Aggleton P, Cover R, Leahy D, Marshall D, Rasmussen ML, editors. Youth, sexuality and sexual citizenship. Abingdon: Routlege; 2018. pp. 168–83.
21 Albury K, McCosker A, Pym T, *et al.* Dating apps as public health 'problems': cautionary tales and vernacular pedagogies in news media. *Health Sociol Rev* 2020; 29(3): 232–48. doi:10.1080/14461242.2020.177788514461242.2020.177788514461242.2020.1777885
22 Attwood F, Hakim J, Winch A. Mediated intimacies: bodies, technologies and relationships. *J Gender Stud* 2017; 26(3): 249–53. doi:10.1080/09589236.2017.1297888
23 Race K. Towards a pragmatics of sexual media/networking devices. *Sexualities* 2018; 21(8): 1325–30. doi:10.1177/1363460718781538

24 Watson A, Lupton D, Michael M. Enacting intimacy and sociality at a distance in the COVID-19 crisis: the sociomaterialities of homebased communication technologies. *Media Int Aust* 2021; 178(1): 136–50. doi:10.1177/1329878X20961568

25 Dredge R, Anderson J. The qualitative exploration of social competencies and incompetencies on mobile dating applications. *Pers Relat* 2021; 28: 627–51. doi:10.1111/pere.12378

26 Hertlein KM. Digital dwelling: technology in couple and family relationships. *Fam Relat* 2012; 61(3): 374–87. doi:10.1111/ j.1741-3729.2012.00702.x

27 Race K. 'Party and Play': online hook-up devices and the emergence of PNP practices among gay men. *Sexualities* 2015; 18(3): 253–75. doi:10.1177/1363460714550913

28 Miles S. Let's (not) go outside: grindr, hybrid space, and digital queer neighborhoods. In: Bitterman A, Hess DB, editors. The life and afterlife of gay neighborhoods. The Urban Book Series. Springer, Cham; 2021. pp. 203–20. doi:10.1007/978-3-030-66073-4_9

29 Amundsen R. Hetero-sexting as mediated intimacy work: 'Putting something on the line'. *New Media Soc* 2020; 24: 122–37. doi:10.1177/1461444820962452

30 Robards B, Churchill B, Vivienne S, *et al.* Twenty years of 'cyberqueer': the enduring significance of the internet for young LGBTIQ+ people. In: Aggleton P, Cover R, Leahy D, Marshall D, Rasmussen M, editors. Youth, sexuality and sexual citizenship. Routledge; 2018. pp. 151–67.

31 Chamas Z. Victoria has introduced a curfew and stage 4 coronavirus restrictions for Melbourne, and stage 3 restrictions for regional Victoria. Here's what that means. ABC News, 2 August 2020. Available at https://www.abc.net.au/news/2020-08-02/victorias- latest-coronavirus-restrictions-explained/12516182.

32 Tibbetts M, Epstein-Shuman A, Leitao M, *et al.* A week during COVID-19: online social interactions are associated with greater connection and more stress. *Comput Human Behav Rep* 2021; 4: 100133. doi:10.1016/j.chbr.2021.100133

33 Watchirs Smith L, Guy R, Degenhardt L, *et al.* Meeting sexual partners through internet sites and smartphone apps in Australia: national representative study. *J Med Intern Res* 2018; 20(12): e10683. doi:10.2196/10683

34 Richters J, de Visser RO, Badcock PB, *et al.* Masturbation, paying for sex, and other sexual activities: the Second Australian Study of Health and Relationships. *Sex Health* 2014; 11(5): 461–71. doi:10.1071/SH14116

35 Chen X, Liu T. On 'never right-swipe whites' and 'only date whites': gendered and racialised digital dating experiences of the Australian Chinese diaspora. *Inf Commun Soc* 2021; 24(9): 1247–64. doi:10.1080/1369118X.2019.1697341

36 Lennes K. Queer (post-) migration experiences: Mexican men's use of gay dating apps in the USA. *Sexualities* 2020; 24: 1003–18. doi:10.1177/1363460720944591

37 Dhoest A. Complicating cosmopolitanism: ethno-cultural and sexual connections among gay migrants. *Pop Commun* 2018; 16(1): 32–44. doi:10.1080/15405702.2017.1413190

38 Jamieson L. Personal relationships, intimacy and the self in a mediated and global digital age. In: Orton-Johnson K, Prior N, editors. Digital sociology. Springer; 2013. pp. 13–33.

39 Whitty MT. Liberating or debilitating? An examination of romantic relationships, sexual relationships and friendships on the net. *Comput Hum Behav* 2008; 24(5): 1837–50. doi:10.1016/ j.chb.2008.02.0092008.02.0092008.02.009

40 Bardi CA, Brady MF. Why shy people use instant messaging: loneliness and other motives. *Comput Hum Behav* 2010; 26(6): 1722–6. doi:10.1016/j.chb.2010.06.021

41 Elder AM. What words can't say: emoji and other non-verbal elements of technologically-mediated communication. *J Inf Commun Ethics Soc* 2018; 16(1): 2–15. doi:10.1108/JICES-08-2017-0050

42 Janssen JH, Ijsselsteijn WA, Westerink JHDM. How affective technologies can influence intimate interactions and improve social connectedness. *Int J Hum Comput Stud* 2014; 72(1): 33–43. doi:10.1016/j.ijhcs.2013.09.007

43 Pym T, Byron P, Albury K. 'I still want to know they're not terrible people': negotiating 'queer community' on dating apps. *Int J Cult Stud* 2021; 24(3): 398–413. doi:10.1177/1367877920959332

44 Craig SL, McInroy L. You can form a part of yourself online: the influence of new media on identity development and coming out for LGBTQ youth. *J Gay Lesbian Ment Health* 2014; 18(1): 95–109. doi:10.1080/19359705.2013.777007

45 Miller RA. "My voice is definitely strongest in online communities": students using social media for queer and disability identity-making. *J Coll Stud Dev* 2017; 58(4): 509–25. doi:10.1353/csd.2017.0040

46 Paradis E. Searching for self and society: sexual and gender minority youth online. In: Paradis E, editor. LGBTQ voices in education. London: Routledge; 2016. pp. 117–31.

47 Miles S. Still getting it on online: thirty years of queer male spaces brokered through digital technologies. *Geogr Compass* 2018; 12(11): e12407. doi:10.1111/gec3.12407

48 Hanckel B, Morris A. Finding community and contesting heteronormativity: queer young people's engagement in an Australian online community. *J Youth Stud* 2014; 17(7): 872–86. doi:10.1080/13676261.2013.878792

49 Elia JP, Eliason M. Discourses of exclusion: sexuality education's silencing of sexual others. *J LGBT Youth* 2010; 7(1): 29–48. doi:10.1080/19361650903507791

50 Ezer P, Kerr L, Fisher CM, *et al.* Australian students' experiences of sexuality education at school. *Sex Educ* 2019; 19(5): 597–613. doi:10.1080/14681811.2019.1566896

51 Welles CE. Breaking the silence surrounding female adolescent sexual desire. *Women Ther* 2005; 28(2): 31–45. doi:10.1300/ J015v28n02_03

52 Saville Young L, Moodley D, Macleod CI. Feminine sexual desire and shame in the classroom: an educator's constructions of and investments in sexuality education. *Sex Educ* 2019; 19(4): 486–500. doi:10.1080/14681811.2018.1511974

53 Paasonen S. Grains of resonance: affect, pornography and visual sensation. *Somatechnics* 2013; 3(2): 351–68. doi:10.3366/soma. 2013.0102

54 McKee A, Albury K, Lumby C. The porn report. Melbourne: Melbourne University Publishing; 2008.

55 Setty E. Meanings of bodily and sexual expression in youth sexting culture: young women's negotiation of gendered risks and harms. *Sex Roles* 2019; 80(9): 586–606. doi:10.1007/s11199-018-0957-x

56 Jacobo J. New York teacher who says she was fired "lost everything" over topless selfie. ABC News, 5 April 2019. Available at https://abcnews.go.com/US/york-teacher-fired-lost-topless-selfie/story?id= 62176028.

57 Jacobs E. Katie Hill sues ex-husband, media outlets over "nonconsensual porn". New York Post, 23 December 2020. Available at https://nypost.com/2020/12/23/katie-hill-sues-ex- husband-media-outlets-over-nude-photos/.

58 O'Connor K, Drouin M, Davis J, *et al.* Cyberbullying, revenge porn and the mid-sized university: victim characteristics, prevalence and students' knowledge of university policy and reporting procedures. *High Educ Q* 2018; 72(4): 344–59. doi:10.1111/hequ.12171

59 Serpe C, Brown C. The objectification and blame of sexually diverse women who are revenge porn victims. *J Gay Lesbian Soc Serv* 2021: 1–23. doi:10.1080/10538720.2021.1911901

60 Nadim M, Fladmoe A. Silencing women? Gender and online harassment. *Soc Sc Comput Rev* 2021; 39(2): 245–58. doi:10.1177/0894439319865518

61 Suzor N, Seignior B, Singleton J. Non-consensual porn and the responsibilities of online intermediaries. *Melbourne University Law Review* 2017; 40(3): 1057–97.

62 Parker R. Sexuality, culture and society: shifting paradigms in sexuality research. *Cult Health Sex* 2009; 11(3): 251–66. doi:10.1080/13691050701606941

63 Allen L, Rasmussen ML, Quinlivan K. The politics of pleasure in sexuality education: pleasure bound. Abingdon Oxon: Routledge; 2013.

64 Fine M, McClelland S. Sexuality education and desire: still missing after all these years. *Harv Educ Rev* 2006; 76(3): 297–338. doi:10.17763/haer.76.3.w5042g23122n6703

65 Harvey SM, Bird ST, Galavotti C, *et al.* Relationship power, sexual decision making and condom use among women at risk for HIV/STDs. *Women Health* 2002; 36(4): 69–84. doi:10.1300/J013v36n04_06

OPEN ACCESS

Regulating tech-sex and managing image-based sexual abuse: an Australian perspective

Anne-Maree Farrell, Nicole Shackleton, Elizabeth Agnew, Samantha Hopkins and Jennifer Power

ABSTRACT

A range of technologies now exist to facilitate sexual desire, pleasure and intimacy. Colloquially known as tech-sex, the growth in the use of such technologies has created a range of new opportunities for sexual expression and connection. Alongside these benefits are harms arising out of their non-consensual use. Drawing on a case study examining management of image-based sexual abuse as part of Australia's recently reformed online safety laws, we argue for a regulatory approach that is both facilitative in showing due respect for adult sexual agency and protective in mitigating harm caused to affected individuals. Operating along a facilitative-protective regulatory axis, such an approach offers the potential to be suitably responsive to both the opportunities and challenges faced by adult individuals who engage with such technologies.

Introduction

In recent years, a range of technologies have become available to facilitate or enhance sexual desire, intimacy and pleasure.[1] Colloquially known as tech-sex, the use of these technologies is growing exponentially in the context of a burgeoning global market for such products facilitated by a range of digital environments, including the internet, computers and smartphones. They have created previously unimaginable opportunities for intimate communication across time and place, transforming the ways in which people seek and engage with their own sexuality, as well as sexual partners.[2] Accompanying

[1]Jennifer Power et al, 'Traversing Tech-Sex: Benefits and Risks in Digitally-Mediated Sex and Relationships' (2022) 19(1) *Sexual Health* 55.

[2]Examples include the production and dissemination of (intimate) images and videos, bluetooth-enabled teledildonics and other sex toys, as well as sexbot technology, enhanced by the use of artificial intelligence. For an overview, see Robert Sparrow, 'Robots, Rape, and Representation' (2017) 9(4) *International Journal of Social Robotics* 465; John Danaher, 'Robot Betrayal: A Guide to the Ethics of Robotic Deception' (2020) 22 *Ethics and Information Technology* 117; Emma Renold and Jessica Ringrose, 'Selfies, Relfies and Phallic Tagging: Posthuman Participations in Teen Digital Sexuality Assemblages' (2017) 49(11) *Educational Philosophy and Theory* 1066; James EB Elsey et al 'The Impact of Virtual Reality versus 2D Pornography on Sexual Arousal and Presence' (2019) 97 *Computers in Human Behavior* 35; Jennifer Power and Andrea Waling (eds), 'New Technologies are Changing Sex, Intimacy and Health' (2020) 29(3) *Health Sociology Review* 129.

This is an Open Access article distributed under the terms of the Creative Commons Attribution-NonCommercial-NoDerivatives License (http://creativecommons.org/licenses/by-nc-nd/4.0/), which permits non-commercial re-use, distribution, and reproduction in any medium, provided the original work is properly cited, and is not altered, transformed, or built upon in any way.

such developments has been an increase in identified harms arising from their non-consensual use, including dating and sextortion scams, and what has been described as image-based sexual abuse (IBSA).[3] Where such harms have occurred, it has disproportionately impacted women and people of colour, as well as sexual and ethnic minorities.[4]

Examination of the legal issues at stake in a range of common law jurisdictions has focused predominantly to date on the role of the criminal law in addressing the non-consensual use of tech-sex,[5] identifying existing shortcomings with potential civil remedies,[6] and recommending a strengthened role for regulators in addressing online harms.[7] In this article, we contribute to this literature by arguing for a state-sponsored regulatory approach to mitigating harm suffered by affected individuals in digital environments. By way of example, we focus on regulatory reform that has recently taken place in one common law jurisdiction, namely Australia, to address harms arising from non-consensual use of intimate images, such as IBSA. We argue for a regulatory approach which operates on a facilitative-protective axis to address such harms, and which is suitably responsive to the opportunities and challenges for adult individuals who engage with tech-sex. In this regard, the preferred regulatory approach should be facilitative in respecting adult sexual agency, accompanied by the need to balance the exercise of such agency with the risks of harm faced by individuals who engage with such technologies. The protective mode will make use of both prevention and remediation strategies as part of this approach. In relation to the former, this will involve education for digital sexual literacy, particularly for at-risk groups; with the latter, it will involve the provision of quick, low-cost redress for harms caused to affected individuals, such as IBSA.

To explore these arguments, the article first positions our approach to regulating tech-sex, as well as harms such as IBSA arising from their non-consensual use. It is an approach which draws on the regulatory theory on the grounds that it invites a holistic, as well as contextualised, approach to understanding the social, legal, market and cultural factors impacting on the design of regulation on both a national and trans-jurisdictional basis. We then examine the issue of consent, including how this is primarily understood in

---

[3]Image-Based Sexual Abuse (IBSA) encompasses a variety of actions, including photographing or recording still or moving intimate images without consent, distributing intimate images without consent, or threatening to distribute intimate images. Intimate images include images of a person's private parts or a person engaged in a sexual act, including digitally altered images, which make it appear that a person is naked or that they are engaging in a sexual act. It covers three principal behaviours: first, the non-consensual taking of nude or sexual images, second, the non-consensual sharing of nude or sexual images, and third, threats to share nude or sexual images, see Nicola Henry et al, *Image-based Sexual Abuse: A Study in the Causes and Consequences of Non-Consensual Nude or Sexual Imagery* (Routledge, 2020) 4.

[4]Australian Government, 'Sextortion Email Campaign Impacting Australians', *Australian Cybersecurity Centre* (9 April 2020) <https://www.cyber.gov.au/acsc/view-all-content/alerts/sextortion-email-campaign-impacting-australians> accessed 12 August 2022; Maya Oppenheim, 'Tens of Thousands of Sextortion Attacks Blocked in the UK' (*The Independent*, 22 February 2021) <https://www.independent.co.uk/news/uk/home-news/sextortion-attacks-block-lockdown-b1805816.html> accessed 12 August 2022; Clare McGlynn et al, '"It's Torture for the Soul": The Harms of Image-Based Sexual Abuse' (2021) 30(4) *Social & Legal Studies* 541, 543–5.

[5]See eg, Clare McGlynn and Erika Rackley, 'Image-Based Sexual Abuse' (2017) 37(2) *Oxford Journal of Legal Studies* 534; Robert Sparrow and Lauren Karas, 'Teledildonics and Rape by Deception' (2020) 12(1) *Law Innovation and Technology* 175.

[6]Nicholas Suzor, Bryony Seignior and Jennifer Singleton, 'Non-Consensual Porn and the Responsibilities of Online Intermediaries' (2017) 40 *Melbourne University Law Review* 1057; Daithí Mac Síthigh, 'The Road to Responsibilities: New Attitudes Towards Internet Intermediaries' (2020) 29(1) *Information & Communications Technology Law* 1.

[7]See eg, Commonwealth of Australia, Senate Standing Committee on Legal and Constitutional Affairs Reference Committee, *Phenomenon Colloquially Referred to as Revenge Porn*, 25 February 2016, ch 5, recs 4, 5; Suzor, Seignior and Singleton (n 6) 1083–7.

the context of sexual offences within the criminal law in common law jurisdictions. This provides important background context concerning the way in which non-consensual use of intimate images is understood in countries such as Australia, ahead of presenting our case study examining the management of IBSA as part of its current national online safety regime. In the final section, we assess this online safety regulatory model by reference to our proposed approach, before offering our concluding comments.

For present purposes, we focus solely on the non-consensual production and/or dissemination of intimate images by adult individuals aged 18 years and over. Although we recognise that specific legislative definitions of the term 'intimate image' exist and vary by jurisdiction, we adopt a broad definition of the term for present purposes. This includes images (and video) involving (partial) nude selfies, live-streaming, webcams and amateur pornography, whose use may be facilitated via a range of digital environments including the internet, computers or smartphones on a local or trans-jurisdictional basis. Our preference in this article is to use the terms 'individuals' and 'users' to refer to those harmed by non-consensual use of intimate images, given that our predominant focus is on the regulatory jurisdiction. In doing so, we nevertheless recognise and support the use of other descriptors, such as 'victim-survivors' for those who have suffered harm through IBSA.

Regulating tech-sex

Our understanding of the role of regulation in mitigating harms arising out of the use of tech-sex, including IBSA, draws on insights from the regulatory studies literature. In this literature, the term 'regulation' is used to refer to a range of political, social and legal processes which impact behaviour, institutions and governance arrangements.[8] We consider this approach captures more fully the shifting nature of the state's relationship with actors, interests, markets and institutions in the context of increasing fluid and interdependent boundaries.[9] This can be exacerbated in the context of national political systems, where there are various constitutional arrangements, differing approaches to criminal, civil and regulatory laws, and separate institutional arrangements for regulating specific policy sectors. Within this literature, law – both hard and soft – is also viewed as one instrument amongst others, in facilitating regulatory governance.[10] Situating the role of law within the broader conceptual range offered by this analytical lens offers the opportunity to better understand its relationship with institutional, political, technological, human rights and public-private factors impacting regulatory processes.

Beyond the nation-state, regulatory processes are recognised as decentred, characterised by fragmentation, complexity and heterarchy.[11] Against this background, a dilemma that is particularly relevant for national online safety regulators is how best to manage non-consensual use of intimate images, where the business activities of the regulatees (e.g. webhosting services and social media platforms) are trans-jurisdictional in operation.

[8]For an overview, see Peter Drahos (ed), *Regulatory Theory: Foundations and Applications* (Canberra: ANU Press, 2017).

[9]Colin Scott, 'Regulation in the Age of Governance: The Rise of the Post Regulatory State' in Jacint Jordana, and David Levi-Faur (eds.), *The Politics of Regulation: Institutions and Regulatory Reforms for the Age of Governance* (Edward Elgar, 2004) 145–74; David Levi-Faur, 'Regulatory Capitalism' in Peter Drahos (ed) (n 8) 289–302.

[10]Bronwen Morgan and Karen Yeung, *An Introduction to Law and Regulation: Text and Materials* (Cambridge University Press, 2007).

[11]Julia Black, 'Decentring Regulation: Understanding the Role of Regulation and Self-Regulation in a "Post-Regulatory" World' (2001) 54(1) *Current Legal Problems* 103.

This may involve corporate oversight of such activities being based in a different jurisdiction to where operational activities take place. These types of trans-jurisdictional arrangements may lead to situations where, for example, an intimate image is posted online in Russia, viewed instantaneously by someone in the UK, shared with someone in Australia and then commented on by a person based in South Korea. Depending on a country's constitutional arrangements, regulatory remit confined to national boundaries can hamper efforts to mitigate harm arising from the non-consensual use of such images.[12] In the circumstances, the need to take account of the complexities raised by these 'polycentric regulatory regimes' can make it difficult for online safety regulators to develop repeat regulator-regulatee interactions which may generate an ongoing commitment to adhere to the aims and objectives of the domestic regulatory regime,[13] in addition to implementing successful compliance and enforcement strategies.[14]

In this regard, differing approaches are offered within the regulatory studies literature as to how best to facilitate such strategies. The deterrence approach focuses on employing formal mechanisms of punishment to sanction poor behaviour by regulatees, as well signalling to other regulatees, actors and organised interests that this is the way in which breach of the regulatory regime will be dealt with.[15] Another option for a national regulator with bounded jurisdictional reach is an 'advise and persuade' compliance strategy, which focuses on preventing harm rather than on punishment. This strategy is focused on conciliation, rather than confrontation. This is done in order to realise the overarching aims of the regulatory regime, rather than focusing on imposing sanctions for breach.[16] In circumstances where neither strategy works, a responsive regulatory approach may be preferred.[17] This would involve employing a mix of compliance and enforcement strategies to ensure appropriate regulatee behaviour, which could escalate towards a more punitive approach in the event that such behaviour does not improve in line with the aims and objectives of the regulatory regime.[18] We consider this strategic mix in more detail later in the article, when we examine by way of case study the national regulatory approach to managing IBSA in Australia.

In the context of new technologies, such as tech-sex, as well as harms such as IBSA arising from their non-consensual use, further questions arise: will existing regulatory models facilitate compliance and enforcement, or will a new approach be required? In this regard, a perennial problem recognised in the regulatory theory literature has been how best to maintain 'regulatory connection' in the face of such technological

[12]For specific concerns that have been raised in relation to IBSA, see Nicola Henry, Asher Flynn and Anastasia Powell, 'Policing Image-Based Sexual Abuse: Stakeholder Perspectives' (2018) 19(6) *Police Practice and Research: An International Journal* 565; see generally Julia Black, 'Constructing and Contesting Legitimacy and Accountability in Polycentric Regulatory Regimes (2008) 2(2) *Regulation & Governance* 137.

[13]See generally Christine Parker, 'The "Compliance Trap": The Moral Message in Responsible Regulatory Enforcement' (2006) 40(3) *Law & Society Review* 591.

[14]Black, 'Constructing and Contesting Legitimacy' (n 12).

[15]Kristina Murphy, 'Regulating More Effectively: The Relationship Between Procedural Justice, Legitimacy, and Tax Non-Compliance' (2005) 32(4) *Journal of Law and Society* 562, 564–5.

[16]Keith Hawkins, *Environment and Enforcement* (Oxford University Press, 1984); Brigid Hutter, 'Regulating Employers and Employees: Health and Safety in the Workplace' (1993) 20 *Journal of Law and Society* 452.

[17]Ian Ayres and John Braithwaite, *Responsive Regulation: Transcending the Deregulation Debate* (Oxford University Press, 1992).

[18]For an overview, see Neil Gunningham, 'Enforcement and Compliance Strategies' in Robert Baldwin, Martin Cave and Martin Lodge (eds), *Oxford Handbook of Regulation* (Oxford University Press, 2010) 120–45.

innovation.[19] One suggested option has been to focus on the new technology itself as the regulatory target, with a potential outcome being the use of 'regulation by design', in which restrictions or harm mitigation are built into the design of the technology itself.[20] However, academic commentators such as Bennett Moses have pointed out that we need to think more deeply about whether moral concerns exist regarding the new technology itself, the social conduct that it facilitates and how this impacts existing legal and institutional arrangements for managing sociotechnical change more generally.[21] Applying such considerations to the case of IBSA, we can ask: is regulation seeking to address concerns arising from first, the sexualised use of technologies that may facilitate this harm; or second, the technologisation of new ways of facilitating sexual expression, connection and intimacy? In the former case, the regulatory focus would be on addressing problematic social behaviour that results in IBSA; whereas in the latter case, it would be on managing the (un)intended consequences resulting from the newness of technologies that facilitate this type of harm.

In reflecting on the appropriate focus for national online safety regulators, it is important to take account of the social context in which new technologies, such as tech-sex, are used. While academic commentators have acknowledged that there is a role for regulation to play in managing risks and harms arising from the use of tech-sex,[22] it is also important to consider the complexities created by our hyper-connected, visual culture in which such regulation is situated.[23] As Henry et al. have observed, 'contemporary digital culture can be characterised by a fixation on visuality – on both the technological artefact that captures or broadcasts the visual, and the material subject/object which can be "seen" and monitored', examples of which include 'reality television, "selfies", live-streaming, webcams and amateur pornography'.[24] For many people, digital sex practices, such as sexting, produce pleasure or a sense of intimacy with another person despite, or in some cases *because of*, the risks. Such risks certainly exist, with potential negative outcomes (both short- and long-term) including poor mental health, loss of opportunities (e.g. jobs), loss of sexual agency and impact upon family/peer relationships.[25]

However, abstinence or 'just say no' approaches to educating people about the risks of practices such as sexting are unlikely to be effective given the ubiquity of such practices in modern sex and dating cultures.[26] Sexual cultures, relationships, desire and pleasure are not things that people consider in isolation from the risks associated with sexual

---

[19] See Roger Brownsword, *Rights, Regulation and the Technological Revolution* (Oxford University Press, 2008) chapter 6.

[20] Lawrence Lessig, *Code: And Other Laws of Cyberspace* (Basic Books, 1999); Karen Yeung, 'Towards an Understanding of Regulation by Design' in Roger Brownsword and Karen Yeung (eds), *Regulating Technologies: Legal Futures, Regulatory Frames and Technological Fixes* (Hart, 2008) 79–108.

[21] Lessig (n 20) 5–6; see also Lyria Bennett Moses, 'Regulating in the Face of Sociotechnical Change' in Roger Brownsword, Eloise Scotford and Karen Yeung (eds), *The Oxford Handbook of Law, Regulation and Technology* (Oxford University Press, 2017) 573–596.

[22] Suzor, Seignior and Singleton (n 6) 1069–73, drawing on the Manila Principles which highlight the use of harm mitigation strategies need to take account of freedom of speech and due process in line with tests of necessity and proportionality, see Global Civil Society, 'Manila Principles on Intermediary Liability' (24 March 2015) <https://manilaprinciples.org/index.html> accessed 12 August 2022; see also Nathan Hodson et al., 'Editorial: Defining and Regulating the Boundaries of Sex and Sexuality' (2019) 27(4) *Medical Law Review* 541, 542.

[23] Henry et al (n 3) 88.

[24] *ibid.*

[25] Henry et al (n 3); McGlynn et al (n 4).

[26] Kath Albury, 'Just Because It's Public Doesn't Mean It's Any of Your Business: Adults' and Children's Sexual Rights in Digitally Mediated Spaces' (2017) 19(5) *New Media & Society* 713.

practices.[27] Indeed, the use of tech-sex offers opportunities to meet, or engage sexually, with others in ways that are not available to them in 'real life'.[28] This includes the use of online platforms and digital technologies which have been used to initiate and maintain intimate relationships (including the sending of intimate images), establish and maintain friendships,[29] as well as operating as a safe place to express one's sexuality.[30] All of these factors are relevant to any understanding of the choices and actions people take with respect to sex, including those that are mediated via digital environments.[31]

Therefore, any attempt at regulating the use of tech-sex must confront such complexities rather than relying on a harm mitigation approach that is grounded in stark, binary or prohibitory terms.[32] It requires a regulatory approach which takes account of how harm is contextualised by socio-cultural, economic and political forces which inform broader digital cultural practices, but that also recognises that such harm is disproportionately suffered on a gendered and intersectional basis. Indeed, feminist and intersectional scholars have long noted the dysfunctional and biased approach taken in regulating risk and dealing with harmful consequences for certain individuals and groups arising from long-standing social, economic, gender, racial or ethnic biases and other inequalities.[33] While it is beyond the remit of this paper to examine such critiques in detail, we nevertheless recognise the importance of taking this into account in seeking to address harms such as IBSA. We now turn in the next section of the article to consider the question of consent, given that much of the regulatory focus in common law jurisdictions regarding the dissemination of intimate images in digital environments has focused on harms suffered arising from their non-consensual use.

A question of consent and image-based sexual abuse

Indeed, consent (and the lack thereof) has long been seen as an important control mechanism for individuals in the exercise of their sexual agency, informing whether and if so how they will enjoy embodied sexual experiences, as well as with whom they will engage in sexual relations. In general terms, consent can be characterised as both substantial and procedural in legal terms. It is substantial in that it refers to an individual evidencing autonomous choice and action; it is procedural in that it usually requires certain

[27]Sara McClelland and Michelle Fine, 'Education and Desire: Still Missing After All These Years' (2006) 76(3) *Harvard Educational Review* 297; Richard Parker, 'Sexuality, Culture and Society: Shifting Paradigms in Sexuality Research' (2009) 11(3) *Culture, Health & Sexuality* 251.

[28]Justin R Garcia et al, 'Sexting Among Singles in the USA: Prevalence of Sending, Receiving, and Sharing Sexual Messages and Images' (2016) 13(5) *Sexual Health* 428; Emily Setty, 'Meanings of Bodily and Sexual expression in Youth Sexting Culture: Young Women's Negotiation of Gendered Risks and Harms' (2019) 80(9) *Sex Roles* 586.

[29]Joris Ouytsel, Michel Walrave and Koen Ponnet, 'Sexting within Adolescents' Romantic Relationships: How Is It Related to Perceptions of Love and Verbal Conflict' (2019) 97 *Computers in Human Behaviour* 216–221.

[30]David Gudelunas, 'There's an App for That: The Uses and Gratifications of Online Social Networks for Gay Men' (2012) 16 *Sexuality and Culture* 347.

[31]Kane Race, 'Party and Play: Online Hook-Up Devices and the Emergence of PNP Practices Among Gay Men' (2015) 18(3) *Sexualities* 253.

[32]Mary Jane Mossman, 'Feminism and Legal Method: The Difference It Makes' (1987) 3 *Wisconsin Women's Law Journal* 147.

[33]See eg, Carol Smart, *Feminism and the Power of the Law* (Taylor & Francis, 1989) 32–34; Diane Kirkby (ed), *Sex, Power and Justice: Critical Perspectives on Law in Australia* (Oxford University Press, 1995) xiv-vi; Monique Mulholland, 'Walking a Fine Line: Young People Negotiate Pornified Heterosex' (2015) 18(5–6) *Sexualities* 731, 733; Sumi Cho, Kimberlé Williams Crenshaw and Leslie McCall, 'Toward a Field of Intersectionality Studies: Theory, Applications, and Praxis' (2013) 38(4) *Signs* 785; Danielle Citron 'Sexual Privacy' (2019) 128 *Yale Law Journal* 1870, 1890; Henry et al (n 3) 11, 124.

steps to be taken in order to verify consent before any potential infringement on the right to bodily integrity. Once consent is obtained, it legitimises certain activities and prohibits others as between the parties engaged in the process. In short, consent is employed as the proverbial red line determining what constitutes acceptable, or conversely unacceptable, interference with individuals' decision-making and their bodies.

Although we recognise that differing approaches exist in a range of jurisdictions,[34] the legal understanding of consent in common law jurisdictions such as Australia (and a lack of consent as it applies in the IBSA context), has been predominantly grounded in the criminal law.[35] Legal consent under the criminal law requires both the capacity to give consent and that such consent is given freely. A lack of consent therefore establishes whether a (sexual) offence has taken place and often features as a key element of the offence in common law jurisdictions.[36] In certain circumstances, a defence of reasonable belief in relation to the victim's consent may be available which, if established on the available evidence, can exonerate the accused.[37] This conceptualisation of consent appears to have in large part been translated into digital environments, particularly with respect to the non-consensual sharing of intimate images.

In considering the potential range of regulatory responses to non-consensual use of intimate images in digital environments, there has been a tendency in the relevant policy and academic literatures in common law jurisdictions to understand its scope and impact by reference to how it is understood within the criminal law.[38] In normative terms, this may be attributable to the (perceived) significance of the criminal law in controlling anti-social behaviour and for setting standards, as well as to the fact that their non-consensual use is often linked to sexual and family violence offending. While the criminal law clearly has its place in this regard, it operates as a slow, reactive and blunt instrument for addressing a range of harms caused to individuals, including persistent problems downstream with regard to enforcement.[39] Existing civil law options, including for breach of privacy, copyright, defamation, harassment or negligence, as well as broader questions of liability in relation to online intermediaries, also suffer from similar problems, as well as being costly and therefore out of reach for many individuals who suffer harms such as IBSA.[40]

---

[34] Amnesty International, 'Let's Talk About "Yes": Consent Laws in Europe' (17 December 2020) <https://www.amnesty.org/en/latest/campaigns/2020/12/consent-based-rape-laws-in-europe/> accessed 12 August 2022.

[35] Examples of common law jurisdictions include the United Kingdom, Ireland, Australia, Canada and New Zealand. For an overview, see McGlynn and Rackley (n 5); Henry et al (n 3).

[36] See Rachael Burgin and Asher Flynn, 'Women's Behaviour as Implied Consent: Male 'Reasonableness' in Australian Rape Law' (2019) 21(3) *Criminology and Criminal Justice* 334; Rachel Killean, Anne-Marie McAlinden and Eithne Dowds, 'Sexual Violence in the Digital Age: Replicating and Augmenting Harm, Victimhood and Blame' (2022) *Social & Legal Studies* 1–22 <https://d oi.org/10.1177/09646639221086592> accessed 12 August 2022.

[37] See Burgin and Flynn (n 36); Ashlee Gore, 'It's All or Nothing: Consent, Reasonable Belief, and the Continuum of Sexual Violence' (2021) 30(4) *Social & Legal Studies* 522.

[38] McGlynn and Rackley (n 5); Tyrone Kirchengast and Thomas Crofts, 'The Legal and Policy Contexts of "Revenge Porn" Criminalisation: The Need for Multiple Approaches' (2019) 19(1) *Oxford University Commonwealth Law Journal* 1; Henry et al. (n 3).

[39] Sentencing Advisory Council, *Sentencing Image-Based Sexual Abuse Offences in Victoria* (27 October 2020) <https://www.sentencingcouncil.vic.gov.au/publications/sentencing-image-based-sexual-abuse-offences-in-victoria> accessed 12 August 2022; Erika Rackley et al., 'Seeking Justice and Redress for Victim-Survivors of Image-Based Sexual Abuse' (2021) 29 *Feminist Legal Studies* 293.

[40] McGlynn and Rackley (n 5); Suzor, Seignior and Singleton (n 6); Mac Síthigh (n 6); Giancarlo Frosio (ed), *The Oxford Handbook of Online Intermediary Liability* (Oxford University Press, 2020).

In the circumstances, this raises broader policy concerns with respect to access to, as well as equality of, justice for harmed individuals in the regulatory jurisdiction, particularly on a gendered and intersectional basis. It also means taking account of how consent may need to be understood in the context of a 'continuum of coercion'[41] that can exist within sexual violence cases and which also can be linked to a broader range of socio-economic factors.[42] While there may be a prominent social media dating narrative involving the consensual sharing of such images, which is seen as an acceptable expression of adult sexual agency,[43] the disparate social reality in which women and minoritised groups find themselves results in their being held socially (if not legally) responsible for all harms caused as a result of IBSA, where such images are shared in digital environments with third parties without their consent. The difficulties faced by such individuals in terms of pursuing legal action in common law jurisdictions arising from IBSA has led to increased political interest and law reform activity in the area. This is explored in more detail in the next section, where we present a case study examining law reform involving Australia's national online safety regulatory regime, and how it has sought to address the problem of IBSA.

Regulating online safety in Australia

In recent years, much of the Australian political and legislative response to non-consensual use of intimate images has focused on addressing IBSA. Although not a new phenomenon,[44] internet and smartphone technology has caused an explosion in the capture of, distribution of, and threat to distribute intimate images. Australia's legislative response to IBSA is among the most advanced globally,[45] the activity having been prohibited in various forms under the criminal law at federal, state and territorial levels in recent years.[46] While laws differ across Australian states and territories,[47] there is a good degree of commonality in approach. For example, there is no legal requirement for the prosecution to prove harm or to prove that the perpetrator intended to cause harm to the victim.[48] Instead, it is accepted that IBSA would be reasonably expected to cause harm or distress to the victim.[49] As such, the prosecution must only prove the accused's intention to distribute, create or threaten to create or distribute a sexually explicit image.[50] Recognising the agency of adults to participate in certain intimate acts as

[41]Liz Kelly, *Surviving Sexual Violence* (Polity Press, 1988).
[42]Vanessa Munro, 'An Unholy Trinity: Non-Consent, Coercion and Exploitation in Contemporary Legal Responses to Sexual violence in England and Wales' (2010) 63(1) *Current Legal Problems* 45.
[43]*ibid*, 118–9.
[44]Henry et al (n 3) 1.
[45]Asher Flynn and Nicole Henry, 'Image-Based Sexual Abuse: An Australian Reflection' (2021) 31(4) *Women & Criminal Justice* 313, 318.
[46]Within the Australian jurisdiction of the Australian Capital Territory (ACT), for example, intimate images include 'a still or moving image, in any form – (ii) for a female or a transgender or intersex person who identifies as a female—of the person's breasts', making these laws more inclusive of trans and non-binary individuals. In addition, the visual capture – in photographic or video form of a person engaged in a sexual act, the distribution of these images, and threats to distribute these images, are also prohibited across all Australian jurisdictions; see also *Enhancing Online Safety (Non-consensual Sharing of Intimate Images) Act 2018* (Cth); *Criminal Code 1995* (Cth) s 474.17A.
[47]See, eg, upskirting laws in the Australian state jurisdiction of Victoria include 'observation of genital or anal region' (i.e. *Summary Offences Act 1966* (Vic) s 41A), whereas the same laws in NSW are incorporated into the revenge porn laws and include 'record intimate images without consent' (*Crimes Act 1900* (NSW) s 91P).
[48]See, eg, *Crimes Act 1900* (ACT) s 72C; Flynn and Henry (n 45) 7.
[49]Flynn and Henry (n 45) 320; McGlynn et al (n 4).
[50]See *Crimes Act 1900* (ACT) s 72C; Flynn and Henry (n 45) 320.

long as consent is provided,[51] all criminal laws include consent as a defence which has traditionally been understood as person- and situation-specific, and which is a process which can be subject to change and withdrawal at any time.[52] Given that issues of coercion, control and power impact consent across all sexual offences, academic commentators have argued that questions of sexual consent are often too focused on the victims, rather than the accused, underpinned by a range of myths and stereotypes, of which previous mention has been made. In the circumstances, it has been argued that consent should either be irrelevant, or that all Australian laws dealing with sexual consent should make it clear that the onus is on the accused to establish that the victim consented.[53]

Notwithstanding a shift in public, political and legal attitudes towards sexual consent in this context, a key issue of concern remains enforcement. In the Australian state of Victoria, a recent report examined sentencing practices following the prosecution of IBSA-related offences.[54] It found that there were very few cases where such offences were prosecuted on their own; rather, most prosecutions involved charges for a number of other non-IBSA offences.[55] The majority of cases were linked to family violence,[56] with the most common alleged offence pursued in these circumstances being the actual or threatened distribution of intimate images. Even in the very few cases where a prosecution took place, IBSA-related offending usually received low sentences, even in cases where serious harm was caused.[57] The report's findings on the types of and rates of prosecution for IBSA offences corresponds with academic research in the area,[58] against a background where the discretion to prosecute is infrequently exercised.

As noted previously, this reflects a wider social issue which is rooted in entrenched gender and intersectional inequalities.[59] This state of affairs remains despite technological innovation or engagement with digital environments.[60] In the circumstances, a regulatory approach which offers a quick, low-cost method for mitigating harm from IBSA represents a welcome additional or alternative redress option for affected individuals.[61] In Australia, this has been facilitated by the recent adoption of a new national regulatory regime for online safety, set out in the Online Safety Act 2021 (OSA 2021).[62] The regime is overseen

---

[51] See for example in the Australian state jurisdiction of New South Wales, *Hansard*, Legislative Assembly, 24 May 2017, 20 (Mark Speakman, Second Reading Speech, *Crimes Amendment (Intimate Images) Bill 2017*).

[52] Killean, McAlinden and Dowds (n 36) 11.

[53] Michelle Evans, 'Regulating the Non-Consensual Sharing of Intimate Images ('Revenge Pornography') via a Civil Penalty Scheme: A Sex Equality Analysis' (2019) 44(3) *Monash University Law Review* 602, 620. Note recent developments in certain Australian jurisdictions, which now require affirmative consent, see Tamsin Rose, 'NSW Affirmative Consent Laws: What Do They Mean and How Will They Work?' (*The Guardian New South Wales*, 1 June 2022) <https://www.theguardian.com/australia-news/2022/jun/01/nsw-affirmative-consent-laws-what-do-they-mean-and-how-will-they-work> accessed 12 August 2022.

[54] Sentencing Advisory Council (n 39).

[55] *ibid* xi.

[56] See also Flynn and Henry (n 45) 322.

[57] *ibid.*

[58] Henry et al (n 3); McGlynn et al (n 4).

[59] Henry et al (n 3) 420.

[60] See Nicola Henry and Anastasia Powell, 'Sexual Violence in the Digital Age: The Scope and Limits of Criminal Law' (2016) 25(4) *Social & Legal Studies* 397; Tatjana Hörnle, '#MeToo - Implications for Criminal Law?' (2018) 6(2) *Bergen Journal of Criminal Law and Criminal Justice* 115; Rachel Killean, Eithne Dowds and Anne-Marie McAlinden (eds), *Sexual Violence on Trial* (Routledge, 2021).

[61] See Henry et al (n 3) 148–50.

[62] See the Online Safety Act 2021 (Cth) (OSA 2021), which came into force on 23 January 2022. For background information on the Act, see Explanatory Memorandum, Online Safety Bill 2021 (Cth).

by a national independent regulatory body, known as the Office of the eSafety Commissioner (eSafety), which coordinates a whole-of-government approach on the issue, as well as having a broader policy remit to promote safer and more positive online experiences.[63] This includes the development of core principles setting out expectations regarding online safety, the conduct of research, as well as the promotion of educational and awareness activities that promote online safety.[64]

Originally established in 2015, eSafety's regulatory remit was initially focused on safeguarding children from online risks and harm. In support of such remit, it was provided with a range of enforcement powers to deal with cyberbullying and abusive online materials, which were targeted at children. Over time, its powers have been extended to include various aspects of online safety involving both children and adults. Following the adoption of the OSA 2021, its powers have now significantly expanded to include regulatory oversight of social media services,[65] relevant electronic services,[66] hosting service providers and designated internet services (services and providers),[67] as well as individual persons who post materials via these services and providers.[68]

eSafety also oversees a range of specific schemes designed to address specific areas of concern involving online safety.[69] This includes its image-based abuse scheme, with its regulatory powers in relation to administering the scheme set out under the OSA 2021.[70] It should be noted that the preference in legislative terms, as well as on the part of eSafety, is to use the term 'image-based abuse', rather than IBSA, which can be attributed to the desire to avoid association with colloquial terms such as 'revenge porn'.[71] As part of overseeing the scheme,[72] eSafety engages in education activities, which includes social

[63]eSafety Commissioner, 'Our Structure' (2022) <https://www.esafety.gov.au/about-us/who-we-are/our-structure> accessed 12 August 2022.

[64]eSafety Commissioner, 'Who We Are' (2022) <https://www.esafety.gov.au/about-us/who-we-are> accessed 12 August 2022.

[65]OSA 2021 (n 62) s 13.

[66]OSA 2021 (n 62) s 13A.

[67]OSA 2021 (n 62) s 14.

[68]See, eg, OSA 2021 (n 62) s 70.

[69]This now includes a world-first adult cyber abuse scheme for adults, where it has powers to require the removal of adult cyber abuse material if it meets the threshold criterion of having been posted with the likely intention of causing serious harm. An updated online content scheme has been established, which enables eSafety to take action against illegal or restricted online content that is likely to cause significant harm. This includes child sexual abuse material and 'abhorrent violent material', regardless of where such materials are hosted, see OSA 2021 (n 62) s 8, pt 9; see also for an overview, eSafety Commissioner, 'Abhorrent Violent Conduct Powers - Regulatory Guidance, eSC RG 5' (December 2021) <https://www.esafety.gov.au/sites/default/files/2021-12/OSA-AVCP-Regulatory-Guidance.pdf> accessed 12 August 2022 ; eSafety Commissioner, 'Online Content Scheme - Regulatory Guidance, eSC RG 4' (December 2021) <https://www.esafety.gov.au/sites/default/files/2021-12/eSafety-Online-Content-Scheme.pdf> accessed 12 August 2022.

[70]OSA 2021 (n 62) pt 6. Note that for the purposes of the application of Act to an intimate image or private sexual material, 'consent' means the following: 'consent that is express, voluntary and informed but does not include consent given by a child; or consent given by an adult who is in a mental or physical condition (whether temporary or permanent) that makes the adult incapable of giving consent or substantially impairs the capacity of the adult to give consent', see OSA 2021 (n 62) pt 1 s 21.

[71]Clare McGlynn, Erika Rackley and Ruth Houghton, 'Beyond "Revenge Porn": The Continuum of Image-Based Sexual Abuse' (2017) 25 *Feminist Legal Studies* 25; Julie Inman Grant, '"Revenge Porn", By Another Name' (eSafety Commissioner, 27 February 2017) <https://www.esafety.gov.au/newsroom/blogs/revenge-porn-another-name> accessed 12 August 2022.

[72]In terms of how the scheme works in practice, see eSafety Commissioner, 'Image-based Abuse' (Australian Government, 2022) <https://www.esafety.gov.au/key-issues/image-based-abuse/take-action/report-to-esafety-commissioner> accessed 12 August 2022.

media campaigns to raise awareness about the scheme.[73] It hosts an online portal which provides comprehensive information regarding online safety, cyberbullying, online abuse targeting women, domestic violence, stalking and IBSA. The portal also contains information about how to communicate with online platforms hosting intimate images and persons who have intimate images in their possession, as well as how to collect and report evidence of IBSA to eSafety.[74]

For the purposes of initiating a regulatory response by eSafety under the scheme, an 'intimate image' includes a still or moving visual image, which (appears to) depict(s) a person's genital area or anal area (whether bare or covered by underwear), or one or both breasts of a female, transgender or intersex person. What constitutes 'intimate material' includes a person in a state of undress, using a toilet, showering, having a bath, or engaged in a sexual act of a kind not ordinarily done in public, in circumstances in which an ordinary reasonable person would reasonably expect to be afforded privacy. This is in addition to images that depict a person without religious attire, if they consistently wear that attire because of their religious or cultural background.[75] Originally established in 2018,[76] the key features of the eSafety scheme have been retained in the OSA 2021, albeit that eSafety now has enhanced powers to deal more rapidly with complaints by affected individuals against services and providers, as well as the person(s) responsible for posting the images.[77] This includes requiring services and providers to remove hosted intimate images within 24 h of receiving a removal notice issued by eSafety,[78] reduced from 48 h under the previous regime. eSafety can also now obtain basic subscriber account information from services and providers, thus making it easier to deal with the problem of anonymous accounts which post and share intimate images online.[79]

There are also a range of enforcement options under the scheme. In addition to informal removal action against services and providers, options include the issuing of formal warnings, remedial directions and infringement notices, as well as obtaining court orders for injunctive relief or the imposition of a (financial) civil penalty.[80] A review of data published in eSafety's Annual Reports in the 2019–2021 period showed a substantial rise in the reporting of abuse across all schemes managed by eSafety, with women being disproportionately at risk of having suffered harm in digital environments. This included young women aged 13–17 years, who were identified as being the 'primary targets' of cyberbullying, with adult women making the majority of requests for assistance with cyberbullying. Similarity in both patterns of behaviour and platforms were noted in reports of

---

[73]This has included the issuing of digital packs to Australian Universities, which contain information designed to reduce the incidents of image-based abuse amongst students, see Australian Communications and Media Authority, eSafety Commissioner, 'Annual Report 2020-21', (Australian Communications and Media Authority, 2021) <https://www.esafety.gov.au/sites/default/files/2021->10/ACMA%20and%20eSafety%20annual%20report%202020-21_0.pdf> accessed 12 August 2022.

[74]eSafety Commissioner, 'How to Report Image-Based Abuse' (Australian Government, 2022) <www.esafety.gov.au/report/image-based-abuse> accessed 12 August 2022.

[75]OSA 2021 (n 62) s 15(4).

[76]See *Enhancing Online Safety (Non-consensual Sharing of Intimate Images) Act 2018* (Cth) (now repealed).

[77]OSA 2021 (n 62) pt 3, div 3, ss 34–5, pt 6, div 3, pt 10.

[78]OSA 2021 (n 62) ss 77–9.

[79]OSA 2021 (n 62) s 194. For an overview of the issues, see eSafety Commissioner, 'Anonymity and Identity Shielding' (Australian Government, 2022) <https://www.esafety.gov.au/industry/tech-trends-and-challenges/anonymity> accessed 12 August 2022.

[80]The civil penalty order would be sought by the eSafety Commissioner pursuant to powers granted pursuant to *Regulatory Powers (Standard Provisions) Act 2014* (Cth) pt 4. The Federal Court of Australia and the Federal Circuit Court of Australia are the relevant courts for the purposes of seeking such orders under the Act.

cyberbullying involving both young and older women.[81] Apart from sextortion scams impacting men which proliferated during the first wave of the Covid-19 pandemic in 2020,[82] women were overwhelmingly the victims of IBSA (75%). Such abuse included posting intimate images online without consent, threatening to share such images via private means and/or digital environments, peer group sharing, coercive control, the use of impersonation accounts, receipt of unsolicited intimate images and the creation of digitally altered images.[83] No further data was published regarding race, ethnicity, socio-economic status or sexual orientation of individuals reporting IBSA.

eSafety reported making use of three main remediation strategies, all of which involved the use of a 'soft' enforcement approach. First, 'alerting' social media services about accounts that were misused to elicit, share or threaten to share intimate content. Such notifications typically resulted in eSafety deleting such accounts (just under 2,000 in 2020-21; 970 in 2019-20).[84] Second, the taking of 'removal action', which involved contacting services and providers (most of which being overseas-hosted exposé or pornography sites), to request the removal of IBSA materials. Such removal action proved to be remarkably successful, with a success rate in the range of 82% to 90%.[85] Third, where this proved unsuccessful, steps were taken to 'limit the discoverability' of such materials, through having it removed from search engine results.[86]

Despite an increase in reports under the IBSA scheme, there was a noticeable and unexplained decrease in the use of the latter two strategies as between the reporting periods 2019–20 and 2020-21. There was also little, if any use, of what could be described as 'hard' enforcement powers under the scheme. In the 2019–21 period, eSafety issued a total of 8 removal notices (all to overseas-hosted sites); 2 remedial directions, 6 formal warnings to perpetrators; and 3 informal warnings issued where it was considered appropriate to adopt a remedial and educative approach to enforcement.[87] There were no reports of use being made of enforceable notices, injunctions or civil penalty orders. We now turn in the next section to assess the effectiveness of Australia's national online safety regulatory model for managing harms such as IBSA.

---

[81]ACMA, eSafety Commissioner, *Annual Report 2020–21* (n 73) 209–12.

[82]*ibid* 213. As eSafety notes, 'Sexual extortion is a form of blackmail and involves threats to post intimate images of the victim unless demands are met, typically for money. It includes the use of fake accounts to threaten distribution of intimate content recorded via video chat, scam email campaigns where victims are threatened with the release of 'hacked' intimate content and dating/romance scams. Victims of sexual extortion were predominately male'.

[83]*ibid* 213–14. eSafety reported that the image-based abuse took the following forms in the 2020–21 period: sextortion (57%); online child sexual exploitation (11%); posting online without consent (8%); threatening to share (excluding sextortion) (4%); sharing via private means (3%); and 'other' (11%). The 'other' category covered harms such as 'peer group sharing among young people, coercive control, impersonation accounts, receipt of unsolicited intimate images and digitally altered images.' The majority of reports of IBSA related to adult victims, involving 73% of reports received. Age-related data included adults aged 18–24 years comprising the highest percentage of victims (40%), followed by those aged 25 years and over (33%). Apart from 1% where age was not known, 26% of victims were children.

[84]*ibid* 215; see ACMA, Office of the eSafety Commissioner, 'Annual Report, 2019–20' (September 2020) <https://www.esafety.gov.au/sites/default/files/2020-10/ACMA%20and%20eSafety%20annual%20report%202019-20.pdf> accessed 12 August 2022.

[85]In 2019–20, this involved over 4,000 locations, across 248 different platforms, with a success rate of 82%. In 2020–21, this decreased significantly with notices issued to only 2,500 locations (generally URLs) across 141 different platforms, with a 90% success rate, see ACMA, Office of the eSafety Commissioner, 'Annual Report 2019–20' (n 84); ACMA, Office of the eSafety Commissioner, 'Annual Report 2020-21' (n 73).

[86]ACMA, Office of the eSafety Commissioner, 'Annual Report 2019-20' (n 73) 216.

[87]*ibid* 214; ACMA, Office of the eSafety Commissioner, 'Annual Report 2020-21' (n 73) 212–3.

Assessing Australia's regulatory model for managing image-based sexual abuse

In the previous section, we examined key aspects of Australia's regulatory model for online safety, focusing on education activities by eSafety, the national regulator. This was in addition to reviewing threshold criteria for initiating a regulatory response to IBSA, as well as the approach taken to mitigating harm. In terms of its response, eSafety clearly focuses on both prevention and remediation strategies, which we have argued are important aspects of the protective mode of our proposed regulatory approach. In relation to the use of preventive strategies, eSafety pursues a range of education activities to increase IBSA awareness and to highlight how to report instances of such abuse for follow-up with respect to mitigating harm. This is largely in line with a regulatory focus on managing risk as a matter of ensuring safety from harm in online environments. It is narrowly prescribed in line with eSafety's legislatively mandated powers which, in turn, have their origins in longstanding political and public concerns around protecting children in such contexts. This has operated in practice to create 'path dependencies'[88] which continue to influence the way risk is framed in policy and legal terms in relation to regulating online safety involving both children *and* adults.

As we have previously identified, it is a framing which we consider to be insufficiently nuanced to take account of both opportunities and challenges that arise for adults with respect to engaging in current digital sexual cultures. This requires a regulatory approach that is designed to facilitate digital sexual literacy against a background where engagement with such cultures has become central to the mediation of social relations, as well as to how sexual connection and intimacy are enacted, developed, and maintained.[89] Alongside regulatory initiatives to manage harms arising out of IBSA, for example, it is vital that concerns about risk and danger involved in the sharing of intimate images take place in a broader context of education initiatives regarding sexual cultures, relationships and pleasure.[90] Focusing predominantly on risky, problematic or dangerous aspects of sex or relationships which are facilitated in digital environments, does not engage with the reality of most people's sexual relationships or the type of relationship (safe, healthy, pleasurable) they may aim to achieve.[91]

Understanding what people perceive to be the benefits of online sexual engagement, including the risks people take, how these risks are perceived in relation to pleasure and desire, and the choices people make in online environments, is necessary for developing a comprehensive regulatory approach to education about digital sexual health. In the circumstances, a nuanced approach needs to be taken by regulators in developing prevention strategies, which should focus on education initiatives which explore the risks and

---

[88]The 'path dependencies' is used to describe how previous or established ideas, ways of thinking, procedures and processes can influence the way in which a current policy problem is viewed which in turn may impact the design of laws, see Paul Pierson, 'Increasing Returns, Path Dependence, and the Study of Politics' (2000) 94(2) *American Political Science Review* 252.

[89]Rachel Scott et al, 'What and How: Doing Good Research with Young People, Digital Intimacies, and Relationships and Sex Education' (2020) 20(6) *Sex Education* 675, 676.

[90]Kath Albury, Amy Adele Hasinoff and Theresa Senft, 'From Media Abstinence to Media Production: Sexting, Young People and Education' in Louisa Allen and Mary Lou Ramussen (eds), *The Palgrave Handbook of Sexuality Education* (Palgrave Macmillan, 2017) 527–545.

[91]Louisa Allen, Mary Lou Rasmussen and Kathleen Quinlivan (eds), *The Politics of Pleasure in Sexuality Education: Pleasure Bound* (Routledge, 2013); Allison Carter et al, 'Sexual Health Promotion' in Jacqueline Gahagan and Mary K. Bryson (eds), *Sex-and Gender-Based Analysis in Public Health* (Springer, 2021) 113–121.

benefits associated with the use of tech-sex, highlighting both positive and negative experiences for users. Given the range of motivations influencing sexual engagement online and/or via such technologies, this involves educational promotion which is centred on keeping individuals safe from (potential) harms while also respecting their sexual agency and capacity to make their own decisions in this regard.[92]

Specifically in the case of harm such as IBSA, which may materialise arising from non-consensual sharing of intimate images, there is a need for national regulators, such as eSafety, to be mindful of the way in which they present education initiatives which are within their remit. While this may involve the giving of practical tips such as ensuring that when sending such images, they are anonymised or do not include any identifying features,[93] this may lead to a risk assessment model that not only fails to fully capture the complexity of online sexual encounters and engagements, including consensual sharing of intimate images. It may also minimise the harms caused – within a non-consensual context – by placing a level of blame on the person captured in the image.[94] In the case of women, for example, sexual agency is consequently diminished via the chastisement of sexual expression and the normalisation of a highly gendered blame culture.[95] Overcoming these persistent challenges requires a social and cultural shift in how we understand sexual violence, female sexuality, sexual agency and issues of consent. While educational initiatives which promote positive discussions on sexuality are important,[96] this must be accompanied by an appreciation of situated vulnerabilities experienced on a gendered and intersectional basis. While eSafety clearly recognises the gendered aspect of harm in the context of IBSA, it has only recently begun to pay more attention to the intersectional aspects of such harm.[97] An appreciation of the intersectionality of both risk and harm is vital in relation to such initiatives, supported by a comprehensive approach to harm mitigation. This requires a pro-active approach, which should be informed by accurate data collection which is published and evaluated on an annual basis.

In terms of the current approach to managing IBSA, eSafety acknowledges that a wrongful act has been committed, and harm caused to affected individuals, as a result of IBSA. In doing so, it employs a range of remediation strategies which facilitate the rapid removal of intimate images where possible.[98] In this way, eSafety is able to initiate removal action, predominantly through making direct contact with services and providers, which demonstrates it is responsive to the need for quick, no-cost redress on the part of affected individuals.[99] Although eSafety clearly has a wide range of enforcement

[92]Power et al (n 1).

[93]See for example, University of Toronto, 'Intimate Images and Privacy' (*Community Safety Office*) <https://www.communitysafety.utoronto.ca/safety-tip/intimate-images-and-privacy/> accessed 17 Aug 2022.

[94]Diana T Sanchez, Amy K Kiefer and Oscar Ybarra, (2006) 'Sexual Submissiveness in Women: Costs for Sexual Autonomy and Arousal' (2006) 32(4) *Personality and Social Psychology Bulletin* 512; Julia Zauner, 'The Continuum of Symbolic Violence: How Sexting Education Neglects Image-Based Sexual Abuse, Dismisses Perpetrators Responsibility, and Violates Rights to Sexual Autonomy' (2021) 5(3) *Journal of Gender-Based Violence* 483.

[95]Henry et al (n 3); Killean, Dowds and McAlinden (n 60).

[96]Elizabeth Agnew, 'Sexting Among Young People: Towards a Gender Sensitive Approach' (2021) 29 *International Journal of Children's Rights* 3.

[97]eSafety Commissioner, 'Protecting Voices at Risk Online' (2022) <https://www.esafety.gov.au/diverse-groups/protecting-voices-risk-online> accessed 12 August 2022.

[98]eSafety Commissioner, 'Civil Penalties Scheme' (2022) <https://www.esafety.gov.au/key-issues/image-based-abuse/take-action/civil-penalties-scheme#:~:text=The%20Enhancing%20Online%20Safety%20Act,notice)%20to%20the%20eSafety%20Commissioner> accessed 12 August 2022.

[99]See Henry et al (n 3).

powers under the IBSA scheme,[100] the available data from its recent Annual Reports points to a marked preference for a 'soft' rather than 'hard' enforcement approach. While a remediation strategy may involve the successful removal of IBSA materials from digital environments, it is not clear that this constitutes an effective prevention strategy on its own vis-à-vis persons that post such materials, or services and providers that host and/or share such materials.[101] Indeed, we would suggest that enhanced effectiveness of such prevention strategies would result from a greater preparedness on the part of national online safety regulators, such as eSafety, to make use of the full range of enforcement powers in the event of (persistent) non-compliance.

As the designated national regulator for online safety, eSafety must necessarily weigh up which approach, or combination of approaches, is likely to strike the right balance in the context of facilitating optimum regulator-regulatee relations, as well as ensuring that suitable remediation is provided to individuals harmed by IBSA. This may be made more complex by the fact that the regulatees with which national online safety regulators engage may operate on a trans-jurisdictional basis. In the circumstances, this may make it much more difficult to develop the sort of regular regulator-regulatee interactions which could generate a sense of corporate social responsibility in seeking to minimise the occurrence of IBSA on hosting services or platforms. Against this background, one option, of which previous mention has been made, is to adopt a deterrence approach which focuses on employing formal mechanisms of punishment to sanction poor behaviour, as well as signalling to other regulatees that this is the way in which breaches of the online safety regulatory regime will be dealt with.[102]

In the case of eSafety, the choice to employ a deterrence approach in seeking to manage IBSA may turn on a number of factors: type of regulatees (i.e. small, medium or large entities);[103] whether the dynamic of the regulated sector is such that regulators consider regulatees to be 'amoral calculators' with respect to the cost of compliance;[104] and with which regulatory cultures regulatees may be most familiar. In the case of services and providers that host and share intimate images, they may be incorporated or managed in overseas jurisdictions, a feature which has been highlighted in eSafety's own data on enforcement activity in relation to the scheme. Where services and providers are based in the U.S., for example, they operate in a regulatory culture which offers immunity from liability based on 'safe harbour' laws,[105] in the context of a more legally contested approach to challenging regulatory decision-making.[106]

---

[100] eSafety Commissioner, 'Civil Penalties Scheme' (n 98).

[101] eSafety's under-utilisation of the full range of enforcement powers pursuant to the civil penalty scheme has already been the subject of adverse commentary, see Henry et al (n 3) 148.

[102] Murphy (n 15) 564–5; see generally Gunningham, 'Enforcing Environmental Regulation' (2011) 23(2) *Journal of Environmental Law* 169.

[103] Fiona Haines, *Corporate Regulation: Beyond 'Punish or Persuade'* (Clarendon Press, 1997).

[104] Robert Kagan and John T Scholz, 'The "Criminology of the Corporation" and Regulatory Enforcement Strategies' in Keith Hawkins and John M Thomas (eds), *Enforcing Regulation* (Kluwer-Nijhoff, 1984) 67.

[105] Note that U.S. law is likely to give 'safe harbour' to online intermediaries which 'knowingly host cyber stalking or revenge porn', for example, although this has been limited somewhat for websites that facilitate sex trafficking (see § 230 Communications Decency Act 1996, U.S.C. § 230). For an overview, see Natalia Homchick, 'Reaching Through the "Ghost Doxer": An Argument for Imposing Secondary Liability on Online Intermediaries' (2019) 76(3) *Washington and Lee Law Review* 1307, 1329. As Henry et al (n 3) notes at 158, these 'safe harbour' laws present difficulties for victim-survivors of IBSA to hold online intermediaries to account.

[106] Robert Kagan, *Adversarial Legalism: The American Way of Law* (Harvard University Press, 2003).

Taking account of how regulatory cultures operate in a given jurisdictional setting where services and providers are based, may also be an important consideration to be taken into account by regulators, such as eSafety, in relation to the choice of enforcement strategies. In the circumstances, an 'advise and persuade' compliance strategy, which focuses on conciliation, rather than confrontation, to facilitate the overarching aims of the regulatory regime, rather than on imposing sanctions for breach,[107] would appear to be the current preferred approach by eSafety. The danger with such an approach is that it can lead to what has been described as the 'compliance trap', with a more cooperative approach to facilitating compliance which on the one hand is likely to assist with developing and maintaining regulator-regulatee relations, but may operate in practice to discourage improved behaviour, particularly where it is observed that poor behaviour goes unpunished.[108]

As noted previously, an alternative approach would be to navigate a middle line between the two approaches based on a responsive regulatory approach, which employs a mix of compliance and enforcement strategies to ensure appropriate behaviour on the part of those subject to the regulatory regime.[109] This would involve escalating towards a more punitive approach in the event that such behaviour does not improve in line with the aims and objectives of the regulatory regime.[110] Indeed, a more responsive regulatory position may be preferred in terms of its relations with the technology industry as eSafety develops into a more mature online safety regulator over time.[111] Although it remains to be seen, this may also be facilitated as a result of eSafety's expanded regulatory remit under the OSA 2021, which now requires that it reviews and registers industry codes and standards, with the objective of achieving responsible industry processes and procedures for dealing with online safety and content issues.[112] Where this objective is not achieved, then eSafety is then better placed to escalate its compliance strategy to impose industry-wide standards in place of agreed codes, investigate complaints arising from alleged breaches of such codes, and impose civil penalties and obtain injunctive orders.[113]

In seeking to strike the right balance in the use of compliance and enforcement strategies against a well-resourced technology industry with global reach, it is also vital that national online safety regulators, such as eSafety, are able to mobilise political and social support to encourage industry commitment to the online safety regulatory regime.[114] In the absence of political support, it is likely to prove difficult to pursue compliance enforcement activities successfully, particularly where it may involve influential

[107]Hawkins (n 16); Hutter (n 16).

[108]Sidney A Shapiro and Randy S Rabinowitz, 'Punishment versus Cooperation in Regulatory Enforcement: A Case Study of OHSA' (1997) 49(4) *Administrative Law Review* 713; Parker (n 13).

[109]Ayres and Braithwaite (n 17).

[110]Gunningham (n 18) 120.

[111]An example of industry collaboration is highlighted by the Safety by Design initiative which involves industry collaboration with eSafety to promote safety, rights and ethics in design processes for online products and services, see eSafety Commissioner, 'Safety by Design' (2022) <https://www.esafety.gov.au/industry/safety-by-design> accessed 12 August 2022.

[112]OSA 2021 (n 62) pt 4.

[113]See OSA 2021 (n 62) ss 48, 50, 53, 57, 60. eSafety Commissioner, 'Learn About the Online Safety Act' (2022) <https://www.esafety.gov.au/whats-on/online-safety-act> accessed 12 August 2022. Industry compliance is also likely to be incentivised through the need to meet the Australian government's Basic Online Safety Expectations (BOSE) Direction 2022, overseen by eSafety, For an overview, see eSafety Commissioner, 'Basic Online Safety Expectations' (2022) <https://www.esafety.gov.au/about-us/who-we-are/basic-online-safety-expectations> accessed 12 August 2022.

[114]Parker (n 13) 593; Gunningham (n 102) 201.

transnational corporate actors.[115] However, where there is a political will, there is clearly a political way through, with the Australian government showing a greater preparedness in recent times to take on 'tech giants' in relation to the hosting and/or sharing of (defamatory) material on their platforms.[116] It is therefore important to keep in mind that politics matters in the national and international regulation of online intermediaries, as well as digital environments more generally. This includes whether, and if so how, harms such as IBSA are to be addressed in such environments, in addition to who is prioritised for redress in the circumstances.

Conclusion

The use of tech-sex in offering a range of opportunities for the pursuit of sexual desire, pleasure and intimacy is to be welcomed. While such developments should be celebrated as a positive step in support of adult sexual agency, we also need to be mindful of the fact that harm may arise from their non-consensual use. The preferred approach in regulatory terms should involve showing due respect for adult sexual agency while also seeking to mitigate harm through the use of prevention and remediation strategies, which are sensitive to the differential impact of harm on a gendered and intersectional basis. Operating along a facilitative-protective axis, this is a regulatory approach that recognises the need for a more nuanced understanding of both the opportunities and challenges involved in managing risk and benefits arising from the use of tech-sex.

While recent regulatory reforms for enhancing online safety are to be welcomed in common law jurisdictions, such as Australia, there is a need to be cautious about framing regulatory design predominantly, or solely, around questions of safety which may promote a top-down regulatory response to managing risk which is overly narrow, prescriptive and largely prohibitory in approach. In the case of tech-sex, we consider it vital that a suitable balance be struck between facilitation and protection in regulatory design and implementation, which recognises the importance that sex and relationships have in individuals' lives and, by extension, the technologies that are now commonly used to facilitate this in our current digital cultures. This involves recognising that managing risk is part of engaging with such technologies. However, such recognition should be accompanied by education activities by national online safety regulators which seek to enhance digital sexual literacy, as well as offering quick, low-cost remediation strategies in order to mitigate harms such as IBSA, where appropriate.

Disclosure statement

No potential conflict of interest was reported by the author(s).

[115]Matías Dewey and Donato Di Carlo, 'Governing Through Non-Enforcement: Regulatory Forbearance as Industrial Policy in Advanced Economies' (2021) *Regulation & Governance* <https://doi.org/10.1111/rego.12382> accessed 12 August 2022, 1–22.

[116]Michelle Meagher, 'Australia's Move to Tame Facebook and Google Is Just the Start of a Global Battle' (*The Guardian* 24 February 2021) <https://www.theguardian.com/commentisfree/2021/feb/24/australia-facebook-google-global-battle-governments-journalism> accessed 12 August 2022; Rob Harris, 'New Australian Laws to Unmask Anonymous Online Trolls and Make Tech Giants Pay' (*Sydney Morning Herald* 28 November 2021) <https://www.smh.com.au/politics/federal/new-australian-laws-to-unmask-anonymous-online-trolls-and-make-tech-giants-pay-20211128-p59csb.html> accessed 12 August 2022.

Funding

Research for this article was undertaken as part of the project, 'The Technological Transformation of Sex: Improving Australia's Response', which is funded by the Australian Research Council (DP190102027). The project research team includes the five authors, as well as Emeritus Professor Gary Dowsett, Dr Alexandra James, Ms Lily Moor and Dr Andrea Waling. Jayne Lucke made a generous contribution to the conceptualisation and design of the project. The project is supported by the Australian Research Centre in Sex, Health and Society at La Trobe University and Edinburgh Law School, University of Edinburgh.

ORCID

Anne-Maree Farrell http://orcid.org/0000-0001-9522-6528
Nicole Shackleton http://orcid.org/0000-0002-1236-2346
Elizabeth Agnew http://orcid.org/0000-0001-5855-5744
Samantha Hopkins http://orcid.org/0000-0002-9609-224X
Jennifer Power http://orcid.org/0000-0002-6566-3214

OPEN ACCESS

Rethinking risk in adults' engagement with sexual digital imagery

Jennifer Power, Gary W. Dowsett, Andrea Waling, Alexandra James, Lily Moor, Nicole Shackleton and Anne-Maree Farrell

ABSTRACT

Introduction Camera-equipped smartphones and other devices allow people to capture and share images directly with others in ways that are spontaneous, instant and relatively inexpensive. Such sharing is a common part of modern sexual intimacies, despite media and educational discourses warning of potential risks. **Methods** This paper reports on a qualitative study in which we interviewed 23 Australian adults about the ways in which they used with digital sexual imagery in their sex lives. The study aimed to explore participants' experiences of digital sexual self-image creation and sharing and the ways discourses of risk and safety shape these experiences. **Results** Findings showed that participants tended to view the creation and exchange of sexual images as a form of sexual play that built intimacy, sexual tension and eroticism into their relationships and expanded their sexual and relationship experiences in positive ways. Participants were aware that sending sexual or nude images left them vulnerable to potential harm or unwanted sexual exposure and were concerned that some people would view such practices as foolish or irresponsible given these risks held such high profile. These concerns meant participants were often secretive about their experiences although the sense of risk and vulnerability in these exchanges enhanced intimacy or eroticism for some participants. **Conclusions** Educational approaches to managing digital risk should recognise that people often have positive digital sexual experiences that can lead them to disengage from fear-based messaging. **Policy implications** As digital technologies evolve, their integration with human sexual intimacy will continue to change and develop in unforeseen ways. Educational and regulatory responses will require ongoing scrutiny and innovation to acknowledge users' positive experiences and desires while responding to risks and challenges.

This article is licensed under a Creative Commons Attribution 4.0 International License, which permits use, sharing, adaptation, distribution and reproduction in any medium or format, as long as you give appropriate credit to the original author(s) and the source, provide a link to the Creative Commons licence, and indicate if changes were made. The images or other third party material in this article are included in the article's Creative Commons licence, unless indicated otherwise in a credit line to the material. If material is not included in the article's Creative Commons licence and your intended use is not permitted by statutory regulation or exceeds the permitted use, you will need to obtain permission directly from the copyright holder. To view a copy of this licence, visit http://creativecommons.org/licenses/by/4.0/.

Modern, camera-equipped, smartphones allow people to capture and share images directly with others or via social media and websites in a way that is spontaneous, instant, and relatively inexpensive. The ubiquity of digital cameras means communication using digital images (photographs and video) is now part of everyday intimacies. People send images to each other, view the Instagram feeds of their friends and family, and communicate via video stream (Madianou, 2016; Watson et al., 2021). Furthermore, digital images and digital technologies are increasingly integrated into people's sex lives. Digitally mediated sexual intimacy that involves imagery—'sexting', 'sexual selfies', 'sex tapes', webcamming, or amateur pornography—is a common part of contemporary sex lives (Amundsen, 2020; Gesselman, Druet, & Vitzthum, 2020).

As these technologies have become more commonplace, so has recognition of the potential risks and dangers they pose, including non-consensual sharing of imagery (sometimes called revenge pornography) and other forms of online sexual harassment and abuse (Henry et al., 2020; Henry & Powell, 2016; Henry, Powell, & Flynn, 2017b). In this paper, we explore the impact of the awareness of such risk on adults' experiences of creating, sending, and/or receiving digital sexual images. Our aim is not to determine how people manage or try to mitigate risks; rather, we explore ways people make sense of risk and how this informs and shapes practices of digital sexual imagery use. In doing this, we hope to develop a nuanced approach to understanding how people navigate risk in the context of pleasures and benefits.

Danger, 'Slut' Shaming, and Possibilities for Pleasure

Recent decades have seen an increasing media focus on the sexualised use of digital technologies, with concerns about 'sexting' (creating or sharing sexual and nude images), particularly amongst young people, and 'revenge pornography' (non-consensual sharing or uploading to websites of sexual or nude images) attracting most attention (Angelides, 2013; Henry et al., 2017b, 2020). Anxieties about digital sexual imagery sit alongside, or within, broader messages about online safety, including scams or deception occurring through hook-up and 'dating' apps and online harassment, stalking, cyber bullying, and 'trolling' (Backe et al., 2018; Tiidenberg & Van Der Nagel, 2020). There is an emerging educational, legal, and regulatory response to these concerns aiming to establish mechanisms for prevention and legal redress for victims of online harm and image-based abuse (Henry et al., 2018). However, the rapidly changing, globalised, digital environment means this is a complex task. The law is often playing 'catch-up' with current practices and technologies, whilst jurisdictional regulation or legal action can have limited reach internationally (Farrell, Shackleton, Agnew, Hopkins, & Power, 2022; Henry, Powell, & Flynn, 2017a; Yar & Drew, 2019). The challenges and limitations of regulatory and legal responses to online harms have meant public education on digital sexual imagery tends toward self-restraint messages, such as 'no sexting is safe', and health promotion and media messages often frame digital sexual image making as inherently risky (Albury & Byron, 2018; Albury et al., 2017, 2020).

Critical scholarship has highlighted the ways in which risk discourses within media or educational messaging have produced digital sexual self-imagery as a politically salient, modern 'sex problem' (Albury et al., 2017, 2020; Angelides, 2013; Tiidenberg & Van Der Nagel, 2020), within in which people engaged in these practices are perceived to be naïve and vulnerable, irresponsible, or malicious. Risk messaging also often draws on gendered and conservative sexual moralising to warn about risk involving sexual exchange or exposure of naked and sexual images (Albury et al., 2017; Ravn et al., 2021). For instance, young people are warned to avoid sexting and digital pornography in order to prevent humiliation, damage to future employment, and potential legal consequences (Angelides, 2013; Hasinoff, 2013), whilst adult women are warned of reputational loss and vulnerability to harassment if their personal sexual images are exposed— the implicit message being that exposure of their naked or sexualised bodies would implicate them as 'slutty' or somehow less worthy (Amundsen, 2020; Setty, 2019). Whilst men are less vulnerable than women to public shaming (Paasonen & Sundén, 2021), many men are aware that they can quickly be labelled a 'creep' if they present as too forward, too explicit, eager, or aggressive in online encounters, yet they also feel pressure to adhere to conventional masculine presentation in online spaces (Ravn et al., 2021; Waling & Pym, 2019; Waling et al., 2022). Critical analysis of discourse surrounding digital sexual practices is not intended to discount the genuinely harmful impact that unwanted sexual exposure or harassment online can cause to victims. Rather, it draws attention to the ways perceived risks from new technologies intersect with gender inequalities and attitudes toward sexuality.

Sitting alongside this research is an emerging body of scholarship exploring the significance of digitally mediated intimacy in contemporary friendships, dating, and intimate relationships (Attwood et al., 2017; Döring, 2009). With respect to digital sexual imagery, this scholarship has attended to the ways smartphones enable people to share images that express sexual desire, pleasure, or affection, and support intimacy and sexual satisfaction (Dredge & Anderson, 2021; Gesselman et al., 2020; Murray & Campbell, 2015; Watson et al., 2021), whilst opening new possibilities for romantic and sexual relationships, and everyday connection and presence over distance (Madianou, 2016; Murray & Campbell, 2015).

In this paper, we report findings from a qualitative study in which we interviewed Australian adults about their experiences of creating and sharing digital sexual images. We aimed to explore the ways people have integrated sexual self-images into their sex lives and relationships and to understand the benefits or pleasures this affords. However, we were also mindful that risk and shame discourses associated with digital sexual images are not inconsequential for people's engagement in these practices. Awareness of risk may, in fact, have profound effects on the ways people choose to engage with digital sexual imagery and how they feel about it. As such, we aimed to explore how people related to discourses of risk and safety as part of practices of digital sexual self-image creation and sharing.

Approach

We approached this study using Nygren and colleagues' (2019) understanding of 'doing risk', which draws on Butler's concept of gender as constituted performatively. Nygren et al. (2019) argue that risk is not an objective reality to be revealed or understood through scientific research. Rather, perceptions of what constitutes 'risky practices' or 'at risk' individuals are produced through the ways we talk about, and respond to, notions of risk in research, in the media, in education, in policy and so forth, in the context of normative ideas about gender, sexuality, age, class, culture, and other structures and processes. Discourses of risk shape, in part, people's experience of these practices and of themselves in relation to digital sexual practices. Risk is, therefore, performative; it is something that is produced in action and interaction, as Nygren et al., (2019, p. 87) explain:

> From our perspective, the act of, for example, not walking home alone at night because of fear of sexual assault, is the doing of risk at the same time as it constitutes respectable femininity. Not performing according to expectations causes anxiety and even fear …, a fear that might be greater and more significant than considering a particular risk, since it is related to subjectification and self-identity.

For our purposes, this framework enables us to make sense of the ways risk discourses relating to sexualised use of technologies are informed by (and reinforce) gendered and sexual stereotypes and inequalities, and to explore how people navigate this in the context of their experiences of sexual pleasure and romantic connection. Our intention is not to downplay or disregard the harm that can be caused by image-based sexual abuse or non-consensual sharing of sexual images. Rather, it is to understand how people relate to the potential for these things to happen as part of their sexual experiences.

A note on language: whilst we recognise that the term 'sexting' is often not used by people in everyday life to describe their practices (Crofts, Lee, McGovern, & Milivojevic, 2016), we use the term in this paper for brevity to refer to creating and sending nude or sexual self-images.

Methods

We report on in-depth interviews with 23 Australian adults aged between 25 and 75 years. Participant recruitment was conducted via a combination of paid Facebook advertising and word-of-mouth promotion though the researchers' networks. Participants were eligible if they lived in Australia, were aged 18 years or older, and had some experience with the creation of sexualised, nude, or erotic images of themselves. Interviews were conducted by one member of the research team in 2020. Australian coronavirus (SARS-CoV-2) pandemic restrictions required all interviews to be conducted either via phone or video (Zoom). Interviews ranged from 30 to 90 min, depending on the length of each participant's responses to the questions. Participants were asked to recount their experiences creating, sharing, and/or receiving amateur sexual imagery, outline their motivations in creating images, describe their relationships with people with whom they shared images, explain the language they used to talk about self-made sexual imagery, and depict the settings, spaces, and social contexts in which they created and shared images. Participants were also asked about their awareness of potential risks associated with digital sexual imagery and how they responded to these. Finally, participants were asked about their perceptions of media reporting on sexting and amateur pornography and how this related to their own experiences. This study received ethics approval from the La Trobe University Human Research Ethics commitee (HEC19432).

Data Analysis

Interviews were recorded, transcribed, and verified. Data were inductively coded using Clarke and Braun's (2018) approach to thematic analysis (see also Braun & Clarke, 2019). We reviewed and coded the data through a framework informed by our theoretical approach to the research topic, attending to the relationship between risk and participants' descriptions of their practices, their feelings about their practices, and feelings about themselves in relation to this. Three members of the research team independently coded the data and discussed findings, checking for consistency and differences in their interpretations of data in order to develop themes (Clarke & Braun, 2018). These themes were further refined through research team discussions and the process of writing and sharing notes, memos, and preliminary drafts of this paper. As themes were developed, researchers revisited data that had previously been analysed with newly identified, or more sharply defined, themes in mind, a method of constant comparison often used to ensure rigour in qualitative data analysis (Boeije, 2002).

Participant Characteristics

Of the 23 participants, three identified as either gay/lesbian (n = 1) or bisexual (n = 2), whilst the rest identified as heterosexual (n = 20). One participant identified as non-binary, and the rest used 'male' (n = 12) or 'female' (n = 10) to identify their gender. No participants identified as trans or gender diverse. Most participants were aged in their 40 s and 50 s (n = 14), with a smaller number in their 30 s (n = 5), 20 s (n = 3), and 70 s (n = 1). All participants resided in Australia. Participants were asked to describe their ethnicity. The majority (n = 13) used terms that indicated a Caucasian Australian background, e.g. Australian, Australian-Caucasian, and British-Caucasian. Other participants identified as Chinese (n = 3), Asian (n = 1), Eurasian (n = 1), Indian (n = 1), or a mix of ethnicities, such as 'English Italian' (n = 4). No participants identified as First Nations people. All participants had received a post-secondary school education, with 12 having an undergraduate qualification, 10 a postgraduate qualification, and one a TAFE/technical training diploma.

Findings

Practices of creating and sharing sexual imagery were described by participants in terms that were largely relational and framed sexual image sharing as a form of mutual exchange, sexual play, flirting, or building sexual tension with another person. Even though viewing photographs or videos was at the centre of these experiences, participants also spoke about sexual gratification and eroticism that came from the process of exchanging images or in creating an image and waiting for a response. Awareness of risk sat within this. Participants knew that sending sexual or nude images left them vulnerable to potential harm or unwanted exposure, and this in part shaped their perception of these practices and experiences, including expectations of reciprocity (mutual exchange of images), perceptions of trustworthiness in others, and feelings of intimacy or eroticism. These broad themes are discussed in more detail below.

Images as Communication, Connection, and Sexual Play

The process of creating and sharing digital sexual images was described by participants as sexual connection and erotic play. Some participants spoke about exchanging images with people they had met online through dating apps (people not known offline), whilst others only created and sent images in the context of an ongoing offline relationship. This included two participants who communicated using sexual imagery with long-distance partners. Two participants spoke about sending nude or sexual images of themselves or other people (such as screen shots from commercial pornography) to certain friends with whom they had no offline sexual relationship but who enjoyed the erotic exchange. Whatever the context, the experience of creating, receiving, and watching self-created sexual images was about sexual communication or play. It was a practice afforded by the simplicity of creating and sharing digital imagery—the digital camera, the small device, Internet connectivity, apps, and messaging services. For example, the timing of a digital image exchange, in which there is a delay between sending an image and receiving a response, amplified the affective experience of these practices for many participants, as Joseph explained:

> There is a sense of excitement from both sending and receiving … First of all, I would spend a good 10, 15 minutes finding the image, cropping the image, and then posting it. Then, I get this excited anxious feeling of, you know, you see the little head icon drop and you think, 'Oh yeah, they've seen it'. And then you wait for the response, and you think how long will it take for them to respond? … It becomes like … an evolving chain reaction, you know, like a tennis match … And that again provides a sense of excitement, you know, a sense of mystery, intrigue … All those emotions and feelings come to play when that happens, yeah. (Joseph, age 48, male, heterosexual)

Participants also described how basic digital technologies (a laptop, the Internet) allowed them introduce sex into everyday exchanges or activities. Linda, for example, described the way the camera's gaze from her laptop eroticised her mundane morning bathroom routine:

> I'd just put the laptop on the little seat in the bathroom and go and have my shower. And I'd come out and I'd be fussing around getting ready for work or whatever I was doing that day. And so, he'd kind of see me from about just under my boobs down to just below my arse. So, he got all pretty much the good bits. And we'd just be yakking away while I cleaned my teeth and did my hair … So, he got to see a fair bit of my time naked. (Linda, age 56, female, heterosexual)

Participants tended to describe their experiences in terms of the excitement or eroticism in the exchange. For many, this was also linked to excitement in the uncertainty of how the sexual images of their bodies, or expression of their sexual desires, would be received. For some, this sense of vulnerability pushed sexual boundaries in ways they found exciting and satisfying. As Michelle's description below illustrates, sending an image, for her, built a sense of sexual agency marked (or brought about) by competing emotions of excitement and uncertainty:

> I guess, like, a little bit of power. It is a bit brave, I think, to [create and send an image], so you feel kind of a bit brave, but also quite anxious because you're, like, are they seeing this photo the way I'm seeing it? … But receiving is, I guess, very exciting for me because, well, partly because there's that sort of trust where you're, sort of, exposing yourself to each other. So, there's that excitement. And that excitement of that person trusting and also, yeah, the visualness of it I enjoy. (Michelle, 35, female, heterosexual)

For Christy, sexting or making videos challenged her sexual boundaries as it allowed her to engage in sex practices not otherwise available, shifting her sense of self as she became more comfortable with practices that she considered risqué:

> I guess [with sexting] you have some nice erotic moments and a bit of self-pleasure … And yeah, I think a bit, for me being able to change my mind-set a bit. I think I would've felt

> I was more conservative than that. And yeah, it's nice to kind of stretch yourself a bit and go 'Oh, I actually am now quite comfortable with that', within assuming you've got a level of, a small level of trust built up already. (Christy, age 51, female, heterosexual)

For participants, sexual imagery operated as a form of erotic communication that was not separate from, or a precursor to, other forms of intimacy, but was part of connecting with another person sexually. Digital sexual practices also offered unique possibilities for pleasure and intimacy due to the function of technologies themselves which, for example, delayed the timing of sending and receiving an image or offered the capacity to look at oneself on screen and enjoy the process of constructing a sexual image. These experiences of pleasure and eroticism provide important context for the following sections in which we focus more directly on the ways risk discourses shaped participants' experiences.

Affective Responses to Risk

Cautionary tales of non-consensual exposure of others' sexual images were common in participants' explanations of the ways they understood risk, although none had experienced such exposures themselves. Participants recalled stories they had read in the media, anecdotes they had heard, or experiences of friends being publicly shamed:

> I have heard, like in the past, there was, particularly in our area, there was a thing all over the news that someone had got hold of a whole heap of videos that people had done and was going to expose people, you know, send them to partners, send them to husbands all that kind of stuff, but yeah, so that … made me think wow, wow, yeah, it, that was quite a while ago, but that sort of made people sort of go, oh, maybe it's not as safe as we think it is. (Laura, age 48, female, heterosexual)

Participants reported many strategies for avoiding unwanted exposure of their images, including cropping their faces or other identifying features and storing data offline. However, management of data or images was a minor theme in participants' narratives about risk. More often, they described the significance of trust and reciprocity in risk management. Receiving an image from someone was an indication that the person was willing to share vulnerability, which was considered a sign of trustworthiness:

> I suppose that's one of the reasons why reciprocation is an important thing for me with this. So, I trust you to send you my photos, but for me to do that and get enjoyment out of it, I need to know that you trust me as well [by sending yours]. (Michelle, age 35, female, heterosexual)

The significance of reciprocity was recognised by heterosexual male participants as important for demonstrating their trustworthiness to women:

> I think it's quite important in the sense that it really shows how much we trust each other, and I really, really value that. If my partner agrees to have those photos and videos done, it really shows a great deal of trust in me, which I think really helps the relationship. (Emil, age 45, male, heterosexual)

The significance of that decision to trust someone became part of the affective and relational experience of sharing images, often producing an enhanced sense of intimacy. Participants spoke about this as a positive outcome of sexting:

> [Exchanging images] can make two people closer together; like, it can make you more intimate … I think it's both because, like, this sort of thing isn't something I would do with just anyone … I think it does bring you together because it is like this special thing that you've done together and you are – it's like a huge amount of trust, I mean, like there was a huge amount of trust. (Jodie, age 42, female, heterosexual)

For some participants, the perceived taboo nature of pornography and the risk of exposure were part of the erotic appeal in creating sexual imagery, particularly videos:

> There's something about seeing yourself, sort of like, live on that little LCD screen that it reminds you that you're, kind of, doing something a little bit naughty. And it adds to that kind of – how can I explain this – I suppose filming yourself there's that kind of forbidden thing about it. (Joe, age 51, male, heterosexual)

Risk discourses shaped the ways participants experienced image exchange as a practice of trust and intimacy or eroticism. The urgency and significance of trusting relationships were enhanced in a situation where sexting could be regarded as dangerous. In the next section, we look more closely at the complexity of participants' responses to risk discourses, revealing the ways individual participants critiqued them, whilst also retaining beliefs about individual responsibility.

Digital Sexual Imagery in Mainstream Media

Most participants were sceptical about mainstream media portrayals of digital sexual imagery (mostly focused on sexting) and regarded as hypocritical the ways that media stories often evoked shame and included warnings of risk and danger to create sensationalist headlines. Elijah, for example, described media reporting as hyperbolic and cynical:

> [There] will, of course, be trashy magazines and newspapers on celebrity sex, and celebrities leak some stuff, and they will profit on it massively … And then, they'll sort of sell it too, [and it will be] glamorised and maybe even slut-shaming, normally shaming the female and – but they'll sell it … And then, there'll do massive scare stories about kids getting involved in it. (Elijah, aged 43, male, bisexual)

Several participants commented that the media's focus on negative stories did not accord with their personal experiences, and also offered few positive solutions to the dangers represented other than shame or worry, as Tomas noted:

> I think it [the media] makes people worry – I think it causes them to, sort of, rethink making those images, or making those productions or whatever. I think it, sort of, changes their perceptions in thinking that what they're doing is a bad thing, or it's not a standard thing other people do. (Tomas, age 26, male, gay)

Participants took a critical stance on the ways media reporting can shame users, as Tomas's comment indicates. However, in the absence of more positive representations of sexting or other strategies for challenging or reframing shame, participants also spoke about risk in terms of poor decision-making and poor judgement of those people being reported on in media. As Arun's response below shows, he was critical of the overall negative media reporting on sexting but saw individual responsibility (not being 'stupid') as the explanation:

> I think [the media is] very negative. So long as you're with somebody you care about, it's not actually harming anybody. You're careful you don't burn yourself. The media highlight on one or two people who are being really stupid about it and they jump on the sensational … So, that it's all sensational headlines and [how it] should be banned and all the other bits and pieces. In reality, it's pleasurable and does no harm. (Arun, age 58, male, heterosexual)

Similarly, Sarah told a story of a friend whose pictures were shared without her consent, acts which Sarah perceived as embarrassing and shameful for her friend, but for which she ultimately thought the friend was responsible due to a poor decision to trust her boyfriend:

> One of my best friends I know takes pictures of herself all the time and sends them. And she's been in a situation where the guy's shown other people that she knows, not distributed it online but definitely shown people within their social circle. And I think that's really sad for her, but then I think why would you trust him? Don't trust him, don't send him that, he's not to be trusted. (Sarah, age 42, female, heterosexual)

Safety in Sarah's mind rested on the ability to know whom to trust, with blame attributed to poor judgement of the woman who naïvely trusted her boyfriend. This approach was reflected in several participant narratives. Good judgement was posited as the solution to manage risk. However, participants were not always clear what such judgement involved. As we explore in the next section, shame extended beyond sexual shaming to include the fear of being shamed for not having good judgement.

Shame and Silence

Participants, on the whole, did not speak with friends about their practices of creating or sharing digital sexual imagery, and some were keen to keep their digital practices secret. In fact, although many participants assumed sexting or making sexual videos is common amongst adults, most participants were not aware whether their friends did this. One participant, Emil (age 45, male, heterosexual), stated that one of his motivations for participating in this study was to find out if his practices were 'normal', noting when asked if he spoke to friends or family about digital sexual practices, 'I don't share at all'. Participants indicated that they chose not to speak about their digital sexual practices as they feared others would think they were foolish or irresponsible for sexting when the risks are so well known. As Lia said:

> Years ago, I think Vanessa Hudgens – the actress in 'High School Musical'? – she sent like a nudge to Zac Efron, and then it got leaked and everyone found out and she was all of a sudden, like, shamed for doing that. And I feel that that's, kind of, the implication that media give when like people sext. Although [sexting] does happen, I feel like people don't talk about it … like, I don't talk about it with my friends. My friends don't really talk about it with me. I don't really know if they do it or not. (Lia, age 27, female, heterosexual)

Similarly, Christy (age 51, female, heterosexual) said that she did not talk about her practices because, 'It goes back to that sense of, oh well, it's [sexting] not a bit dirty, but you know, that it's a foolish thing to do'. Participants were well aware that 'you should not do this' was the strategy most commonly advocated to manage risk:

> I think it's definitely different because more often than not I think you hear about images of women. And they're told, well, you shouldn't do that. (Michelle, 35, female, heterosexual)

Although participants assumed sexting was common and provided this study with nuanced accounts of their own practices and experiences, the only other stories on sexting they had to hand, based on experiences of other people they knew or had heard about, were ones of unwanted exposure and public shaming. Consequently, participants were concerned about being judged as irresponsible or exercising poor judgement in sharing sexual images, in addition to their concerns about unwanted exposure. Discourses of risk and shame served mainly to create silence on digital sexual image making.

Discussion

Risk and safety messages about digital sexual imagery often mirror public health messages that emphasise harm whilst promoting individual responsibility for avoiding risky situations (Albury & Crawford, 2012; Albury et al., 2017; Angelides, 2013). Our aim for this paper was to explore how participants felt about discourses of risk and safety in relation to digital sexual practices, and the ways knowledge of risk discourses shaped their actions, experiences, and feelings about their practices. We wanted to capture the breadth of people's digital sexual experiences or the ways in which individual strategies to deal with sexual risk and safety are developed in the context of seeking pleasure, human connection, or other experiences (Albury, 2018). Our participants provided complex accounts of handling risk and safety in which risk interacted with, and was productive of, pleasure, trust, reciprocity, and connectedness. For many participants, trust and intimacy were related to their sense of risk, not something that occurred despite risks. In these online settings, the development of a sense of intimacy was often accelerated and amplified because, given potential risks, it was so significant to the exchange.

The complexity in the ways people experience pleasure and manage risk has been widely recognised in sexuality and sexual health research (Cameron-Lewis & Allen, 2013; Carballo-Diéguez et al., 2011; Vance, 1984), as well as in more recent studies of people's management of online safety (Pym et al., 2021). Pleasure and risk are not mutually exclusive. In sexual or romantic encounters, people often use many strategies to balance, hold, or sometimes foreground, emotional and physical risk as part of enhancing eroticism, pleasure, and connection (Bollen & McInnes, 2004). The challenge for researchers, educators, or policy makers is to acknowledge and explore this complexity and not reduce people to irresponsible subjects, or disregard or denigrate pleasures, that draw on risk or danger (Vance, 1984).

Contemporary research on sexual health education and promotion has emphasised the ineffectiveness of fearbased messaging and its potential for stigmatising affected communities or individuals (Fairchild et al., 2018). People will be better equipped to enjoy safe sexual relationships if they develop a sense of agency and the confidence to talk with potential online partners about sex and safety, so they can clarify what they do and do not want to do (Cense, 2019; Fine, 1988). However, individual, fearbased messaging is often the approach taken to address complex, gender-based, structural violence. For example, as Hall (2004) observed, gender-based sexual assault is often regarded as an intractable problem to solve due to structural inequality. Approaches to rape prevention that focus on risk reduction for individual women (e.g. advising women to avoid walking alone at night) are more achievable for sexual assault prevention, in the short term, than creating structural change. However, such strategies often come at the expense of women, instilling victim blaming and shaming of women who do not adhere to prevention messages. The Internet is often perceived in similarly complex terms with digital image-based sexual risk and abuse embedded in broader cultures of gender-based and sexual violence (Henry & Powell, 2016), whilst the digital environment— global, amorphous, and often underground—is complex and difficult to regulate using conventional processes, such as legislation or standard law enforcement (Henry & Powell, 2016; Henry & Witt, 2021; Jurasz & Barker, 2021). Consequently, people using digital technologies to explore their sexual interests are forced to choose between not using these technologies or exploring them and trusting the people they encounter there, despite knowing this is far from risk-free.

Drawing from Nygren and colleagues' (2019) concept of 'doing risk', these findings show the ways in which notions of what it means to be safe or morally responsible online are integrated with participant's affective experiences—of eroticism or intimacy—and actions regarding trust and reciprocity. Participants were aware of the moral dimensions of online risk—evident in their judgement of other people for being naïve or stupid and their own fear of being shamed for sending sexual images. However, participants also held a critical stance toward portrayals of online risk and danger, particularly in relation to gender and media shaming of people who engage sexually online (Giritli Nygren et al., 2017). Narratives of trust and reciprocity were a strategy for managing these complexities whilst creating space for sexual pleasure. Being selective with who they trusted, or engaging in acts of reciprocity and seeking or expressing cues of trustworthiness when sharing images, was a strategy for participants to mitigate potential for unwanted exposure. This was by no means a foolproof strategy to prevent harm, and participants were not naïve to this, but it enabled them to hold knowledge of potential harm and still view themselves (in their own eyes and those of others) as responsible adults and ethical online sexual citizens. Participants could therefore embrace awareness of risk and concerns about irresponsibility alongside a critical awareness of media messaging, their enjoyment of risk and danger, and a sense of agency in their sexual practices. Within this nuanced and complex engagement with risk, participants both upheld and challenged normative ideas about the relationship between sex, pleasure, safety, and responsibility.

Recognising this complexity may provide a way forward for opening conversations about the nature of online safety. In this study, participants were reluctant to talk to offline friends about their practices as they feared being judged or regarded as irresponsible. These findings would suggest that a focus on risk alone can contribute more to shame, silence, and avoidance of discussions on safety, than inviting conversations, online and offline, about risk and pleasure.

Finally, it is worth highlighting that participants in our study were not young people. Most of our participants were aged in their 30 s, 40 s, and 50 s and were all actively engaged in creating and sharing digital sexual imagery. We should always remember that the digital world is not the exclusive domain of young people.

Conclusion

In this project, we explore risk relating to production and exchange of sexualised digital images not as an easily definable set of negative outcomes to be avoided, but as set of discourses and practices that shape the ways people make sense of, and engage with, digital sexual intimacy. In doing this, we were able to explore the multiple effects of risk discourses on people's experiences but also note a disengagement from those discourses in participants' online sexual lives. This is not to disregard the reality that the online environment can lead to significant harms for people in some circumstances and there is a need to educate people about ways to mitigate such harms. However, this education needs to occur with reference to the breadth of experiences people may be having online and also in ways that do not contribute to shame or silences about practices considered risky.

Recent decades have seen, to some extent, a shift from moralising or sex-negative sexual health promotion and education. This occurred largely in response to the HIV pandemic, in which successful HIV programmes involved social networks and sexual cultures of, first, gay and bisexual men and, soon thereafter, sex workers and other sex and gender minorities, and focused on creative and sexpositive approaches to health promotion and disease prevention (Brown et al., 2014; Dowsett, 2009, 2014; Dowsett et al., 2001). There has also been growing recognition of the significance of pleasure, desire, and human connectedness in comprehensive sexuality education, including consent-focused sexuality education (Allen, 2004; Gilbert, 2018). However, this approach has not often, yet, extended to digital sexual practices or education about online safety (Albury et al., 2017). Such technologies, especially those that involve sexually explicit imagery, are often uncritically framed in sexual health promotion and education as only potentially dangerous and to be avoided (Byron, 2015; Hollingshead et al., 2020; Marwick, 2008; Tiidenberg & Van Der Nagel, 2020). Findings from this study confirm that an approach that emphasises risk and shame can adversely affect individuals and create a silence that undermines open conversation on online sex practices. Sex-positive approaches to digital safety are important, as is ensuring that producers and distributers of these and emerging technologies are accountable for safety, rather than responsibility resting only with individual users. As digital technologies evolve, their integration with human sexual intimacy will continue to change and develop in unforeseen ways. Any educational and regulatory responses to this evolution will require ongoing scrutiny and innovation to remain salient to the sexual experiences and desires of digital technologies users.

Acknowledgements

Professor Jayne Lucke assisted with the development of the project, funding acquisition, and development of the survey.

Author Contribution

JP conducted data analysis and wrote the manuscript. AW and AJ conducted data analysis and contributed to the manuscript. GWD worked closely with JP to design the study and write the manuscript. All authors met fortnightly to discuss progress of the project, provide insight into findings, and determine the direction for the discussion and conclusion. All authors reviewed several versions of this manuscript.

Funding

Open Access funding enabled and organized by CAUL and its Member Institutions. This project was funded by an Australian Research Council Discovery Grant (DP190102027).

Data Availability

To protect participant's confidentiality these data have not been made publicly available. Inquiries about data access should be directed to the corresponding author.

Declarations

Competing Interests The authors declare no competing interests.

Publisher's Note

Springer Nature remains neutral with regard to jurisdictional claims in published maps and institutional affiliations.

ORCID

Jennifer Power https://orcid.org/0000-0002-6566-3214

References

Albury, K. (2018). Young people, digital media research and counter-public sexual health. *Sexualities, 21*(8), 1331–1336.

Albury, K., & Byron, P. (2018). Taking off the risk goggles: Exploring the intersection of young people's sexual and digital citizenship in sexual health promotion. In P. Aggleton, R. Cover, D. Leahy, D. Marshall & M. L. Rasmussen (Eds.), *Youth, sexuality and sexual citizenship* (pp. 168–183). Abingdon: Routlege.

Albury, K., & Crawford, K. (2012). Sexting, consent and young people's ethics: Beyond Megan's story. *Continuum, 26*(3), 463–473.

Albury, K., Hasinoff, A. A., & Senft, T. (2017). From media abstinence to media production: Sexting, young people and education. In L. Allen & M. Ramussen (Eds.), *The Palgrave handbook of sexuality education* (pp. 527–545). Springer.

Albury, K., McCosker, A., Pym, T., & Byron, P. (2020). Dating apps as public health 'problems': Cautionary tales and vernacular pedagogies in news media. *Health Sociology Review, 29*(3), 232–248.

Allen, L. (2004). Beyond the birds and the bees: Constituting a discourse of erotics in sexuality education. *Gender and Education, 16*(2), 151–167.

Amundsen, R. (2020). Hetero-sexting as mediated intimacy work: 'Putting something on the line'. *New Media & Society*, 1461444820962452.

Angelides, S. (2013). 'Technology, hormones, and stupidity': The affective politics of teenage sexting. *Sexualities, 16*(5–6), 665–689.

Attwood, F., Hakim, J., & Winch, A. (2017). Mediated intimacies: Bodies, technologies and relationships. *Journal of Gender Studies, 26*(3), 249–253.

Backe, E. L., Lilleston, P., & McCleary-Sills, J. (2018). Networked individuals, gendered violence: A literature review of cyberviolence. *Violence and Gender, 5*(3), 135–146.

Boeije, H. (2002). A purposeful approach to the constant comparative method in the analysis of qualitative interviews. *Quality and Quantity, 36*(4), 391–409.

Bollen, J., & McInnes, D. (2004). Time, relations and learning in gay men's experiences of adventurous sex. *Social Semiotics, 14*(1), 21–36.

Braun, V., & Clarke, V. (2019). Reflecting on reflexive thematic analysis. *Qualitative Research in Sport, Exercise and Health, 11*(4), 589–597.

Brown, G., O'Donnell, D., Crooks, L., & Lake, R. (2014). Mobilisation, politics, investment and constant adaptation: Lessons from the Australian health-promotion response to HIV. *Health Promotion Journal of Australia, 25*(1), 35–41.

Byron, P. (2015). Troubling expertise: Social media and young people's sexual health. *Communication Research and Practice, 1*(4), 322–334.

Cameron-Lewis, V., & Allen, L. (2013). Teaching pleasure and danger in sexuality education. *Sex Education, 13*(2), 121–132.

Carballo-Diéguez, A., Ventuneac, A., Dowsett, G. W., Balan, I., Bauermeister, J., Remien, R. H., & Mabragaña, M. (2011). Sexual pleasure and intimacy among men who engage in "bareback sex." *AIDS and Behavior, 15*(1), 57–65.

Cense, M. (2019). Rethinking sexual agency: Proposing a multicomponent model based on young people's life stories. *Sex Education, 19*(3), 247–262.

Clarke, V., & Braun, V. (2018). Using thematic analysis in counselling and psychotherapy research: A critical reflection. *Counselling and Psychotherapy Research, 18*(2), 107–110.

Crofts, T., Lee, M., McGovern, A., & Milivojevic, S. (2016). *Sexting and young people*. Hampshire: Palgrave McMillan.

Döring, N. M. (2009). The Internet's impact on sexuality: A critical review of 15 years of research. *Computers in Human Behavior, 25*(5), 1089–1101.

Dowsett, G. W. (2009). Dangerous desires and post-queer HIV prevention: Rethinking community, incitement and intervention. *Social Theory & Health, 7*, 218–240.

Dowsett, G. W. (2014). Dirty work'down under: A comment on Janice Irvine's 'Is sexuality research "dirty work"? *Sexualities, 17*(5–6), 657–661.

Dowsett, G. W., Bollen, J., McInnes, D., Couch, M., & Edwards, B. (2001). HIV/AIDS and constructs of gay community: Researching educational practice within community-based health promotion for gay men. *International Journal of Social Research Methodology, 4*(3), 205–223.

Dredge, R., & Anderson, J. (2021). The qualitative exploration of social competencies and incompetencies on mobile dating applications. *Personal Relationships, 28*, 627–651.

Fairchild, A. L., Bayer, R., Green, S. H., Colgrove, J., Kilgore, E., Sweeney, M., & Varma, J. K. (2018). The two faces of fear: A history of hard-hitting public health campaigns against tobacco and AIDS. *American Journal of Public Health, 108*(9), 1180–1186.

Farrell, A.-M., Shackleton, N., Agnew, E., Hopkins, S., & Power, J. (2022). Regulating tech-sex and managing image-based sexual abuse: An Australian perspective. *Information & Communications Technology Law*, 1–18.

Fine, M. (1988). Sexuality, schooling, and adolescent females: The missing discourse of desire. *Harvard Educational Review, 58*(1), 29–54.

Gesselman, A. N., Druet, A., & Vitzthum, V. (2020). Mobile sex-tech apps: How use differs across global areas of high and low gender equality. *PloS one, 15*(9), e0238501. https://doi.org/10.1371/journal.pone.0238501

Gilbert, J. (2018). Contesting consent in sex education. *Sex Education, 18*(3), 268–279.

Giritli Nygren, K., Öhman, S., & Olofsson, A. (2017). Doing and undoing risk: The mutual constitution of risk and heteronormativity in contemporary society. *Journal of Risk Research, 20*(3), 418–432.

Hall, R. (2004). "It can happen to you": Rape prevention in the age of risk management. *Hypatia, 19*(3), 1–19.

Hasinoff, A. A. (2013). Sexting as media production: Rethinking social media and sexuality. *New Media & Society, 15*(4), 449–465.

Henry, N., Flynn, A., & Powell, A. (2018). Policing image-based sexual abuse: Stakeholder perspectives. *Police Practice and Research, 19*(6), 565–581.

Henry, N., McGlynn, C., Flynn, A., Johnson, K., Powell, A., & Scott, A. J. (2020). *Image-based sexual abuse: A study on the causes and consequences of non-consensual nude or sexual imagery*: Routledge.

Henry, N., & Powell, A. (2016). Sexual violence in the digital age: The scope and limits of criminal law. *Social & Legal Studies, 25*(4), 397–418.

Henry, N., Powell, A., & Flynn, A. (2017a). Not just 'revenge pornography': Australians' experiences of image-based abuse. *A summary report. Melbourne: RMIT University.*

Henry, N., Powell, A., & Flynn, A. (2017b). *Not Just 'revenge pornography': Australians' experiences of image-based abuse: A summary report*. Melbourne.

Henry, N., & Witt, A. (2021). Governing image-based sexual abuse: Digital platform policies, tools, and practices. In J. Bailey, A. Flynn, & N. Henry (Eds.), *The Emerald international handbook of technology-facilitated violence and abuse* (pp. 749–768). Bingley Emerald Publishing Limited.

Hollingshead, B. M., Dowsett, G. W., & Bourne, A. (2020). 'It's like getting an Uber for sex': Social networking apps as spaces of risk and opportunity in the Philippines among men who have sex with men. *Health Sociology Review, 29*(3), 264–278.

Jurasz, O., & Barker, K. (2021). Sexual violence in the digital age: A criminal law conundrum? *German Law Journal, 22*(5), 784–799.

Madianou, M. (2016). Ambient co-presence: Transnational family practices in polymedia environments. *Global Networks, 16*(2), 183–201.

Marwick, A. E. (2008). To catch a predator? The MySpace moral panic. *First Monday, 13*(6). Retrieved from https://firstmonday.org/ojs/index.php/fm/article/download/2152/1966

Murray, C. E., & Campbell, E. C. (2015). The pleasures and perils of technology in intimate relationships. *Journal of Couple & Relationship Therapy, 14*(2), 116–140.

Nygren, K. G., Olofsson, A., & Öhman, S. (2019). *A framework of intersectional risk theory in the age of ambivalence*. Cham Springer.

Paasonen, S., & Sundén, J. (2021). Shameless dicks: On male privilege, dick pic scandals, and public exposure. *First Monday, 26*(4). https://doi.org/10.5210/fm.v26i4.11654

Pym, T., Byron, P., & Albury, K. (2021). 'I still want to know they're not terrible people': Negotiating 'queer community' on dating apps. *International Journal of Cultural Studies, 24*(3), 398–413.

Ravn, S., Coffey, J., & Roberts, S. (2021). The currency of images: Risk, value and gendered power dynamics in young men's accounts of sexting. *Feminist Media Studies, 21*(2), 315–331.

Setty, E. (2019). Meanings of bodily and sexual expression in youth sexting culture: Young women's negotiation of gendered risks and harms. *Sex Roles, 80*(9), 586–606.

Tiidenberg, K., & Van Der Nagel, E. (2020). *Sex and social media*. Bingely Emerald Group Publishing.

Vance, C. S. (1984). Pleasure and danger: Toward a politics of sexuality. In C. Vanver (Ed.), *Pleasure and danger: Exploring female sexuality* (pp. 1–29).

Waling, A., Kerr, L., Bourne, A., Power, J., & Kehler, M. (2022). 'It's nice to be appreciated': Understanding heterosexual men's engagements with sexting and sharing dick pics. *Sexualities, 25*(3), 198–221.

Waling, A., & Pym, T. (2019). 'C'mon, no one wants a dick pic': Exploring the cultural framings of the 'Dick Pic' in contemporary online publics. *Journal of Gender Studies, 28*(1), 70–85.

Watson, A., Lupton, D., & Michael, M. (2021). Enacting intimacy and sociality at a distance in the COVID-19 crisis: The sociomaterialities of home-based communication technologies. *Media International Australia, 178*(1), 136–150.

Yar, M., & Drew, J. (2019). Image-based abuse, non-consensual pornography, revenge porn: A study of criminalization and crime prevention in Australia and England & Wales. *International Journal of Cyber Criminology, 13*(2), 578–294.

Dating apps as public health 'problems': cautionary tales and vernacular pedagogies in news media

Kath Albury, Anthony McCosker, Tinonee Pym and Paul Byron

ABSTRACT

In this paper we examine how popular media reporting positions dating and hookup app use as a 'social problem' that impacts on health and wellbeing. The paper adopts a mixed-methods media studies approach to create and analyse a dataset of over 6,000 international news articles published within a 12-month period, drawing on thematic content analysis and inductive and deductive techniques. These analyses are framed in relation to online consultations with Australian sexual health professionals and app users. Applying Briggs and Hallin's theory of biocommunicability (2007) – which proposes that contemporary health professionals' scientific framing of public health problems are, in part, shaped by popular media discourses – we identify a significant category of supportive discussions of safer app use within social news and lifestyle reporting. This discursive space features what we have termed 'vernacular pedagogies' of app use, revealing app users' safety strategies, and their experiences of pleasure and playfulness. We argue that an analysis of popular media can provide valuable insights into how everyday experiences of safety, risk and wellbeing are being shaped and contested with dating and hookup app use, and that these insights can be used to develop meaningful health promotion strategies.

Introduction

As dating and hookup apps (such as Tinder and Grindr) have become increasingly ubiquitous, media commentary and debate about their use has proliferated. For example, a 2017 Australian news story headlined '*Asking for trouble*': *Dating app warning amid rising STI cases* cites a sexual and reproductive health clinician's view that 'STI transmission is entirely down to human behaviour and people need to think twice when using dating apps for hook-ups' (Australian Associated Press, 2017).

At the same time, health researchers and public health organisations are seeking to better understand the way app use impacts on users' sense of sexual and emotional health and wellbeing. In this paper we examine how popular media reporting positions dating and hookup app use as a 'social problem' that impacts on health and wellbeing. We also identify a significant category of supportive discussions of safer app use –

involving pleasure and playfulness – within social news and lifestyle reporting. We adopt a mixed-methods media studies approach to create and analyse a dataset of over 6,000 international news articles published within a 12-month period, drawing on thematic content analysis (Krippendorff, 2013) combining inductive and deductive techniques to identify patterns in the dominant themes and concepts identified within news reports. We consider this analysis in the context of a larger research project that also involves consultations with Australian sexual health professionals seeking better ways to deliver sexual health outreach, and qualitative research activities with a diverse population of dating app users. We seek to map – and better understand – the dominant media accounts of dating and hookup apps to help inform health promotion and other sexual health professionals and researchers, who increasingly need to address this sphere of mostly hidden sexual health activity. This is a first step in opening a dialogue that might reconfigure different forms of knowledge and expertise among those improvising with safe sexual health practices in dating app use.

Applying Briggs and Hallin's theorisations of biocommunicability (2007) – that is, the argument that contemporary health professionals' scientific framing of public health problems are, in part, shaped by popular media discourses – we identify a discursive space that we have termed 'vernacular pedagogies' of app use. This space is significant for understandings new media technologies because it establishes the parameters through which health literacies (Nutbeam, 2008) can develop – both for health professionals and educators, and app users. That is, vernacular pedagogies not only set persistent frameworks for health professionals' understandings of app users' health and wellbeing concerns, but can provide guidance or templates for entertaining and engaging health promotion and health education approaches that may begin to break down the risk-oriented and stigmatising frameworks that pair apps with danger and health risks. Our analysis does not seek to discount the value of popular media discourse as an influence in health research and public health agendas. On the contrary, we suggest that media content featuring first-person accounts of app-use can provide valuable insights into peer-to-peer information sharing in digital cultures, which inform meaningful health promotion strategies.

Background

Multidisciplinary research approaches have illustrated how popular and user-generated media content addressing health issues and experiences interconnect with 'expert' discourses produced and circulated by health researchers, practitioners, and health service providers. Drawing on Briggs and Hallin's (2007, 2016) concept of 'biocommunicability', we suggest that professionals developing health campaigns, resources or interventions relating to dating and hookup app use can usefully draw on what we have termed the 'vernacular pedagogies' of safe and pleasurable dating app and hookup use – that is, the kinds of observational reportage commonly shared in opinion columns, feature articles and social media posts. Briggs and Hallin (2007) propose the term 'biocommunicability' as a means of thinking about how biopolitics operate within the sphere of health reporting. They argue that this occurs through three primary frameworks through which prevailing discourses come to be established, often driving research agendas and public investment (Briggs & Hallin, 2007). They note that the field of public health (particularly health promotion) tends to frame its end-user or 'target' as an individual subject in need of authoritative information that allows them to make 'good choices' in relation to their health and wellbeing.

While some forms of health reporting follow what the authors term a 'biomedical authority' model, in which medical experts are framed by journalists as the natural 'owners' of health knowledge, this is not always the case (Briggs & Hallin, 2007). A significant number of health and wellbeing stories revolve around expert health consumers, who actively seek out information online or from 'credible' media sources, a discursive framing that Briggs and Hallin refer to as 'the patient-consumer' model (Briggs & Hallin, 2007, pp. 51–54). Elsewhere, Briggs and Hallin identify the 'public sphere' model (Briggs & Hallin, 2010) which centres the perspectives of health activists and advocates, and prioritises peer-to-peer communication as opposed to foregrounding expert sources. Moving beyond what they see as a uni-directional 'transmission' model of health promotion, Briggs and Hallin's framework provides a lens for viewing the specific power relations that emerge via the production, circulation, consumption and understanding of media content relating to health and wellbeing (Briggs & Hallin, 2007). For emergent health issues and contexts, such as the introduction of new platforms for mediating intimate relationships, this is the groundwork through which health literacies are established (Nutbeam, 2008).

Biocommunicability has been adopted by a number of researchers investigating the intersections of news reporting, digital technologies, and health. For example, in their review of recent literature in the social sciences addressing the relationships between digital technologies and young people's mental health, Fullagar, Rich, Francombe-Webb, and Maturo (2017) and Fullagar, Rich, and Francombe-Webb (2017) observe that while there are increasing calls to recognise the social and relational aspects of health (and ill health), many formal digital health 'interventions' still tend towards individualised and medicalised understandings of health, illness, and wellbeing. Holland (2017) explores the tensions between journalistic and expert narratives prevalent in a national mental health 'awareness-raising' campaign, and the critiques offered by opinion writers and bloggers who were themselves mental health service consumers. In this emerging literature, biocommunicability provides a means of reflecting on ways media practices produce, reinforce and undermine shared understandings of social value and 'authority' in relation to health and medical issues. It has further value for conceptualising the ways social issues come to be constituted as public health 'problems' (Bacchi, 2016).

As Briggs and Hallin (2016) observe, news reporting does not simply convey 'myths' or 'facts' regarding health and wellbeing. Health researchers, health policy-makers, health care providers, and laypeople alike define health 'problems' (and their potential solutions) with reference to media narratives. This process is most striking in relation to the reporting of epidemics and public health crises – such as HIV or Ebola – but is also evident in 'lifestyle' reporting of health and wellbeing issues. Following Briggs and Hallin, we suggest that an analysis of both 'legacy' news reporting and 'digital first' media genres can help us better understand the ways that dating apps are associated with health and wellbeing concerns.

Our analysis focuses on the dominant media sources that generate a significant space for public discussion – producing and circulating shared knowledge, anxieties, and experiences. These scenes of public discourse both reflect and shape how audiences (including health professionals, laypeople, and app users) are oriented to think about dating and hookup apps and their social impact through news and online media content. Additionally, a number of 'born-digital' social news sites like *BuzzFeed* are included in our analysis. Hurcombe, Burgess, and Harrington (2019) observe that social news sites tend toward editorial policies that depart from traditional news values such as objectivity and 'balance', leaning instead towards a 'strong and explicit positionality' (Hurcombe et al., 2019, p. 1). As a form of 'spreadable' or shareable media (Jenkins, Ford, & Green, 2018), social news items allow subject matter like dating – and dating apps – to be treated both as reportage and as 'relatable' social content on social media platforms.

As Byron and Albury (2018) have noted, while interactions on social platforms such as Instagram, Twitter, and Facebook are (in the main) publicly accessible, the nuance of everyday practices of chat and picture exchange on dating and hookup apps are only visible to app users. Where non-app users have little or no access to everyday cultures of dating app use, they are likely to be reliant on other publicly mediated platforms for information. With this in mind, we suggest that vernacular media have much to offer health promotion professionals and health educators who seek to develop culturally appropriate messaging for dating app users in the context of what Race (2009) has termed 'counterpublic health' – that is, health messaging that actively engages with the pleasurable and at times playful aspects of dating and hooking up online (Race, 2009, pp. 159–160).

Methods

Our analysis of media reportage of dating and hookup apps supported a larger mixed methods inquiry into Australian 18–35-year-olds' experiences of digital dating app cultures. The project was approved by Swinburne's Human Research Ethics committee (HREC 2018/159), with additional approvals from partner organisation review boards. In order to ensure relevance for local health promotion organisations, we held four online consultations with a professional reference group over a 14-month period.

The group's 20 participants included representatives of government and non-government health organisations, as well as professionals in the fields of mental health, sexuality education, tertiary student support services, and youth work. While all members of the reference group agreed that an understanding of dating and hookup app cultures was important for them – both as individuals and in an organisational context – the majority did not have personal experience of app use. Consequently, we also held three online consultations with 18–35-year-old app users of diverse genders and sexualities, who provided input into our research design and preliminary analyses (Albury et al., 2019). In the early stages of the project, we invited these groups to share their perceptions of media reportage of dating and hookup apps, asking them to describe a 'typical' news story – which most imagined in terms of cautionary tales:

> Generally victim blaming for using the app in the first place or how this generation of young people have gone "wild" for sex.
>
> An assault of some description, for example sexual assault, stalking or physical assault.
>
> Bad experiences of dating apps and how we have lost our ability to converse with people in "real life".

I think that they would focus on the safety issue, maybe latching on to sexual assault stories or dramatic escapes …

Our media analysis sought to test these perceptions of 'typical' narratives, to better understand the ways apps might be framed as a health 'problem', and to more broadly explore the ways that apps and app-use might report within the context of safety, risk, and wellbeing. Recent approaches to media content analysis acknowledge the increasing complexity of the digital media ecosystem and seek to track the production and flow of ideas, information (and misinformation), attention, and public engagement across a wide range of channels. To efficiently extract and explore digital media content addressing dating and hookup apps, our study used Media Cloud in combination with NVivo qualitative analysis software. As an open-source platform for studying media ecosystems, Media Cloud contains a collection of more than 1.1 billion stories imported via their sources' RSS feeds, with 568,000 stories added to the collection daily.

The research questions for the analysis are as follows:

- **RQ1**: What are the dominant themes for articles substantially discussing dating apps and their uses?
- **RQ2**: How are risk, safety, and wellbeing characterised in news media conversations?
- **RQ3**: How have the concepts 'dating app' and 'hookup app' permeated more broadly as a cultural referent for digitally mediated relationships?

While our collaborations with health professionals are grounded in the context of Australian policy and practice, we are mindful of both the syndication of news stories across wire services such as AAP, and the informal sharing practices of news consumers via global social media platforms such as Twitter and Facebook. Consequently, we map common themes occurring in public English language media conversations about dating and hookup app uses in media outlets based in Australia, the United States, and the United Kingdom. Sources are managed in Media Cloud through a number of national collections to help targeted analysis. The Australian National Collection contains 61 media sources, the U.S. Top Online News, 2017 Collection contains 31 sources, and the U.K. National Collection contains 82 sources reflecting a larger pool of news media.

Source articles were collected between 1 May 2017 and 30 April 2018. The analysis is deliberately restricted to provide a contemporary snapshot of current perspectives and discussions. The keyword set was developed through iterative search processes to best capture core relevant content and variations, and identify exclusions where necessary. Only the most popular dating apps at the time of this research were used as search terms (Tinder, Grindr, and Bumble) to maintain a relatively narrow search net. Search terms were: 'dating app*', Tinder AND dating OR date*, Grindr, 'hook-up app*' OR 'hookup app*', Bumble AND dating OR date*. While these terms returned some non-relevant data, they were chosen to ensure the best possible coverage of media discussion of dating and hookup apps.

The total number of articles extracted was 6108: Australia (526); United States (1971); United Kingdom (3611). A sample of 300 articles were selected systematically from the full dataset for qualitative coding using QSR NVivo software. The sample was derived by taking 1 in every 30 articles from the U.K. dataset ($n = 100$); 1 in every 20 articles from the U.S. dataset ($n = 96$); and 1 in every 5 articles from the Australian dataset ($n = 104$) (subscriber-only articles were excluded). Media content from the three countries of origin was combined for an overview analysis that sought to describe the dominant themes, and to draw out broad patterns at a global level. However, the stratified sample also enabled analysis by country. The sample was chosen according to keywords, as opposed to genre. The overall dataset primarily consisted of news reportage or feature articles (authored by professional journalists), with the minority of articles consisting of opinion and/or editorial content.

The analytical approach applies thematic content analysis (Krippendorff, 2013), incorporating both inductive and deductive processes, to identify patterns and develop core themes or concepts that best characterise the way dating and hook-up apps are accounted for in the sample. While our second research question requires these qualitative approaches to characterise and explain the various accounts of dating and hook-up apps, the first research question could best be answered by quantifying the dominant themes covered by articles in the data set. Figure 1 visualises the hierarchical categories and proportion of associated articles, with some exemplary headlines. While this technique remains interpretive, all four authors reviewed and iterated codes with an acceptable level of inter-coder agreement. The final set of five top-level codes and sub-codes were: 'Risk' (crime, harassment, personal data, privacy); 'Wellbeing' (drug use, mental health, sexual health); 'Safety and play' (pedagogies, play, alternative uses, mediated relationships); 'App design and technology' (business models, platform affordances, app company research, other Tinder-like apps). The category of 'app design and technology' was excluded from the analysis to address the research questions' focus on the health implications of app use.

Taking a linguistic approach in our analysis, we explore specific examples and explain two main aspects. Firstly, we address the articles' focus and ideational content or topic (what they are about). Secondly, we analyse their stance on, or evaluation of, dating and hook-up apps and user experiences (Bednarek, 2006). As these articles were published within a 12-month period, they cannot be seen as representative of *all* media reportage on dating and hook-up apps. In some cases, these articles reflect a surge of interest in high-profile incidents such as app-related court cases that occurred at a specific time. For the purposes of this article, we have excluded articles that fell under our themes of 'app technologies' (articles focusing on apps' features or the parent companies' business models), and 'peripheral mentions' (where dating and hook-up apps are mentioned in passing but are not central to the discussion).

Findings

Foregrounding risk

A distinct set of articles associate a number of risks with dating and hook-up app use via headlines such as 'Tinder rapist' or 'Grindr scammer'. While these headlines paint an unambiguously negative picture of the apps and their use, the stance adopted within each article varies greatly. While some articles attribute blame to predatory individual app users, many critique apps' corporate owners. Key themes revolve around crime, harassment, and breaches of privacy relating to personal data. Of the first category, 'crime'

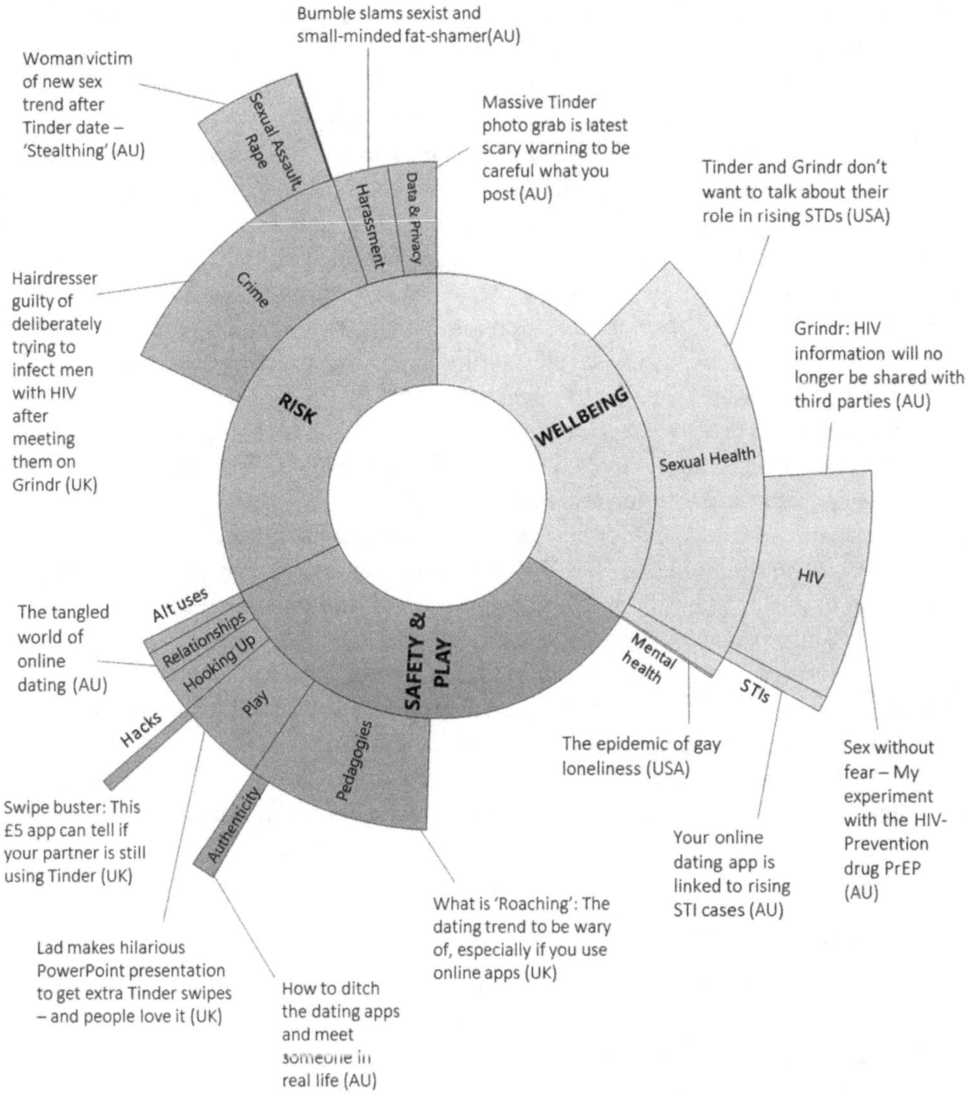

Figure 1. Hierarchical categories showing three key themes and associated subthemes ($n = 300$ articles).

most commonly included 'catfishing', or the use of false profiles used to lure users for a range of purposes, along with extortion and blackmail, stalking, sexual assault, and homophobic violence. Articles about harassment address unsolicited sexual messages and images, and offer first-person perspectives on experiences of abuse via dating apps. Articles on personal data and privacy deal with data breaches by apps discussed disclosure of Grindr users' HIV status to third party apps, and concerns regarding scams.

Crime

A significant number of articles report on crimes associated with app use. Often the articles simply associate app use with violence against women and patterns of abusive behaviour and gendered violence more widely, involving men who were known to their victim. Dating apps were foregrounded in this reporting through headline phrases such as *Stalker back in jail… after failed Tinder date* (Kidd, 2018) and *Woman goes missing after posting about upcoming Tinder date* (Brennan, 2017).

Several articles reported on 'stealthing' (the practice of removing a condom during sex without a partner's consent). In one news article (Golloyan, 2017), stealthing is referred to as a 'new sex trend', linked to Tinder and heterosexual casual sex. Stealthing also appears in coverage of a U.K. case in which a HIV positive man was charged with deliberately infecting partners he met through Grindr (Keay, 2017; Thompson & Mills, 2017). One U.S. opinion article (Cracker, 2017) discusses stealthing the context of gay men's sexual cultures and 'the psychic fallout of the AIDS epidemic more broadly'.

A cluster of news articles cover cases of extortion, blackmail, and violence against gay men. Two Australian cases feature here: one involving a group of Perth teenagers who met with gay men from Grindr to rob and bash them (WA Today, 2017), and the high-profile case of a teenager who used Grindr for extortion, leading to the suicide of one of his targets (ABC News, 2017; Dingwall, 2017). A U.K. newspaper reports on a vigilante group entrapping a man on Grindr (Smith, 2017). Entrapment was presented across a range of scenarios as a risk associated with the geo-locational functionality of apps.

Revenge porn, or image-based abuse, was also reported in cases of extortion and blackmail. In one Australian article, coverage of a proposal to legislate against image-based abuse (Gorey, 2017) referenced the extortion of gay men on Grindr. Discussions of image-based abuse most commonly referred to the practice of 'catfishing', which was represented in headlines such as *The terrifying Tinder scam catching out countless Australians* (Foster, 2018).

Discrimination and harassment

A number of news and human-interest articles outlined cases of women receiving unsolicited sexual messages and 'dick pics' on Tinder (Hartley-Parkinson, 2017; A. Jones, 2017), with the latter also being sent via Apple's Airdrop (Bluetooth) feature (Dunn, 2017). A range of first-person opinion articles offered insight into experiences of harassment and discrimination online, including sexual racism and HIV stigma on gay apps (Nichols, 2017), and using Tinder as a trans woman (Dawson, 2017) or as a person with a chronic health condition (Young, 2017).

Considering wellbeing and health

Articles in this category associated dating and hook-up apps with a range of issues concerning sexual health and mental health, along with reference to drugs and drug use, and health research relating to app use. Generally, articles focusing on sexual health linked apps with increased diagnoses of STIs among heterosexual and non-heterosexual app users. Articles linking apps to HIV transmission primarily related to gay and bisexual men's app use. Mental health was raised as an issue for many app users in relation to anxiety, loneliness, and depression, and as a barrier to authenticity, intimacy, and sociality.

Sexual health

Our sample period coincided with public health trials in Australia, the United States, and the United Kingdom, in which pre-exposure prophylaxis medications (PrEP) were made available to HIV-negative men. Unsurprising, a number of articles associated PrEP with cultures of dating, sex, and hook-up app use (Cracker, 2017). In a long-read (or feature article) titled *Sex without fear – my experiment with the HIV-prevention drug PrEP* (Cain, 2017), a U.K. journalist explored in-app conventions for discussing HIV status.

Sexual health was most commonly reported by linking dating app use with susceptibility to sexually transmitted infections (STIs) such as gonorrhoea (Graham, 2018; S. Jones, 2017). Typically, 'online dating' or the use of dating and hook-up apps is taken as one headline factor amongst others linked to increased STI rates, including the rise in the number of visitors to Australia (e.g. 'with over 640,000 backpackers' who are thought to engage in 'risky' practices such as 'having multiple sexual partners without protection while using drugs and alcohol') (S. Jones, 2017). One article called for app-based health promotion campaigns under the headline *Tinder and Grindr don't want to talk about their role in rising STDs* (Belluz, 2017).

Mental health

Many articles explore the negative emotional and mental health experiences associated with dating apps, hooking up, and contemporary mediated relationships in general. Common themes include gay men's vulnerability to body dissatisfaction or unhappiness about their appearance, and pressure from within the community, said to be fuelled by porn and Grindr profile pictures (e.g. '40 percent of the images on the site were of faceless, buffed torsos') (Romensky, 2017). In a range of first-person think pieces, hook-up apps are linked to a decline in 'gay community', which is associated with a perceived loss of social support. A widely-shared long-read article in the *Huffington Post* (Hobbes, 2017) explores what it defines as *The epidemic of gay loneliness* through a number of firsthand accounts, as well as through reference to a range of research findings highlighting high rates of mental ill-health among LGBTQ+ people. The author attributes a decline in gay community to the 'shocking primacy of hook-up apps in gay life … For many of us, they have become the primary way we interact with other gay people' (Hobbes, 2017).

Heterosexual dating cultures were also associated with anxiety, negativity, and mental health issues. Articles highlight pressures on single people around Valentine's Day and urge safety and restraint in Tinder use (O'Neill, 2018). One warns that 'swiping through [Tinder] makes you unhappy about your body' (Weston, 2017), linking the app to low self-esteem among heterosexual users. Anxieties regarding heteronormativity are also present in a piece in *The Sun* which describes Tinder as 'toxic' to heterosexual men, claiming that access to sex without commitment makes them feel 'burnt out, bored – and lonely' and 'like prostitutes' (Daubney, 2017).

Safety and play in app cultures

We define this cluster of articles in relation to 'safety and play' because they directly or indirectly aim to create shared knowledge about cultures of app use, helping readers to understand the design features and cultures of use on different apps. This is often achieved through the context of play, humour, or 'relatable' entertainment. This category contained less news reportage and more 'lifestyle' or entertainment-focused features. These include 'how to' articles and 'listicles' documenting recognisable tropes of off-putting behaviour on dating apps, usually written by women who date men. Examples of this genre include a satirical glossary of men's off-putting Tinder biographies (Bastow, 2017), and satire of heterosexual men's profile-pictures: *I am a Tinder guy holding a fish and I will provide for you* (Collier, 2017). Gendered entitlement in dating app cultures is exemplified in stories such as the man who sent a woman a bill for their first Tinder date after she did not reply to his messages (Knox, 2018). Dating app platforms themselves play a role in offering methods for understanding cultures of app use. Some articles reported on app companies taking a clear stance in relation to acceptable user behaviour, such as Bumble's open letter to a 'sexist' user who was barred after sending abusive messages (Mullin, 2017).

A significant number of articles in this category offer positive advice on how to use apps well. *BuzzFeed* in the United States, along with U.K. tabloids, offers many articles taking this 'pedagogical' stance, appealing to younger readers likely to use apps and open to such tips. Some articles celebrate playful or creative uses of dating apps, such as 'funniest chat-up lines' and profiles (Chan, 2017). They also outline stories of unusual uses of the app, such as the young man who made a self-deprecating PowerPoint presentation for his profile (Petcar, 2018).

Pedagogical articles may also claim apps have 'changed the rules' for dating and hooking up (Lawton, 2017). In these articles, dating apps are positioned as producing unique problems with communication and relationships. These articles often work to generate a sense of expertise or literacy to better understand technologised dating and hook-up cultures, foregrounding digital practices such as emoji use, referenced in several articles reporting on a set of custom 'gaymoji' launched by Grindr (Trebay, 2017).

Discussion

The findings presented here show how dating and hook-up apps are currently presented in popular media settings through competing frames. While these frames do not necessarily determine practices and experiences of app use, we take the approach of characterising the scenes of public discourse that circulate around these apps for several reasons. Firstly, articles that frame app use as a public health problem are clearly aimed at non-app users, either ignoring or actively obscuring actual experiences of app use. The dataset offers us a means of reflecting on how non-users of apps (including educators and health service providers) are likely to perceive both app users and the cultures of dating and hook-up app use. Secondly, we sought to better understand how public conversations about dating and hook-up app use (and non-use) are contested and shaped in popular media settings, with the aim of discovering new models for sexuality education and health promotion practice. These discursive frames, in other words, can be used to develop tools to establish effective health literacies and cultures of care (Hurley, 2002) around dating and hook-up app use.

Accounts of coercion, abuse, sexual violence, sexual racism, and discrimination are common in the dataset. We acknowledge the importance and complexity of these issues (both in terms of primary prevention and in relation to the need to support victims to recover and seek justice), as is conveyed in a number of recent research projects examining these aspects of digital media culture (Carlson, 2019; Henry & Powell, 2018; Lee, 2019; March, Grieve, Marrington, & Jonason, 2017; Thompson, 2018; Vitis & Gilmour, 2017). Additionally, we note an established (and growing) body of research in our home discipline of media studies addressing the diverse everyday uses of apps – including the use of dating platforms as social media networks to facilitate connections within diasporic communities, and across social/ethnic boundaries (for example Cassidy & Wang, 2018; Ferris & Duguay, 2019; Shield, 2016).

A relatively small but prominent set of investigative articles in our dataset brushed the surface of the question of wellbeing in app use, particularly in relation to mental health. Questions are raised of apps in their exacerbation of loneliness, poor social connection, stigma, and mental ill health. While links between app use and mental ill-health can easily be sensationalised, they raise under-researched issues that deserve further scrutiny. Other online channels of communication have been investigated for their ability to facilitate positive peer-to-peer mental health support (McCosker, 2018; Naslund, Aschbrenner, Marsch, & Bartels, 2016). However, not enough is yet known about the potential for dating and hook-up apps to facilitate such supportive interactions, relieve anxieties around establishing social and sexual connection with others or, conversely, the pressures they may add to the mental wellbeing of some users.

Additionally, while we have not imposed overall measures of 'quality' or 'accuracy' on our data, we note that a number of media reports linked the increased use of dating apps with increased diagnoses of STIs in Australia and elsewhere. As Albury, Burgess, Light, Race, and Wilken (2017) have noted, global public health organisations have, in recent years, sought to access dating and hook-up app data and metadata to assist in public health surveillance and interventions. However, significant concerns have been raised regarding the ethical implications of such actions, particularly where there is a potential to share data with law enforcement agencies (2017, p. 8). To our knowledge, no epidemiological study to date has found causal links between app use and increases STI or HIV diagnoses. Despite this lack of evidence, spokespeople for Australian public health services and international health promotion organisations have made a number of public statements speculating that such a link exists (Reeders, 2018). We suggest that such statements are examples of biocommunicability in action. That is, where journalists and editors invite public health professionals to speculate on health and wellbeing issues, and health spokespeople agree to provide speculative commentary, a perception may grow amongst health professionals that actual evidence exists beyond hypotheses.

For the remainder of this discussion, we focus on the health promotion potential of accounts of 'safety and play', which featured prominently in the Australian sources we reviewed. Many articles in this category not only entertain, but explicitly offer strategies for participating in dating and hookup app cultures. As McKee (2017; 2012) has argued, entertainment media producers can offer valuable insights to sexuality education and health promotion professionals seeking to produce engaging content. That is, young people need information about safe sex practices that are 'presented in ways that are clearly relevant to their own experiences and interests' (McKee, 2012, p. 503). Similarly, Albury (2019) suggests that the Australian sexual health promotion workforce could increase capacity for both understanding and deploying digital technologies and platforms by looking to successful examples of news and entertainment-based digital content. This 'counterpublic' approach to sexual health promotion is well-established in the field of gay men's health but is less common in content targeting other audiences (Race, 2009; Warner, 2002). Sexual health promotion has to negotiate the tension that emerges in our dataset, between asserting authority when presenting health information about new technologies and sexual practices, and 'deferring' to the experiences of those who are actively engaged in using those technologies for relationships and sexual encounters.

Our analysis identified a category of media reports that adopt a playful approach to dating and hookup app use, deploying humour and empathetic storytelling techniques. This category of articles foregrounds the expertise of dating app users, featuring the kinds of peer-to-peer information sharing Briggs and Hallin identify as the 'public sphere' model of biocommunicability (2010). In this model, media audiences are framed not as 'patient-consumers' of health information, but as agentic citizens in a dialogic space of public health communication that also includes health service providers, health educators, policy-makers, and regulators (Briggs & Hallin, 2010). Accounts of dating apps that take this perspective could be understood as counter-reactions or even byproducts to more authoritative risk or 'problem' oriented pieces. Within our dataset, the voices of professional expertise were less likely to appear in reportage on the everyday aspects of dating app use, in which first-person experience was foregrounded.

These pedagogical stories appeared most prominently in digital-first 'social news' stories, in keeping with what Hurcombe (2019, p. 4) has dubbed the 'social news logics' of 'sociability' – in which news content is crafted for maximum shareability and 'personalisation' – foregrounding first-person voice and intimate, highly subjective positioning. Building a dialogue between these alternatives in public accounting requires firstly, accepting the knowledge that pedagogical, first-person and even sociable stories of app use can offer. Secondly, as exemplified in some approaches to health promotion in relation to HIV, health agencies can better leverage forms of vernacular knowledge and 'learning by doing' to inform campaigns and push back against unfounded but authoritative accounts of app use.

Many such articles deploy what we have termed 'vernacular pedagogies', sharing not only cautionary tales, but instructions for safe and pleasurable practices of app use. These articles describe strategies for optimising in-app encounters, including guidelines for selecting profile pictures, composing in-app biographies, and engaging in chat with other app users. They also offer tips for interpreting other users' profiles, and identifying 'red flags'. The pedagogical articles in our dataset adopt familiar lifestyle and entertainment news genres (including social news genres such as the listicle) to communicate etiquette, debate ethical practice, and offer 'how tos' for dating and hookup app use.

We have labelled these practices 'vernacular pedagogy' to build on Burgess and Green's notion of 'vernacular creativity', which describes the ways that early YouTube content creators draw on established and easily recognisable media genres (such as movie trailers) to create their own versions of shareable entertainment (Burgess & Green, 2018). The term vernacular pedagogy also invokes Escoffier's (1998) account of the early days of the HIV epidemic, which documents the ways that 'vernacular knowledge' about safe-sex practices first emerged via practices of 'learning through doing' in gay men's sexual communities, and only later became formalised as 'health communication' (see also Martos, 2016). Just as gay men's vernacular knowledge was adapted by health organisations in their development of formal safer sex health communication content in the 1980s and 1990s, we suggest that emergent vernacular dating and hook-up app pedagogies offer a useful model for contemporary health communicators developing content and resources for both app users and non-users.

Conclusion

Our review of media reporting relating to dating and hook-up app use uncovered public conversations of criminal activity and unethical approaches to sexual consent and sexual health. This was expected – both because news reporting intrinsically favours 'bad news', and because dating and hook-up apps are still considered by many to be novel (and therefore risky) technologies. The headlines for risk-themed articles show a heavy focus on harassment, scams, or privacy breaches, and wellbeing-themed articles cover STI outbreaks, 'epidemics' of mental ill-health, or loneliness associated with dating apps. However, our analysis uncovered the equally dominant presence and popularity of articles that take a pedagogical stance, offering insights into how to negotiate or master app use, which we defined as relating to 'safety and play'. Building on Briggs and Hallin's (2007) exploration of public (and counterpublic) spheres within biocommunicability, we have reflected on what we have termed the 'vernacular pedagogies' that emerge in both social news items, and 'legacy' news genres such as opinion columns, first-person lifestyle, and entertainment content.

These articles primarily adopt a first-person approach, describing both positive and negative experiences with dating and hook-up apps in order to explore new forms of intimacy and relationality associated with digital cultures. These stories are not always focused on the apps themselves, but on the way social media platforms and digital devices impact on intimate practices and relationships. Where they do focus on apps, they reflect on the ways that the technical properties of digital apps and devices (such as the capacity for geolocation) effect user's experiences of safety, play, and wellbeing. That is, they provide insights into cultures of app use, allowing us to think creatively about the role digital technologies play in everyday life.

Disclosure statement

No potential conflict of interest was reported by the author(s).

Funding

This work was supported by the Australian Research Council [project ID LP160101687].

ORCID

Kath Albury http://orcid.org/0000-0001-9043-8126
Anthony McCosker http://orcid.org/0000-0003-0666-3262
Tinonee Pym http://orcid.org/0000-0001-6731-4475
Paul Byron http://orcid.org/0000-0001-6591-3060

References

Albury, K. (2019). 'Recognition of competition' versus the will to app: Rethinking digital engagement in Australian youth sexual health promotion policy and practice. *Media International Australia*, *171*(1), 38–50.

Albury, K., Burgess, J., Light, B., Race, K., & Wilken, R. (2017). Data cultures of mobile dating and hook-up apps: Emerging issues for critical social science research. *Big Data & Society*, *4*(2), 1–11. doi:10.1177/2053951717720950

Albury, K., Byron, P., McCosker, A., Pym, T., Walshe, J., Race, K., … Dietzel, C. (2019). *Safety, risk and wellbeing on dating apps: Final report*. Melbourne: Swinburne University of Technology. doi:10.25916/5dd324c1b33bb

Bacchi, C. (2016). Problematizations in health policy: Questioning how "problems" are constituted in policies. *SAGE Open*, *6*(2), 1–16. doi:10.1177/2158244016653986

Bednarek, M. (2006). *Evaluation in media discourse: Analysis of a newspaper corpus*. London: Continuum.

Briggs, C. L., & Hallin, D. C. (2007). Biocommunicability: The neoliberal subject and its contradictions in news coverage of health issues. *Social Text*, *25*(4), 43–66. doi:10.1215/01642472-2007-011

Briggs, C. L., & Hallin, D. C. (2010). Health reporting as political reporting: Biocommunicability and the public sphere. *Journalism*, *11*(2), 149–165. doi:10.1177/1464884909355732

Briggs, C. L., & Hallin, D. C. (2016). *Making health public: How news coverage is remaking media, medicine, and contemporary life*. Abingdon: Routledge.

Burgess, J., & Green, J. (2018). *Youtube: Online video and participatory culture*. Cambridge: Polity Press.

Byron, P., & Albury, K. (2018). 'There are literally no rules when it comes to these things': Ethical practice and the use of dating/hook-up apps. In A. Dobson, B. Robards, & N. Carey (Eds.), *Digital intimate publics and social media* (pp. 213–229). London: Palgrave Macmillan.

Carlson, B. (2019). Love and hate at the cultural interface: Indigenous Australians and dating apps. *Journal of Sociology*. doi:10.1177/1440783319833181

Cassidy, E., & Wang, W. Y. (2018). Gay men's digital cultures beyond Gaydar and Grindr: LINE use in the gay Chinese diaspora of Australia. *Information, Communication & Society*, *21*(6), 851–865. doi:10.1080/1369118X.2018.1437201

Escoffier, J. (1998). The invention of safer sex: Vernacular knowledge, gay politics and HIV prevention. *Berkeley Journal of Sociology*, *43*, 1–30.

Ferris, L., & Duguay, S. (2019). Tinder's lesbian digital imaginary: Investigating (im)permeable boundaries of sexual identity on a popular dating app. *New Media & Society*, *22*(3), 489–506. doi:10.1177/1461444819864903

Fullagar, S., Rich, E., & Francombe-Webb, J. (2017). New kinds of (ab) normal?: Public pedagogies, affect, and youth mental health in the digital age. *Social Sciences*, *6*(3), 99. doi:10.3390/socsci6030099

Fullagar, S., Rich, E., Francombe-Webb, J., & Maturo, A. (2017). Digital ecologies of youth mental health: Apps, therapeutic publics and pedagogy as affective arrangements. *Social Sciences*, *6*(4), 135. doi:10.3390/socsci6040135

Henry, N., & Powell, A. (2018). Technology-facilitated sexual violence: A literature review of empirical research. *Trauma, Violence, & Abuse*, *19*(2), 195–208. doi:10.1177/1524838016650189

Holland, K. (2017). Digital media and models of biocommunicability in health journalism: Insights from the production and reception of mental health news. *Australian Journalism Review*, *39*(2), 67–77.

Hurcombe, E. (2019). *The logics of social news: How BuzzFeed, Junkee and Pedestrian.tv are making news more engaging, sociable and personal* [Doctoral dissertation, Queensland University of Technology]. QUT EPrints. https://eprints.qut.edu.au/132172/

Hurcombe, E., Burgess, J., & Harrington, S. (2019). What's newsworthy about 'social news'? Characteristics and potential of an emerging genre. *Journalism*. doi:10.1177/1464884918793933

Hurley, M. (Eds.). (2002). *Cultures of care and safe sex among HIV positive Australians. Papers from the HIV Futures I and II surveys and interviews* (ARCSHS Monograph Series Number 43). The Australian Research Centre in Sex, Health and Society, La Trobe University.

Jenkins, H., Ford, S., & Green, J. (2018). *Spreadable media: Creating value and meaning in a networked culture*. New York: New York University Press.

Krippendorff, K. (2013). *Content analysis: An introduction to its methodology* (3rd ed.). Carbondale: Sage.

Lee, J. (2019). *Talking about race and gender with Tinder: Raced and gendered visibility of non-white women* [Doctoral dissertation, Southern Illinois University at Carbondale]. OpenSIUC. https://opensiuc.lib.siu.edu/dissertations/1719/

March, E., Grieve, R., Marrington, J., & Jonason, P. K. (2017). Trolling on Tinder® (and other dating apps): examining the role of the Dark Tetrad and impulsivity. *Personality and Individual Differences, 110*, 139–143. doi:10.1016/j.paid.2017.01.025

Martos, A. J. (2016). Vernacular knowledge and critical pedagogy: Conceptualising sexual health education for young men who have sex with men. *Sex Education, 16*(2), 184–198. doi:10.1080/14681811.2015.1088434

McCosker, A. (2018). Engaging mental health online: Insights from beyondblue's forum influencers. *New Media & Society, 20*(12), 4748–4764. doi:10.1177/1461444818784303

McKee, A. (2012). The importance of entertainment for sexuality education. *Sex Education, 12*(5), 499–509. doi:10.1080/14681811.2011.627727

McKee, A. (2017). Learning from commercial entertainment producers in order to create entertainment sex education. *Sex Education, 17*(1), 26–40. doi:10.1080/14681811.2016.1228528

Naslund, J. A., Aschbrenner, K. A., Marsch, L. A., & Bartels, S. J. (2016). The future of mental health care: Peer-to-peer support and social media. *Epidemiology and Psychiatric Sciences, 25*(2), 113–122. doi:10.1017/S2045796015001067

Nutbeam, D. (2008). The evolving concept of health literacy. *Social Science & Medicine, 67*(12), 2072–2078. doi:10.1016/j.socscimed.2008.09.050

Race, K. (2009). *Pleasure consuming medicine: The queer politics of drugs*. Durham: Duke University Press.

Reeders, D. (2018, January 30). An epidemic of bullshit. *Overland*. https://overland.org.au/2018/01/an-epidemic-of-bullshit/

Shield, A. D. J. (2016). New in town: Gay immigrants and geosocial media. In A. Dhoest, L. Szulc, & B. Eeckhout (Eds.), *LGBTQs, media and culture in Europe* (pp. 244–261). Abingdon: Routledge.

Thompson, L. (2018). "I can be your Tinder nightmare": Harassment and misogyny in the online sexual marketplace. *Feminism & Psychology, 28*(1), 69–89. doi:10.1177/0959353517720226

Vitis, L., & Gilmour, F. (2017). Dick pics on blast: A woman's resistance to online sexual harassment using humour, art and Instagram. *Crime, Media, Culture, 13*(3), 335–355. doi:10.1177/1741659016652445

Warner, M. (2002). Publics and counterpublics. *Public Culture, 14*(1), 49–90.

News Articles Cited

ABC News. (2017, May 12). Grindr scammer sentenced to six months' detention for blackmail. *ABC News*. https://www.abc.net.au/news/2017-05-12/teen-sentenced-to-six-months-in-detention-for-grindr-blackmail/8521748

Australian Associated Press. (2017, February 11). 'Asking For Trouble': Dating app use on the rise amid rising STI cases. *The Age*. https://www.theage.com.au/national/queensland/asking-for-trouble-dating-app-warning-amid-rising-sti-cases-20170211-guams9.html

Bastow, C. (2017, March 15). Here's a glossary of Tinder bio terms to help you decide which way to swipe. *The Sydney Morning Herald*. https://www.smh.com.au/lifestyle/life-and-relationships/heres-a-glossary-of-tinder-bio-terms-to-help-you-decide-which-way-to-swipe-20170315-guyn8y.html

Belluz, J. (2017, November 13). Tinder and Grindr don't want to talk about their role in rising STDs. *Vox*. https://www.vox.com/science-and-health/2017/11/13/16620286/online-dating-stds-tinder-grindr

Brennan, C. (2017, November 23). Woman goes missing after posting about upcoming Tinder date. *New York Daily News*. https://www.nydailynews.com/news/national/woman-missing-posting-upcoming-tinder-date-article-1.3652436

Cain, M. (2017, June 22). Sex without fear – my experiment with the HIV-prevention drug PrEP. *The Guardian*. https://www.theguardian.com/society/2017/jun/22/sex-without-fear-my-experiment-with-hiv-preventative-drug-prep

Chan, E. (2017, October 5). Love at first swipe? Tinder users reveal the funniest (and most cringe-worthy) chat-up lines used on the dating app. *The Daily Mail.* https://www.dailymail.co.uk/femail/article-4951620/Tinder-users-reveal-funniest-chat-lines.html

Collier, A. (2017, May 1). I am a Tinder guy holding a fish and I will provide for you. *The New Yorker.* https://www.newyorker.com/humor/daily-shouts/i-am-a-tinder-guy-holding-a-fish-and-i-will-provide-for-you

Cracker, M. (2017, June 1). Stealthing is a disturbing aspect of gay sexual culture. But calling it a clear-cut crime won't solve the problem. *Slate.* https://slate.com/human-interest/2017/06/stealthing-in-gay-sexual-culture-needs-careful-discussion-not-criminalization.html

Daubney, M. (2017, November 2). Why Tinder is "toxic" to men … by three blokes who claim they get TOO MUCH sex via the app that leaves them "lonely" and "feeling like prostitutes". *The Sun.* https://www.thesun.co.uk/fabulous/4828858/why-tinder-is-toxic-to-men-too-much-sex/

Dawson, J. (2017, May 19). 'I can't be a 24-hour sexual fantasy': Juno Dawson on dating as a trans woman. *The Guardian.* https://www.theguardian.com/society/2017/may/19/juno-dawson-cant-be-24-hour-sexual-fantasy-dating-trans-woman

Dingwall, D. (2017, June 13). Canberra teen avoids imprisonment for role in Grindr extortion scam. *Brisbane Times.* https://www.brisbanetimes.com.au/national/act/canberra-teen-avoids-imprisonment-for-role-in-grindr-extortion-scam-20170613-gwq1vs.html

Dunn, M. (2017, August 15). Apple's Airdrop feature used to send penis pics to people on the same train in new trend. *News.com.au.* https://www.news.com.au/technology/gadgets/mobile-phones/apples-airdrop-feature-used-to-send-penis-pics-to-people-on-the-same-train-in-new-trend/news-story/0092c1efd34625a5b7e899e86c984753

Foster, A. (2018, April 2). The terrifying Tinder scam catching out countless Australians. *News.com.au.* https://www.news.com.au/lifestyle/relationships/dating/the-terrifying-tinder-scam-that-countless-australians-are-being-caught-out-by/news-story/81db374b44be3f554a78063cb172d41c

Golloyan, C. (2017, May 5). Woman victim of new sex trend after Tinder date. *News.com.au.* https://www.news.com.au/lifestyle/relationships/sex/i-was-a-victim-of-stealthing/news-story/65214fd296a64cf0a88a515673fd46a7

Gorey, M. (2017, May 10). ACT Greens urge government action to combat image abuse and "revenge porn". *The Sydney Morning Herald.* https://www.smh.com.au/national/act/act-greens-urge-government-action-to-combat-image-abuse-and-revenge-porn-20170510-gw19ir.html

Graham, B. (2018, January 16). Gonorrhoea and syphilis on the rise in Melbourne. *ABC News.* https://www.abc.net.au/news/2018-01-16/gonorrhoea-and-syphilis-on-the-rise-in-melbourne/9332636

Hartley-Parkinson, R. (2017, June 2). Mother says she is 'one pervert away from joining a nunnery' over dirty messages. *Metro.* https://metro.co.uk/2017/06/02/mother-says-she-is-one-pervert-away-from-joining-a-nunnery-over-dirty-messages-6679274/

Hobbes, M. (2017, March 2). The epidemic of gay loneliness. *The Huffington Post.* https://highline.huffingtonpost.com/articles/en/gay-loneliness/

Jones, A. (2017, November 4). Hook-ups, sexting and unwanted threesomes: First-time dating in the age of Tinder. *The Guardian.* https://www.theguardian.com/lifeandstyle/2017/nov/04/hookups-sexting-unwanted-threesomes-first-time-dating-age-tinder

Jones, S. (2017, August 16). Your online dating app is linked to rising STI cases. *International Business Times.* https://www.ibtimes.com.au/your-online-dating-app-linked-rising-sti-cases-1558232

Keay, L. (2017, October 17). Alleged victim of hairdresser accused of deliberately infecting lovers with HIV was "starstruck" by him and "let his guard down". *The Daily Mail.* https://www.dailymail.co.uk/news/article-4986172/Victim-HIV-hairdresser-starstruck-him.html

Kidd, R. (2018, February 15). Stalker back in jail after sending man hundreds of texts after failed Tinder date. *News.com.au.* https://www.news.com.au/lifestyle/relationships/dating/stalker-back-in-jail-after-sending-man-hundreds-of-abusive-texts-after-failed-tinder-date/news-story/eed5770f94497f9dc3d05210b982814d

Knox, P. (2018, April 17). Man sends US woman a bill for their first and only date after she didn't text him back. *News.com.au*. https://www.news.com.au/finance/money/costs/man-sends-us-woman-a-bill-for-their-first-and-only-date-after-she-didnt-text-him-back/news-story/ab37229daa5a7ab220754cf37e3ff56b

Lawton, G. (2017, September 9). Is it wrong to resent going Dutch on a Tinder date? *The Guardian*. https://www.theguardian.com/lifeandstyle/2017/sep/09/is-it-wrong-to-resent-going-dutch-on-a-tinder-date

Mullin, G. (2017, December 15). Bumble slams "sexist and small-minded" fat-shamer in scathing open letter. *The Sun*. https://www.thesun.co.uk/news/5146822/bumble-dating-app-sexist-fatshamer-open-letter/

Nichols, J. M. (2017, July 9). People read horrific messages HIV-positive people receive on Grindr. *The Huffington Post*. https://www.huffingtonpost.com.au/entry/hiv-positive-people-grindr_n_595fb234e4b0615b9e911a0b?ri18n=true

O'Neill, M. (2018, February 13). Watch out for 'zombie bots' this Valentine's Day: IBM security experts warn botnet campaign targeting lonely singles is on the rise. *The Daily Mail*. https://www.dailymail.co.uk/sciencetech/article-5382505/Watch-zombie-bots-Valentines-Day.html

Petcar, S. (2018, February 20). Lad makes hilarious PowerPoint presentation to get extra Tinder swipes – and people LOVE it. *The Sun*. https://www.thesun.co.uk/news/5625749/tinder-powerpoint-extra-swipes-sam-dixey-leeds-student/

Romensky, L. (2017, October 25). Why gay porn is helping to fuel body dissatisfaction for gay men. *ABC News*. https://www.abc.net.au/news/2017-10-17/body-dissatisfaction-linked-to-gay-porn/9054856

Smith, A. (2017, August 28). 'Paedophile hunting' vigilante group live stream capture of pervert. *Metro*. https://metro.co.uk/2017/08/28/paedophile-hunting-vigilante-group-live-stream-capture-of-pervert-6885099/

Thompson, F., & Mills, K. A. (2017, November 15). Hairdresser guilty of deliberately trying to infect men with HIV after meeting them on Grindr. *The Mirror*. https://www.mirror.co.uk/news/uk-news/hairdresser-guilty-deliberately-trying-infect-11527325

Trebay, G. (2017, March 17). Gaymoji: a new language for that search. *The Sydney Morning Herald*. https://www.smh.com.au/world/gaymoji-a-new-language-for-that-search-20170316-guz7fh.html

WA Today. (2017, December 16). Jail for two who lured gay men to bashings. *WA Today*. https://www.watoday.com.au/national/western-australia/jail-for-two-who-lured-gay-men-to-bashings-20171216-h05rjn.html

Weston, P. (2017, August 5). Why Tinder makes you sad: Users of the dating app have lower self-esteem because they focus too much on their appearance. *The Daily Mail*. https://www.dailymail.co.uk/sciencetech/article-4761478/Swiping-Tinder-makes-unhappy-body.html

Young, B. (2017, November 6). What it's like dating with alopecia. *News.com.au*. https://www.news.com.au/lifestyle/health/health-problems/what-its-like-dating-with-alopecia/news-story/712c96df32904c5a711a372a10ee1c46/news-story/712c96df32904c5a711a372a10ee1c46

'I don't think my torso is anything to write home about': men's reflexive production of 'authentic' photos for online dating platforms

Andrea Waling, Michael Kehler, Jennifer Power, Lucille Kerr and Adam Bourne

ABSTRACT

This paper explores men's use of dating apps with an emergent body image focus, addressing cisgender, heterosexual men's feelings about dating app profile pictures. Drawing from interviews with 15 cisgender, heterosexual men residing in Australia about their use of dating applications including Tinder, Hinge, and Bumble, this paper examines how cisgender, heterosexual men construct their dating app profile pictures, and the decisions they make about the content of images they use for dating profile pictures. Utilizing concepts of self-presentation, authenticity, and bodily reflexive practices, this paper argues that the men in the study are attempting to present authentic and real selves in a dating world, while being confronted by concerns regarding body image and perceptions of ideal bodies. They also demonstrate conflicting desires to appear more muscular, fit, and athletic while not presenting as vain or narcissistic. In the process of creating profiles, these men develop a sense of self drawing on understandings of masculinity and specifically notions of idealized male bodies, which simultaneously run counter to the very authentic images of the self they seek to present.

Introduction

Online dating has seen a marked increase in the millennial years, becoming a common and mainstream social practice aimed at establishing both short and long-term sexual and romantic partnerships (Berkowitz, Tinkler, Peck, & Coto, 2021; Krüger & Spilde, 2020; Shield, 2019; Timmermans & Courtois, 2018). Research has focused on neoliberalism and gamification of dating (Chan, 2018), violence and safety (Pym, Byron, & Albury, 2021), intimacies (Albury, McCosker, & Evers, 2021), body image and self-presentation (Strubel & Petrie, 2017), and the broader social phenomenon of hook up and casual sex cultures (Timmerman & Courtois, 2018). In the online dating format, self-presentation is important. An online dater has to 'market' themselves to secure a potential date (Chan, 2018; Ellison, Hancock, & Toma, 2012; Oakes, Johnson and Parry, 2020). Profile pictures are central in this process, with varying levels of significance depending on the dating app. Tinder and Grindr, for example, are image-based with limited text, while other apps such as okCupid allow for long passages of text in the dating profile. There are variations in how much an individual presents their 'ideal self' relative to their 'authentic self'. However, representations must not be too distant from the 'truth', as online dating may be the first step to having a face-to-face meeting (Ellison et al., 2012).

The practice of falsifying an identity to lure someone into a romantic relationship to achieve financial or identity theft is also not uncommon on online dating platforms (Gibbs, Ellison, & Lai, 2010). Individuals can easily falsify a dating profile and associated profile imagery, giving rise to concerns as to whether profiles are in fact genuine representations of an individual (Duguay, 2017; Gibbs et al., 2010). Photographs are easy to manipulate with photo-editing tools and mobile apps (such as Snapchat®). People may curate a particular image or version of themselves in their online dating profiles, but this is not necessarily an untruth. The 'selfie' (a photo one has taken of oneself usually with a webcam or mobile phone, and often uploaded to social media) is one such way people present themselves – it is through this that people create an idealized, carefully curated version of themselves (Albury, 2015; Hancock & Toma, 2009; Tiidenberg & Gómez Cruz, 2015).

Impression management is a key component of this practice. People upload images with an awareness of how others are likely to perceive them (Vilnai-Yavetz & Tifferet, 2015) in an environment where profile images are a representation of a person's body, identity and personality (Haywood, 2018; Strano, 2008). Given the centrality of the profile picture to the online dating experience, it is not uncommon for photos to be constructed or manipulated in ways that others may consider to be inaccurate or inauthentic representations (Hancock & Toma, 2009; Sedgewick, Flath, & Elias, 2017). In recognition of concerns about this, dating apps such as Tinder rely on cross-engagement with public-facing social networking sites (SNS) such as Facebook to create a more 'authentic' and 'legitimate' dating environment, since Facebook is regarded as a more truthful representation of a person (Duguay, 2017).

Research and theory on dating app profile pictures that look beyond psychological accounts of body image and self-esteem concerns have focused primarily on young cisgender, heterosexual and queer women and trans and gender diverse heterosexual and people (Duguay, Burgess, & Suzor, 2018) or cisgender men who have sex with men (Miller, 2018). Cisgender refers to a person who describes their gender in a way that corresponds to the sex they were assigned at birth. Miller (2018) and Rodriguez, Huemmer, and Blumell (2016) note how gay and bisexual men's dating apps privilege particular representations of masculinity that come through not only the body itself, but also, the language used to describe the body, both in profile descriptions, and in what others desire. Barrett (2020) explores how queer men using dating apps like Grindr experience issues such as transphobia and trans men exclusion, racism, HIV stigma, and fat-phobia among other concerns. Experiences of racism has also been noted in queer women's experiences of dating apps (Li & Chen, 2021). Oakes et al. (2020) note how queer men use strategies of 'selling one's self' and 'the buying of others' in their selection and production of dating profile images.

Few studies have focused on cisgender, heterosexual men's production of, or use of, dating app profile pictures. Some studies have shown that cisgender, heterosexual men are aware of the complex and contradictory ways in which their images are read by others and work to manage this. Ward (2017) writing from a media and communications studies perspective, explored profile dating pictures in some detail, arguing that some cisgender, heterosexual men wanted their photos to be idealized versions of their (masculine) self to secure the best chance of meeting a romantic partner, and yet authentic enough to be regarded as realistic and not disingenuous. The mechanisms by which cisgender, heterosexual men produce profile images are not accounted for, and there is an overall assumption that all cisgender, heterosexual men will actively choose images that present powerful representations of traditional masculinity with little self-reflection regarding these choices (Hess & Flores, 2018). However, Haywood's (2018) work explores the production of cisgender, heterosexual young men's Tinder profile photos in more detail, arguing that their production and selection of self-images highlight a 'reflexive reflexivity' (155), the practice of individuals not only reflecting on developing their profile, but also what they do in respect of how they then evaluate their reflexive capacities. Haywood's (2018) participants engaged this in their attempt to balance the desire to present an aggressive masculine self with a self that is 'a "decent lad" and "genuine lad",, while "not being a dick", and ensuring 'that I am not an idiot or a dozer' (153). This desire comes from within themselves, and from broader cultural perceptions. As Tanner, Maher, and Fraser (2013) note, images of muscularity or those which suggest high investment in appearance and grooming may be read as vain and be negatively regarded. This runs contradictory to assumptions that cisgender, heterosexual men will present idealized versions of masculinity centred on fitness, athleticism, and muscular physiques.

We ask, how do cisgender, heterosexual men make sense of their production, selecting, and posting of photos in dating apps? We also seek to understand how their broader considerations about their bodies and bodily reflexive practices align with their photo choices, as well as how they determine which image/s denote/s a real or authentic self, particularly as it applies to perceptions of masculinity. We explore these questions by investigating what cisgender, heterosexual men consider when they take dating app profile pictures, and moreover, the decisions they make when uploading specific photos to their dating profiles. To do this, we first draw from theories of self-presentation (Giddens, 1991; Goffman, 1959) and authenticity in online dating (Duguay, 2016, 2017), and bodily reflexive practices (Connell, 1995).

Authenticity and identity

Scholars have long considered issues of 'authenticity' and representation of the self, particularly in the digital context (Duguay, 2016). Vannini and Williams (2009) argue that 'authenticity' is a social construct in and of itself but positioned as objective and truthful. When it comes to gender and sexuality, ideas about what is 'real' and what are 'fake' may be socially constructed but end up becoming accepted as truth about what is, and what is not, authentic.

Duguay (2017) notes that a number of studies exploring digital self-presentation draw from the work of Goffman (1959), particularly that concerning 'on-stage' and 'off-stage' performances of identity when thinking through this question of authenticity (Duguay, 2016; Gaden & Dumitricia, 2015; Hogan, 2010). In these cases, digital representations of the self are seen as contemporary manifestations of the 'on-stage' persona that is carefully curated for different audiences (Gaden & Dumitricia, 2015) and may be in conflict or inconsistent with the experience of the 'off-stage' self. However, as Duguay (2017) contends, this application of Goffman's (1959) work is unable to account for the interpersonal and material elements necessary to achieve a coherent sense of their own authentic self, or what she notes, the *stuff* (emphasis added) of authenticity (353). This *stuff* is composed of varied things that might come together in different ways, such as how app settings and interfaces lend themselves to providing additional elements of authenticity to a dating profile app. As Duguay (2017) outlines, Giddens (1991) saw identity development as a continually reflexive project in which people gain a sense of who they are – their authentic self – in relation to everyday action and habits, the opportunities, and choices they have access to, and the material realities of their life. An authentic identity is contextualized in a historic and material reality, but it is not static – it is created and recreated through reflexive action and thus is fluid, ever-changing (Duguay, 2017). Engaging in the creation of a dating profile is part of the reflective presentation of self.

This identity project is compounded with online daters' concerns that digital dating cultures encourage increasingly manipulated and fabricated images, making it impossible to judge what is authentic (Bonner-Thompson, 2017; Ellison et al., 2012; Gibbs et al., 2010; Ward, 2017). In online dating, it is the image or representation of what a person may be like, which precedes any potential reality of that person, or may even determine the perception of their selves. This 'reality' is constituted through varied mediated relations and identity projects that draw from a range of sociocultural and lifestyle choices factors, and individuals may draw upon these resources to curate an online dating profile that speaks to some form of preconstructed 'authenticity' (Duguay, 2017). While all selves can be said to be socially produced, this perception may not be an accurate interpretation.

Considering the concerns of authenticity of profiles reported in research on online dating (Gibbs et al., 2010; Ward, 2017), this has implications for thinking about how cisgender, heterosexual men might grapple with this question of the authentic, considering that it is the simulation of their self that may ultimately determine the reality of the potential for a date or relationship (or lack thereof). In thinking about this question of the *stuff* and authenticity (Duguay, 2017) we turn to a consideration of men's bodies, masculinity, and body reflexive practices.

Men's bodies and body reflexive practices

Bodies as emblematic of forms of masculinity are part of the broader research landscape which requires investigating bodily practices and the connections to the sociology of the body as meaningfully situated and contextually important (Bordo, 1999; Connell, 1995, 2001; Gill, Henwood, & McLean, 2005; Hakim, 2018, 2020; Norman, 2011; Swenson & Allen, 2019; Wagner, 2016). Connell (1995, p. 45) theorized the signification of bodies and gender arguing that 'true masculinity' is believed to proceed from men's bodies or express a natural belief about men's bodies. Bodies thus are constituted as situationally meaningful through social relationships. As Connell explains, body reflexive practices are formed by structures. For example, Hakim's (2018, 2020) work highlights the fit, athletic and muscular male body as a response to austerity in the UK. Hakim (2020) contends that increased precarity in the employment and labour sectors, alongside the individualizing expectations of neoliberalism, means that straight and queer men are now also expected to engage in similar practices to demonstrate their self-worth (see also Oakes et al., 2020). Bodily practices can be understood as responses to a situation that invites or disallows possibilities.

In the case of dating apps, bodies remain central in the conversation, and that such bodies function as forms of capital (Chan, 2018; Hakim, 2018, 2020; Oakes et al., 2020). Generally, it is assumed that cisgender, heterosexual men produce images that will correspond with traditional ideals of masculinity (Hess & Flores, 2018) in order to be valuable on the dating market (Chan, 2018; Haywood, 2018; Oakes et al., 2020). Such ideals include highly muscular physiques, and engaging in traditional displays of masculinity (see Connell, 1995). However, the assumption that masculinity is the only discourse framing cisgender, heterosexual men's production of profile pictures for dating apps assumes that masculinity is the only thing that cisgender, heterosexual men believe women desire, and thus should present. This would include presenting a body that is athletic, muscular, and conventionally masculine. Psychological research suggests that men may feel compelled to achieve a muscular body to attract women (Frederick & Haselton, 2007). However, a recent qualitative focus group study exploring 24 Australian women's perceptions of men's sexualized bodies found that the majority of women are not looking for these qualities when seeking relationships or sexual encounters with men, finding that muscularity or related images (such as, fitness photos) suggest narcissism, vanity, and poor relationship material (Waling, Duncan, Angelides, & Dowsett, 2020a).

Additionally, masculinity has been publicly scrutinized and positioned as problematic in the last decade, and men may be increasingly aware of this in their own projects of masculinity (Waling, 2019a, 2019b, 2020). Yet, masculinity, and ideals around what constitutes a proper masculine physique remain, particularly in studies on young cisgender, heterosexual men and boys, and sports, fitness, and social media cultures (Burns & Kehler, 2014; Drummond, 2020; Drummond & Drummond, 2015; Kehler & Atkinson, 2010). The emergence of concepts like 'toxic masculinity' contribute to a broader discourse that assumes men's subject positions and how they might engage with these ideals (see Waling, 2019b for a critique of this concept; Haywood, 2020 for a critique on masculinity as discourse).

Cisgender, heterosexual men may be grappling with a series of varying and contradictory expectations and possibilities in presenting their selves in online dating profile images that attempt to demonstrate desirable forms of masculinity, alongside presenting their real or authentic selves when seeking emotional or sexual connections. To understand these potential and varying expectations around vulnerability and authenticity, we conducted interviews with 15 cisgender, heterosexual young men who are using, or have used, dating apps. Below, we provide an account of our methodology and method.

Methodology

This work is framed by an *interpretivist paradigm* which 'focuses primarily on recognising and narrating the meaning of human experiences and actions' (Levers, 2013) with a consideration that such experiences are subjective and in which there may be multiple realities. In this paper we focus on cisgender, heterosexual men's production of, or rationale in choosing, public-facing images for dating profiles. A qualitative approach was deemed appropriate to gain a better understanding of the processes that cisgender, heterosexual men engage with in their choosing of profile dating pictures (Morse & Field, 1996). Semi-structured interviews were employed, framed by an emotional reflexive approach (Holmes, 2010) and *interpretative phenomenological analysis* (IPA) approach (Willig, 2013). Emotional reflexivity focuses on the embodied, cognitive and emotional processes in which individuals make sense of their lives and choices (Holmes, 2010). IPA is a methodological framework where researchers aim to understand participants and their perspectives with reference to their physical and cultural realities (Smith, 1996). This involves paying close attention to histories and narratives, affect and feelings, senses, and language as they seek to make sense of their personal lived experience (Willig, 2013).

Methods

Ethical approval for this study was provided by La Trobe University Human Research Ethics Committee (HEC18477). Participants provided informed written consent to participate in this study and to allow their deidentified data to appear in publications. As the study was about understanding how cisgender, heterosexual men make sense of, and engage with, dating apps and production of both non-sexually explicit and sexually explicit imagery, we did not engage in participation observation of dating apps nor analyse participant dating profiles. Covert participant observation of dating apps also involves many ethical concerns, particularly because participants have not consented to having their profiles studied (Shield, 2019).

Data collection

Semi-structured interviews by the lead author were conducted with 15 cisgender, heterosexual young men residing in Australia between the ages of 18 and 30 during the months of January and March 2019. As this study was framed by an IPA approach, 15 interviews was an appropriate number for in-depth analysis of the data (see Smith, 1996; Yardley, 2000). Participant eligibility was determined by their age (18–30), country of residence (Australia), and whether they had been using a dating app in the last two years to seek out romantic and/or sexual encounters. Facebook advertising was used, which linked participants to a recruitment website that outlined details of the study, and a contact option. Participants who were deemed eligible to participate were offered a choice of either a video chat or audio chat interview, phone interview, or IM messaging interview. While not the focus of this paper, we note that these different method options were chosen to provide men opportunity to use a method that best suited them, particularly as methods such as IM messaging allow for anonymity, and can be an empowering and comfortable for participants who may be able to think over their responses more easily (see Pearce, Thøgersen-Ntoumani, & Duda, 2019). Using instant messaging for interviewing participants about online dating may be especially appropriate and relevant, as instant messaging is commonly used during online dating (Malta, 2012). Additionally, it has been noted that IM messaging does not yield less rich data than audio and video or face-to-face options (Shapka, Domene, Khan, & Yang, 2016).

Participants were asked a series of questions about their use of dating apps, reflections on choices around profile dating pictures and body image, reflections on contemporary dating practices, and their engagement in the sending of sexually explicit imagery. In this paper, we focus specifically on their use of dating apps and their production of profile imagery. Elsewhere we have focused on sexting and production of sexually explicit imagery (Waling, Kerr, Bourne, Power, & Kehler, 2020b). Audio-based interviews were professionally transcribed while IM messaging provides an instant transcript upon completion, and participants were offered the opportunity to review their transcripts, to which all declined. Interviews ranged between 45 minutes to an hour and a half. A $50 gift voucher was provided as remuneration for participant time.

Participants

15 cisgender, heterosexual men between the ages of 18 and 30 chose to take part in this exploratory research study.

Table 1 provides a breakdown of participant characteristics. Most identified as Anglo-Celtic Australian (n = 9). Half were between the age of 25 and 30, while the other half were between 18 and 25. The majority of the sample had a undergraduate university degree (n = 11), and had been using dating apps for more than a year (n = 11). All participants noted Tinder as the primary dating app they used currently or had used in the past two years from the point of data collection, followed by Bumble (n = 6). These are two common general dating apps used in Australia. In Australia, the use of dating apps is one of many ways in which individuals may seek out romantic companionship and sexual encounters. Others include meeting people through work, friends or family, through hobbies, or at events, including social events. Eight participants identified as being currently single, and most identified as seeking or preferring monogamous relationships (n = 13) rather than polyamorous (n = 2). Nearly half resided in urban areas of Victoria, the second most populous state of Australia (n = 7).

Analysis

Data analysis occurred in a series of steps using an IPA framework (Smith, 1996). Once transcripts were available, they were checked and verified by the lead author by listening back to the audio recordings and ensuring they matched the transcripts. They were then loaded into NVivo for coding organization. In the first phase the transcripts were read repeatedly, with notes made regarding what was being said. These notes were the basis for top-level descriptive codes to which the data were initially assigned using a codebook. Transcripts were then coded a second time by hand by exploring first-found coding in more depth and detail to explore the emergence of latent and salient themes. These were then clustered where appropriate to establish superordinate themes. All authors engaged in ongoing communication to discuss the findings.

Findings

Below we explore how cisgender, heterosexual men make sense of the process in which they take, or choose, photos for their dating app profile pictures. These include processes of 1) settings, selfies and 'doing' shots; 2) feelings of discomfort, and self-doubt in presenting the body, and 3) negotiating tensions of authenticity and vanity when seeking sexual, romantic, and/or emotional connections.

Table 1. Demographic characteristics (N = 15).

Demographic characteristic	*N*	%*
Age		
18–21	5	33%
22–25	3	20%
26–30	7	47%
Dating apps used*		
Tinder	15	100%
Bumble	6	40%
Hinge	3	20%
okCupid	3	20%
Feeld	2	13%
Blender	1	7%
Change	1	7%
Coffee meets Bagel	1	7%
Education Attained		
Secondary School	1	7%
TAFE Diploma	1	7%
Bachelor's Degree	11	73%
Master's Degree	1	7%
Doctor of Philosophy	1	7%
Ethnicity***		
Anglo-Celtic Australian	9	60%
North African and Middle Eastern	1	7%
North-East Asian	2	13%
South Eastern European	2	13%
Southern and Central Asian	1	7%
Length of time		
Less than a year	4	27%
1 year	3	20%
2 years	3	20%
3 years	2	13%
4+ years	3	20%
Relationship status****		
Single	8	53%
Partnered	5	33%
Casually dating	2	13%
Relationship style		
Monogamous	13	87%
Polyamorous	2	13%
Residential location*****		
Urban	14	93%
Regional	1	7%
State or Territory		
Australian Capital Territory	1	7%
New South Wales	2	13%
Queensland	5	33%
Victoria	7	47%

*Percentages have been rounded to the nearest whole number.
**As some participants used more than one dating app, percentages do not add up to 100%.
***Ethnicity is reported following the *Australian Standard Classification of Cultural and Ethnic Groups 1249.0* (2019), developed by the Australian Bureau of Statistics.
****Some participants identified as polyamorous, and thus may be in relationships while also using dating apps. Others had used the apps in the last two years (as per the study's eligibility criteria), but had stopped when entering an exclusive relationship.
*****Urban is defined by the Australian Bureau of Statistics as having a population of 100,000 or more people.

Settings, selfies and 'doing' shots

Awareness of the body as visual currency was evident in participant's narratives about the ways they evaluated, manipulated or adorned their bodies for photos. Participants were conscious of the way they wanted people to read their bodies and the visual cues (such as interests, hobbies, or lifestyle indicators) that would indicate authenticity. Participants attended to how they looked with a view to appearing authentic, which involved ensuring that they did not look like they had 'tried' with their photographs (Ward, 2017). Nevertheless, they were keenly aware of how their images could be read within the culture of internet dating. This was achieved through being strategic about what settings they located their images in, and ensuring that they had photographs that represented them as actively 'doing' something:

> Most of the photos that I have are incidental or like a friend's been taking it at the time, so there's very little preparation that goes into that. When I do, or when I did take photos, the preparation that would go into that would be setting up the thing, setting up myself like grooming whatnot, I don't know maybe wearing a nice shirt that's ironed or something like that. (Kirk, 24, casually dating)

> So it was a photo of me like out in that, and I'm all wet and soaked through and all that sort of stuff, but I'm just wearing decent clothes and it's a nice photo. And then the other ones are at like, as I've gone out to a concert and things like that and I'm just sort of dressed nice and presentable. (Nick, 25, single)

The tension for some participants was navigating what they saw as strategic placement, working to their strengths to show the best of themselves and the desire to be 'accepted as myself, rejected as myself, [rather] than accepted as some manipulated thingy' (Miguel, 26, single). Participants also noted the importance of active shots in which they are seen doing things. Such strategies often involved picking photos that demonstrated activity of some kind, such as playing a sport, or illustrating an interest in hobbies or other pursuits. This would then demonstrate aspects of their personalities beyond what they may look like to give a sense to a romantic prospect as to who they are as a person. For example, Jacob (29, single), notes he has a few images of him 'doing interesting things like hiking or things like that' and Miguel who explains that 'there was one [photo] where after winning a trivia night there's a photo of me holding the prize, you know, so I like the message of that one'. In these cases, Jacob chooses a photograph to illustrate an athletic aspect of his self, while Miguel chooses an image which illustrates an intellectual aspect of the self.

Active shots were a way to avoid the perceived narcissistic nature of selfies, which were seen about being invested in looks only rather than the whole person. Kirk, for example, describes bathroom selfies as distasteful:

> the worst thing for me is like a bathroom selfie . . . I want it to be tasteful because we're very visual in terms of how we use, or have the social media set up is very visual, most people would just see it for a few seconds and then swipe on, and that's all you really have to grab somebody.

While Kirk refers to the 'grab' in terms of grabbing the attention of others through an attention-grabbing image, in selfie culture this 'grab' is crucial to which steps follow be they pursuit or rejection. The impact of the selfie culture (Tiidenberg & Gómez Cruz, 2015) and the preparation or arguably lack of preparation according to some participants, is evident when Nick remarks on 'in the moment' selfies as opposed to other types of selfies he has taken. He remarks, 'I'm not good with any of, I'm not good with angles and all that sort of stuff, so a lot of the time when I do take a selfie I kind of just don't feel good about it afterwards'. Here, Nick reflects on an insecurity about taking time to do a selfie, recognizing the level of hidden skill necessary to achieve what he feels is an adequate photo, and the resulting feeling of disappointment afterwards. By this, the level of skill required to achieve something that appears 'effortless' and yet takes time, practice, and potentially additional resources such as professional cameras and lighting equipment.

Harry (20, single) was similar, arguing that selfies were 'just too "try hard", I don't know, I put so little effort into my photos'. He further remarks that he just uses photos 'that look nice, me when I'm out' and tries 'to show personality' in his photos. The men in our study are in fact seeking, and moreover provoking what Senft and Baym (2015) describe as 'court[ing] viewer interaction' (1594). Images are posted to invite a particular response, and there is a calculated risk in the process of taking posturing selfies and posting images on dating sites. Even before the image is posted online the participant registers his own sense of self and what the image may convey.

Discomfort and self-doubt

Gill et al. (2005) explain that 'the male (body) has become an object of the gaze rather than simply the bearer of the look' (39). Bodily surveillance and the ability to gaze upon their bodies as well as other men's bodies has implications (Norman, 2011; Wagner, 2016). Jack (26, casually dating) for example does not post torso images of himself because of how he evaluates his own body:

> I think it's – well first of all I don't think my torso is anything to write home about, so I don't think I'd put that on there for the reason that it's not like it's kind of get anyone all riled up and excited.

This was echoed by others:

> I don't think like my body is, like my best part, like my torso is my best part of my body, or something like that. So I don't think it's something I can show off. (Lyle, 20, partnered)

> I don't have the most athletic body either, or should I say I don't have like a body builder kind of body right now, so that's also maybe what is detracting from me doing such a thing. But also clothing the body you choose right, so like I can dress in clothes which I think represent me better than just my body. (Kirk)

The culture of online dating and the conscious decisions these men made about which images to post and what images expressed or conveyed was regularly and consistently connected to how they were able to gaze upon their own bodies. Both Gill et al. (2005) and Norman (2011) argue that 'representational forms' such as dating platforms have increased the discursive repertoire available to men. The historical shift away from cisgender, heterosexual men averting their eyes from looking upon the male body to a concerted and intentional gaze upon men's bodies is striking. Brody (30, single) explains

> I think perhaps maybe I'm a bit body conscious, I think, or it's probably a split between. Like, I think it's I see those [torso shots] and I think they're a bit stupid, and then also I think I'm probably body conscious [. . .] Like, I don't really mind being shirtless in front of someone, but I don't know if I want, like, a picture that's of me shirtless you know. Especially out of context, like it's like yeah okay it's a picture of me and my mates at the beach, but I guess I'm a bit conscious to having it so on display and so public . . . I'm not unfit but I wouldn't say that I look fit, so I'd say that you know it would kind of be like the reaction that I guess I would think that the reaction would be like, why is this guy showing off his dad bod or like, his average body? It's sort of like, you know, there's not really a reason to be shirtless, it's not really much to show off.

In this case, Brody anticipates the reaction he would get. He self-evaluates, imposing external expectations on his body. He decides his body is unworthy on the basis of what he understands about men's bodies and the calculated social exchange or benefit for showing his torso. While he admittedly thinks torso shots are a 'bit stupid', he also acknowledges his own level of body discomfort. Further, he highlights the need for context, that the torso image needs to be within a context of appropriate activity, such as attending the beach, rather than just a photo of the torso. Again, these men evaluated the dating environment and the utility of particular images as well as the meaning associated with posting certain kinds of images, dressed, undressed, and not posting others. His assessment of his body is related to fitness and the devaluing of bodies that are 'average' in a culture that heralds lean muscular bodies.

Dating apps and the visual landscape involved in posting images has provided a context in which men look upon their own bodies as well as the bodies of other men. The current climate and online dating culture has provided a mirror and a legitimate context for cisgender, heterosexual men to speak to and about their bodies. These men remarked, for example, that

> when I look at myself in the mirror and I don't see someone who's very attractive, and I've got a bit of a belly and I'm not necessarily the most skinniest person in ways, … when I kind of strip back to just looking at myself say in the mirror and it's just skin, I don't feel very comfortable, I don't feel like – yeah I feel like sometimes like I disgust myself with how I look … they're going to judge me on is my appearance and I'm not tall and big and manly. (Nick)

When further asked to describe what he saw as the expectations or 'look' that prevailed for men, he explained,

> When a female thinks of a guy and what's attractive [. . .] being broad shouldered [. . .] having a bit of muscle that sort of athletic sort of build [. . .] it's really hard to sort of, I guess, compete with that sort of look. (Nick)

The individual experience of the living body and the managing of that body is directly related to how these men read their bodies in the context of dating apps and social media platforms where their bodies, in whichever manner they choose, are on display for public consumption and evaluation. There was a recurring theme suggesting the bodies of these men were not an asset but rather a potential deficiency.

Vanity and authenticity

The participants were aware of competing discourses of authenticity and desirability as they increasingly engaged with reflections on, and of, their bodies. In this case Miguel explains

> I know it's me that got the 50 matches, you know, but if you do these like manipulated photos like on Photoshop got the 50 matches you know because it's not really you.

He makes a distinction arguing for the 'real you' as opposed to 'manipulated photos'. Jacob was similar, arguing that 'there's a difference between choosing photos of yourself that are flattering with makeup on or nice clothes or whatever versus explicitly staging something that's intended to mislead'. In another conversation Kirk explains that 'I'm not totally photogenic and I definitely get the comments that I'm a lot better looking in real life, when I meet up with someone'. The contradiction between portrayals of the self-captured in photographic images and posted on dating websites is later realized when the young man hears that he is 'better looking in real life'. This is echoed by Jack

> My phone has a lovely thing called a beauty filter on it, which sort of takes, smooths my skin out and like takes a little bit of the blemishes and the redness out of my face and stuff like that. But I try and not to overly use that, so I try and keep it as close to me as possible.

Jack highlights the use of 'filters' to present a nicer version of himself, but highlights that he is concerned about overuse, and that it does not accurately reflect his image. There is a clear evaluative tone to how these men make sense of and 'see' their bodies in the process of posing for photographs and using these images. There is an unmistakable desire to be seen in particular ways and contexts, while maintaining a degree of 'authenticity' in how this is achieved.

The men in our study spent a considerable amount of time thinking about their bodies and gaining understanding about their own bodies in relation to other bodies, particularly the placement and location of other men's bodies, and the participants recognized that images of muscularity and torso shots may send the 'wrong' message. Jack provides further argument and insight into how he understands the posting of particular images and importantly the posting of torso images by other men:

> the photos that you choose to put up kind of say something about who you are and what you're into and what groups you belong to, and putting a selfie up or a torso shot I think kind of signals that I'd be the type of person who'd be – I don't think vain is the right word, but maybe like kind of into that kind of selfie Instagram culture, it's like really conventional, it's really like mainstream – yeah, kind of boring as well I think in my experience, it signals that you're a kind of boring person, and there's nothing else going on in your life apart from your appreciation of yourself.

Jack dismisses both selfie shots and torso images. He is unequivocal in linking the selfie culture to Instagram culture to mainstream, conventional practices of posting. His attention to the choice of pictures as a process imbued with meanings is captured when he suggests that it ultimately 'signals that you're a kind of boring person and there's nothing else going on in your life apart from the appreciation of yourself'.

Kirk also remarks on his disdain for posting images of his body, arguing that 'there's no personality that goes into that [...] there's nothing that makes you stand out'. He instead favoured more social settings so that he would 'appear as fun/friendly/sociable, and to avoid appearing as self-absorbed/gym junkie type'. The men repeatedly expressed similar arguments for not posting torso shots regarding concerns about how that may be perceived. Marshall (30, partnered) for example comments that

> part of it is that isn't the kind of image I'm trying to cultivate, and I look fine but not exceptional with my shirt off.

His purpose and intent are to 'cultivate' a 'kind of image'. At the same time Marshall assesses his own naked body as 'fine but not exceptional'. He later remarks that these types of torso shots would make him appear like a 'meathead' and moreover, he comments that 'it seems like posturing' and he was 'staying away from stereotypes'. Marshall understood the tensions in a culture of online imagery and a visual culture that was underscored by prevailing notions of chiselled, sculpted bodies. In his words 'I don't have any respect for it' and so he refused to participate in 'any form of macho nonsense'. Participants were strategic and indeed thoughtfully engaged in considering how their images as representations of them will be read and interpreted.

Discussion & conclusion

The findings from this study provide new insights into the ways in which the use of dating apps, and construction of profile pictures for these apps, require cisgender, heterosexual men to navigate complex and often contradictory expectations of masculinity, beauty and authenticity. There is a recurring and powerful tension evident among the participants in how they position, manoeuvre, and configure their bodies while being openly anxious about how their bodies were read by the recipient. The choosing of certain kinds of photographs to evoke certain meanings are based on preconceptions about how their image may be read and interpreted, and not based in any actual reality. Prevailing understandings about bodies as emblematic of forms of masculinity were routinely woven into conversations where the participants linked a 'lack in their bodies' or an inadequacy such as an absence of muscularity, to a greater valuing of personality and an outright dismissal of bodies as inadequate, while more authentic, truer selves can be expressed through pictures that convey personality, not appearance *per se*.

There is a contradiction here in relation to the body being the thing that demonstrates one's 'best self' (Hakim, 2020; Oakes et al., 2020) and yet at the same time, it is also seen as vain and narcissistic. These men are caught in a kind of double bind or dualism (Norman, 2011), the body is meant to represent their best self, and this is tied up in complexities around muscular/fit/'healthy' bodies being just that, yet at the same time, they are mindful, aware and uneasy that such notions ascribe to concerns of vanity and narcissism. This is in line with Haywood's (2018) study and other studies on queer men (Chan, 2018; Hakim, 2020; Oakes et al., 2020), where participants were conscious of the meanings and potential interpretations of the images used. We argue that for the men in this study, there was an active and conscious need to navigate between what they perceived as their 'authentic' self, and an underlying apprehension that their 'authentic' image would not be appealing enough in the dating market (Chan, 2018; Hakim, 2018, 2020; Oakes et al., 2020). As dating platforms ask people to effectively rate themselves through the imagined eyes of others (Krüger & Spilde, 2020), these men are conflicted about managing a 'real' self despite their awareness that the stereotypical 'hot guy' is not necessarily effective. There is a very conscious curating of imagery, but there was a resignation as to the limits of this.

Online dating is a distinct cultural practice – within this culture there is a set of normative expectations (Duguay, 2017; Ellison et al., 2012; Sedgewick et al., 2017) in which people's attractiveness and acceptability as a potential sexual or romantic partner is assessed (Duguay, 2017; Krüger & Spilde, 2020). This research contributes a more in-depth understanding regarding how cisgender, heterosexual men choose and display dating profile pictures and pays attention to concerns about body image and vulnerability, as well as how men navigate between desires to be authentic while also being marketable and desired (Chan, 2018; Hakim, 2018, 2020; Oakes et al., 2020). This does not rest on the assumption that men solely reproduce images to curate an ideal of masculinity (Haywood, 2020; Waling, 2019a, 2019b) as others have suggested (Hess & Flores, 2018). Profile images are not assessed simply on the basis of the physical appearance of the person, but on the cultural cues (Hakim, 2018, 2020) within the image. Cisgender, heterosexual men are expected to present an authentic masculine self in their images (Haywood, 2018), even though displaying traditional markers of masculinity in a profile picture (such as showing a muscly body or a naked torse) is often considered inauthentic, vain or crass. Men then continually assess and evaluate how their image will be read as both masculine and appropriate in a world where such images are increasingly under scrutiny and criticized (Waling, 2019b; Waling et al., 2020a). They also continually evaluate their own sense of 'authenticity' within the context of the complex cultural expectations of the online dating environment, and use strategies to mitigate this by selecting images that can speak to aspects of their personality.

As Duguay (2017) and others have noted, the profile picture is a particular piece of architecture. It is one image set within a platform whereby someone is encouraged to make an immediate judgment. To come back to Goffman (1959), the performance of the self (the front stage) on the profile image is static and the interaction between performer and audience is one step removed, in which it is the image that precedes reality. While human interaction is core to online social spaces, technology is a significant part of that interaction and shapes, creates and modifies the interaction (Duguay, 2017). Yet, as Duguay (2017) notes, dating technology is not necessarily equivalent with human interaction or experience, which includes human processes of emotion, insecurity and desire around wanting to be 'good enough' when engaging with dating apps. In the process of creating profiles and developing social relationships through dating apps these men develop a sense of self based on knowledge they have about what ideal male bodies should look like, and yet, simultaneously, note that such ideals can lead to misinterpretations as to who they are *as people*.

Disclosure statement

No potential conflict of interest was reported by the author(s).

Funding

This project was funded by a Research Focus Area: Building Healthy Communities grant from La Trobe University, Bundoora, Australia.

ORCID

Andrea Waling http://orcid.org/0000-0003-1370-5600
Michael Kehlher http://orcid.org/0000-0003-1637-7040
Jennifer Power http://orcid.org/0000-0002-6566-3214
Lucille Kerr http://orcid.org/0000-0002-6171-3106
Adam Bourne http://orcid.org/0000-0001-5299-8835

Data accessibility/data availability statement

Due to the nature of this research, participants of this study did not agree for their data to be shared publicly, so supporting data is not available.

Ethics approval

This research was conducted with the La Trobe University Human Research Ethics Committee (HEC18477) approval as it involves human participants.

Consent to participate

Participants provided informed written consent to participate in this study.

Consent for publication

Participants provided informed written consent to allow their deidentified data to appear in publications.

References

Albury, K., McCosker, A., & Evers, C. (2021). Men seeking women: Awkwardness, shame, and other affective encounters with dating apps. *First Monday, 26*(4). doi:10.5210/fm.v26i4.11637

Albury, K. (2015). Selfies, sexts, and sneaky hats: Young people's understandings of gendered practices of self-representation. *International Journal of Communication, 9*(1), 1734–1745.

Barrett, E. L. R. (2020). Sexing the margins: Homonationalism in gay dating apps. In D. Farris, D. Compton, & A. Herrera (Eds.), *Gender, sexuality and race in the digital age* (pp. 115–136). Cham, CH: Springer.

Berkowitz, D., Tinkler, J., Peck, A., & Coto, L. (2021). Tinder: A game with gendered rules and consequences. *Social Currents, 8*(5), 491–509.

Bonner-Thompson, C. (2017). 'The meat market': Production and regulation of masculinities on the Grindr grid in Newcastle-upon-Tyne, UK. *Gender, Place & Culture*, 24(11), 1611–1625. https://doi.org/10.1080/0966369X.2017.1356270

Bordo, S. (1999). *The male body: A new look at men in public and in private*. New York, NY: Farrar, Straus and Giroux.

Burns, J., & Kehler, M. (2014). Boys, bodies and negotiated school spaces: When boys fail the litmus test. *Culture, Society and Masculinities, 6*(1), 3–18.

Chan, L. S. (2018). Ambivalence in networked intimacy: Observations from gay men using mobile dating apps. *New Media & Society, 20*(7), 2566–2581.

Connell, R. W. (1995). *Masculinities*. Berkeley, CA: University of California Press.

Connell, R. W. (2001). *The men and the boys*. Berkeley, CA: University of California Press.

Drummond, M., & Drummond, C. (2015). It's all about the six-pack: Boys' bodies in contemporary Western culture. *Journal of Child Health Care, 19*(4), 423–431.

Drummond, M. (2020). *Boys bodies: Sport health and physical activity*. London, UK: Palgrave MacMillan.

Duguay, S., Burgess, J., & Suzor, N. (2018). Queer women's experiences of patchwork platform governance on Tinder, Instagram, and Vine. *Convergence, 26*(2), 237–252.

Duguay, S. (2016). "He has a way gayer Facebook than I do": Investigating sexual identity disclosure and context collapse on a social networking site. *New Media & Society, 18*(6), 891–907.

Duguay, S. (2017). Dressing up Tinderella: Interrogating authenticity claims on the mobile dating app Tinder. *Information, Communication & Society, 20*(3), 351–367.

Ellison, N. B., Hancock, J. T., & Toma, C. L. (2012). Profile as promise: A framework for conceptualising veracity in online dating self-presentations. *New Media & Society, 14*(1), 45–62.

Frederick, D. A., & Haselton, M. G. (2007). Why is muscularity sexy? Tests of the fitness indicator hypothesis. *Personality & Social Psychology Bulletin, 33*(8), 1167–1183.

Gaden, G., & Dumitricia, D. (2015). The 'real deal': Strategic authenticity, politics and social media First Monday. Retrieved November 22, 2021, from http://firstmonday.org/ojs/index.php/fm/article/view/4985/4197

Gibbs, J. L., Ellison, N. B., & Lai, C.-H. (2010). First comes love, then comes google: An investigation of uncertainty reduction strategies and self-disclosure in online dating. *Communication Research, 38*(1), 70–100.

Giddens, A. (1991). *Modernity and self-identity: Self and society in the late modern age*. Cambridge, UK: Polity Press.

Gill, R., Henwood, K., & McLean, C. (2005). Body projects and the regulation of normative masculinity. *Body & Society, 11* (1), 37–62.

Goffman, E. (1959). *The presentation of self in everyday life*. Garden City, AT: Doubleday.

Hakim, J. (2018). The spornosexual': The affective contradictions of male body-work in neoliberal digital culture. *Journal of Gender Studies, 27*(2), 231–241.

Hakim, J. (2020). *Work that body: Male bodies in digital culture*. London, UK: Rowman & Littlefield.

Hancock, J. T., & Toma, C. L. (2009). Putting your best face forward: The accuracy of online dating photographs. *Journal of Communication, 59*(2), 367–386.

Haywood, C. (2018). *Men, masculinity and contemporary dating*. London, UK: Palgrave.

Haywood, C. (2020). Looking at men and masculinity: Popular discourse, cultural narratives and the limits of gender. In A. Pardo (Ed.), *Masculinities: Liberation through photography*. 19–25. Munich, GE: Prestel.

Hess, A., & Flores, C. (2018). Simply more than swiping left: A critical analysis of toxic masculine performances on Tinder nightmares. *New Media & Society, 20*(3), 1085–1102.

Hogan, B. (2010). The presentation of self in the age of social media: Distinguishing performances and exhibitions online. *Bulletin of Science, Technology & Society, 30*(6), 377–386.

Holmes, M. (2010). The emotionalisation of reflexivity. *Sociology, 44*(1), 139–154.

Kehler, M., & Atkinson, M. (2010). *Boys' bodies: Speaking the unspoken*. New York, NY: Peter Lang.

Krüger, S., & Spilde, A. C. (2020). Judging books by their covers – Tinder interface, usage and sociocultural implications. *Information, Communication & Society, 23*(10), 1395–1410.

Levers, M.J.D. (2013). *Philosophical paradigms, grounded theory, and perspectives on emergence*. Thousand Oaks, CA: SAGE Open. doi:10.1177/2158244013517243

Li, H., & Chen, X. (2021). From "Oh, you're Chinese ... " to "No bats, thx!": Racialised experiences of Australian-based Chinese queer women in the mobile dating context. *Social Media + Society, 7*(3), 205630512110353.

Malta, S. (2012). Using online methods to interview older adults about their romantic and sexual relationships. In M. Leontowitsch (Ed.), *Researching later life and ageing expanding qualitative research horizons*. 146–172. London, UK: Palgrave Macmillan.

Miller, B. (2018). Textually presenting masculinity and the body on mobile dating apps for men who have sex with men. *The Journal of Men's Studies, 26*(3), 305–326.

Morse, J. M., & Field, P. A. (1996). *Nursing research: The application of qualitative approaches*. Boston, MA: Springer.

Norman, M. E. (2011). Embodying the double-bind of masculinity: Young men and discourses of normalcy, health, heterosexuality, and individualism. *Men and Masculinities, 14*(4), 430–449.

Oakes, H., Johnson, C. J., & Parry, D. C. (2020). "Making myself more desirable": Digital self-(re)presentation on geo-social networking apps for men seeking men Parry, D.C., & Johnson, C.W. (Eds.), In *Sex and Leisure: Promiscuous Perspectives* (pp. 1–18). London, UK: Routledge.

Pearce, G., Thøgersen-Ntoumani, C., & Duda, J. L. (2019). Synchronous text-based instant messaging: Online interviewing tool. In P. Liamputtong (Ed.), *Handbook of research methods in health social sciences* (pp. 1369–1383). Singapore, SI: Springer.

Pym, T., Byron, P., & Albury, K. (2021). 'I still want to know they're not terrible people': Negotiating 'queer community' on dating apps. *International Journal of Cultural Studies, 24*(3), 398–413.

Rodriguez, N. S., Huemmer, J., & Blumell, L. E. (2016). Mobile masculinities: An investigation of networked masculinities in gay dating apps. *Masculinities & Social Change, 5*(3), 241–267.

Sedgewick, J. R., Flath, M. E., & Elias, L. J. (2017). Presenting your best self(ie): The influence of gender on vertical orientation of selfies on tinder. *Frontiers in Psychology, 8*. doi:10.3389/fpsyg.2017.00604

Senft, T., & Baym, N. (2015). What does the selfie say? Investigating a global phenomenon. *International Journal of Communication, 9*, 1588–1606.

Shapka, J. D., Domene, J. F., Khan, S., & Yang, L. M. (2016). Online versus in-person interviews with adolescents: An exploration of data equivalence. *Computers in Human Behavior, 58*, 361–367.

Shield, A. D. (2019). *Immigrants on Grindr*. London, UK: Palgrave Macmillan.

Smith, J. A. (1996). Beyond the divide between cognition and discourse: Using interpretative phenomenological analysis in health psychology. *Psychology & Health, 11*(2), 261–271.

Strano, M. M. (2008). User descriptions and interpretations of self-presentation through facebook profile images. *Cyberpsychology: Journal of Psychosocial Research on Cyberspace, 2*(2), article 1.

Strubel, J., & Petrie, T. A. (2017). Love me Tinder: Body image and psychosocial functioning among men and women. *Body Image, 21*, 34–38.

Swenson, A. R., & Allen, K. R. (2019). My shape: Young men's perceptions of their relationship to their bodies. *Psychology of Men & Masculinities, 20*(4), 585–593.

Tanner, C., Maher, J., & Fraser, S. (2013). *Vanity: 21st century selves*. London, UK: Palgrave MacMillian.

Tiidenberg, K., & Gómez Cruz, E. (2015). Selfies, image and the re-making of the body. *Body & Society, 21*(4), 77–102.

Timmermans, E., & Courtois, C. (2018). From swiping to casual sex and/or committed relationships: Exploring the experiences of Tinder users. *The Information Society, 34*(2), 59–70.

Vannini, P., & Williams, J. P. (2009). *Authenticity in culture, self, and society*. Farnham, UK: Ashgate Publishing.

Vilnai-Yavetz, I., & Tifferet, S. (2015). A picture is worth a thousand words: Segmenting consumers by Facebook profile images. *Journal of Interactive Marketing, 32*, 53–69.

Wagner, P. E. (2016). Picture perfect bodies: Visualising hegemonic masculinities produced for/by male fitness spaces. *International Journal of Men's Health, 15*(3), 235–258.

Waling, A., Duncan, D., Angelides, S., & Dowsett, G. (2020a). 'Damn, Channing Tatum can move!': Women's accounts of men's bodies and objectification in post-feminist times. *Sexualities*, 136346072096765. doi:10.1177/1363460720967657

Waling, A., Kerr, L., Bourne, A., Power, J., & Kehler, M. (2020b). 'It's nice to be appreciated': Understanding heterosexual men's engagements with sexting and sharing Dick Pics. *Sexualities*, 136346072094729. doi:10.1177/1363460720947297

Waling, A. (2019a). Rethinking masculinity studies: Feminism, masculinity, and poststructural accounts of agency and emotional reflexivity. *Journal of Men's Studies, 20*(1), 89–107.

Waling, A. (2019b). Problematising 'toxic' and 'healthy'masculinity for addressing gender inequalities. *Australian Feminist Studies, 34*(101), 362–375.

Waling, A. (2020). *White masculinity in contemporary Australia: The Good Ol' Aussie Bloke*. Abingdon, UK: Routledge Press.

Ward, J. (2017). What are you doing on Tinder? Impression management on a matchmaking mobile app. *Information, Communication & Society, 20*(11), 1644–1659.

Willig, C. (2013). *Introducing qualitative research in psychology* (3rd ed.). New York, NY: McGraw-Hill Education.

Yardley, L. (2000). Dilemmas in qualitative health research. *Psychology & Health, 15*(2), 215–228.

Building community, one swipe at a time: hook-up apps and the production of intimate publics between women

Jonathan Petrychyn, Diana C. Parry and Corey W. Johnson

ABSTRACT

Hook-up apps are an increasingly popular way for women to meet other people for sex, dating, relationships, and more. As a mundane and habitual form of media, the multiple uses of hook-up apps allow for the production of intimacy in surprising and complex ways. This paper draws on narrative interviews with 15 self-identifying women to explore how dating and hook-up apps help produce 'intimate publics' for women. The field of intimate publics available to women users of hook-up apps is broader than those afforded by in-app interactions; there is an entire network of intimacy, sociality, and publicity that forms around hook-up apps. Our findings show that while both queer and straight women use hook-up apps to find sex, hook-ups, dates, and relationships, they are also central to building community, friendship, and sociality between women.

Dating and hook-up apps have exploded in popularity over the last decade and have become a key feature of public and intimate life. While the use of mobile technologies to facilitate intimate connections appears novel, dating apps are part of a long history of communications technologies mediating dating reaching back at least to the first publication of 'Lonely Hearts' advertisements in British newspapers in 1695 (Duguay, Burgess, & Light, 2017). Though the various forms of mediated dating that followed Lonely Hearts ads flirted with shame, stigma, and moral panics, especially following the internet revolution of the 1990s, today hook-up apps have made online dating an increasingly popular and now the most accepted way to meet new people for dates, chat, sex, friendship, and more. With this growing popularity comes a growing diversity of apps and experiences using these apps, especially as affected by one's gender, sexuality, race, social class, and generation. Also with growing popularity comes growing skepticism and unease with their utility. Do these apps actually facilitate lasting intimate connections? Or are they symptomatic of a larger culture of individualism and isolation exacerbated by new digital technologies? Do these apps help or harm our emotional, mental, and physical health?

We agree with Duguay et al. (2017) and think moral concerns about hook-up apps – and technology and intimacy generally – are largely overblown. While users have legitimate concerns about how dating apps affect their health, safety and well-being, our research suggests that they are adept at mitigating and negotiating these risks to seek out and develop the sorts of intimacy they desire. Indeed, we argue that it is this very negotiation of potential risks that is characteristic of the production of what we term 'intimate publics.' Over the past decade, hook-up apps have become a crucial mediator and catalyst for both queer and straight women to create intimate publics.[1] As Albury and Byron (2016) have shown, hook-up apps 'perform multiple functions for young same-sex attracted men and women: promoting a sense of belonging [...], facilitating intimacy and friendship, and serving as a password-protected 'container' for sexual experimentation, picture exchange, and chat' (pp. 1-2). This article builds on this work and seeks to understand how both straight and queer women negotiate the multiple functions hook-up apps offer, and how this supports the creation of intimate publics.

This paper is part of a larger study on the experiences and habits of hook-up app users across the spectrum of gender and sexuality, and draws specifically on our interviews with 15 queer and straight women. While sex, dating, and hooking up are important reasons many women use dating apps, the queer women we talked to indicated the importance of these apps in building community and friendships, while the straight women we spoke to valued using hook-up apps with their friends as a shared social activity. We argue that access to, and production of, these intimate publics is an important feature of these women's enjoyment and well-being during their leisure time, and has important ramifications for women's health.

Background

Apps, as habitual and mundane bundles of code have become central nodes through which to consider questions of digital intimacies and networked publics (Chun, 2016; Morris & Murray, 2018). The habitual mundanity of apps in general is what has allowed dating apps in particular to become such a common and popular way to meet people for sex, relationship, friendships, and more. When apps become habitual, they become intimate. This habitual intimacy is what allows for the creation of publics, communities, and networks to be built around these apps. Hook-up apps operate at the nexus of digital intimacy and networked publics.

Digital intimacies

Access to the multiple forms of intimacy hook-up apps produce is an on-going scholarly concern. Studies of hook-up apps often take up the question of intimacy in one of two ways. The first way is through the framework of 'intimate data' (Weltevrede & Jansen, 2019). This literature discusses the policies and infrastructures that regulate and scaffold the data and information collected and distributed by these apps. Intimate data does not necessarily refer to the specific content of messages exchanged between users, but the paratextual and contextual information that structures these interactions. This includes data gathered from the mobile device itself, like location, but also information gathered from user input, like gender, age, sexual identity, email address, and so on. Much of the literature is concerned with how apps and platforms manage this data and protect user information (Albury, Burgess, Light, Race, & Wilken, 2017; David & Cambre, 2016). This is not only a growing concern of scholars and data security experts, but of users as well: Lutz and Ranzini (2017) note that in their study of privacy concerns on Tinder, many of their participants were more concerned about how hook-up apps sell and manage their intimate data than other users sharing intimate photos or conversations without their consent.

The second way intimacy is taken up in the hook-up app literature is through a discussion of user intimacy, sex, and eroticism. This body of work tends to focus largely on gay men's experiences on apps (Tziallas, 2015), and the complex and varied intimacies between men who have sex with men (MSM). Ahlm (2017) argues that despite Grindr's potential to reinvigorate public sex and public intimacies between men, users tend to negotiate their sexual practices, desires and stigmas in ways that reproduce neoliberal logics of privatisation. Building on this, Møller and Petersen (2018) focus on gay men's non-monogamous intimacies and the ways non-monogamous couples set up rules and boundaries around app use so it does not disrupt their sense of home. Møller and Petersen draw on the work of Berlant (1998) and Jamieson (2011) to articulate intimacy as 'the practices and work done to produce affective domains that *constitute* the private and the sense of home,' (Møller & Petersen, 2018, p. 212) situating the forms of intimacy produced by hook-up apps within the private sphere.

When the impact of hook-up app-produced intimacies on the public is considered, it is often from a public health and epidemiological perspective. Much of the health-focused literature focuses on questions of public sexual health and risk, and largely with MSM populations (Landovitz et al., 2013; Macapagal et al., 2018). Indeed, Hobbs, Owen, and Gerber (2017) note that this perspective dominates the hook-up app literature, though growing interest in hook-up apps within communication and cultural studies is shifting this balance. Health research on hook-up apps has not yet moved past an epidemiological approach that focuses on sexual health the role of hook-up apps in both contributing to transmission and helping researchers track outbreaks of HIV/STIs (Lupton, 2014). There is a nascent literature on hook-up apps and intimacy that implies a health and well-being perspective, but it largely sees hook-up apps as posing barriers to intimacy that users must overcome (David & Cambre, 2016). There is a need for health perspectives on these apps that thinks through how hook-up apps can contribute to general health and well-being beyond epidemiology, and that do not take technology as an *a priori* barrier.

Networked publics

In this way, theories of networked publics can provide a useful framework to decentre negative perspectives of technology (Ito, 2008). A networked public is an 'imagined collective that emerges as a result of the intersection of people, technology, and practice' (boyd, 2010, p. 39). Like their non-networked counterparts, these collectives are sites where public, private, and corporate interests are negotiated (van Dijck, 2012) and depend on a broader sense of community beyond cohabiting together in physical space (Dean, 2010). However, for Papacharissi (2016), what significantly differentiates networked publics are their affective registers: 'networked, affective publics present a departure from the rationally based deliberative protocols of public spheres, and help us reimagine how we may define and understand civic discourse among networked crowds in a digital era' (p. 320). Affective networked publics centre the emotional capacities of publics and how they use digital technologies to make political change.

Papacharissi's (2016) theory centres the civic and political features of affective publics, their broader effects on the functioning of democracy, and 'how we might interpret the civic materiality and gravitas of affective publics' (p. 312). We argue that Papacharissi's theory applies unevenly to the kinds of networked publics formed on dating apps. While the publics formed on dating apps are indeed affective publics, the scale of their civic, democratic, and political gravitas is more intimate than those on Twitter. By shifting our focus from Twitter to Tinder, we want to look at how we might interpret the *intimate* materiality of affective publics. How does this shift toward more intimate affective registers change our understanding of how networked publics are formed?

Intimate publics

As new media technologies that straddle the boundary between public and private, hook-up apps underscore that intimacy *is* a public matter. Plummer (2003) suggests that 'our most intimate decisions are shaped by (and in turn shape) our most public institutions' (p. x). We build on Plummer's (2003) notion of intimate citizenship as well as Berlant's (1997) theory of an intimate public sphere to articulate the mediated intimacies afforded by hook-up apps as productive of intimate publics. Since the 1960s, the division between the public and private has collapsed, and feminist and gay and lesbian liberation movements moved concerns about sex, sexuality, and intimacy forcefully into the public sphere. In the wake of this growing publicity of sex, and the subsequent backlash from conservative forces in the 1980s, Berlant theorised the intimate public sphere as that space where heteronormative intimacies regulate who is permitted to be in public. Berlant argues that the public sphere has shifted away from the Habermasian ideal of a truly democratic space of civic life, to a space where politics, citizenship, and belonging become privatised and individuated.

While Berlant's work is lobbed as a critique against the increasing individualisation and privatisation of public space by neoliberal politics and discourse, it points toward a broader struggle over the role of intimate affairs within public life. This is not only a struggle over the types of sex and sexuality permitted in public (Berlant & Warner, 1998), but the forms of belonging, community, and sociality afforded. As these theories of intimate public sphere and intimate citizenship suggest, there is so much more to our intimate relationships than the simple feeling of closeness (Jamieson, 2011). Intimacy is public, and embeds us, our bodies, and our technologies within public life.

Intimacy allows us to build and be a part of community, a key factor in health and well-being. Building on work on women's health and leisure, we conceptualise health broadly as 'the ability to live life fully' (Parry & Light, 2014, p. 53). Parry, Glover, and Mulcahy (2013) have shown that there can be significant benefits to women who use technology to connect over the basis of shared identity and sexuality. However, Parry and Light (2014) also note that there is

> difficulty in addressing whether technologies are emancipatory or constraining in light of a number of other factors such as, which women are using technology (considering race, ethnicity, class, age, sexual identity, socioeconomic status, etc.) as well as which technologies are being used and in what ways. (p. 43)

Access to new media technologies like hook-up apps is not homogenous and is affected by women's 'history of and current access to social, cultural, and economic capital' (Baum, Newman, & Biedrzycki, 2014, p. 358). Whatever effects hook-up apps have on our intimacies, these effects are unevenly distributed and are affected by who has access to these technologies, for how long, and in what spaces.

Methodology

This paper is part of a larger project in which 45 hook-up app users across varying gender and sexual identities were interviewed about their hook-up app use with the aim of understanding how hook-up apps influence users' identities, relationships, and quality of life. Guided by the framework of appnography (Cousineau, Oakes, & Johnson, 2018), we used narrative interviewing because of its potential to position participants' gendered subjectivities, illuminate examples of agency and cultural contestation, reveal human transformation and promote advocacy through connection with the participants and the readers of the research (Costa & Matzner, 2007). We took an experience-centred approach to interviewing, as it 'assumes that narratives: are sequential and meaningful; are definitely human; "re-present" experience, reconstituting it, as well as expressing it; [and] display transformation and change' (Squire, 2008, p. 42). This approach provides the discursive space 'to demonstrate that local contexts and wider, societal contexts are inextricably linked' (Phoenix, 2008, pp. 65–66).

With ethics approval, the research team used purposive sampling to recruit participants directly through various hook-up apps. Our team members modified their profile descriptions on their personal accounts to stipulate they were seeking to recruit participants. Participants were selectively chosen to achieve diversity across gender (e.g. man, woman, trans, nonbinary) and sexual identity (e.g. lesbian, gay, bisexual, queer, straight). Given that eight team members were conducting interviews, we constructed an interview guide to ensure the interviews would generate rich and consistent data to help us most effectively address our research questions. To promote feelings of mutual trust and safety, as well as to pursue potential leads in conversation that require insider knowledge, interviewers and participants were matched according to gender and sexual identity as closely as possible, a unique methodological decision with implications to be further discussed in Johnson, Petrychyn, and Parry (2020).

For the purposes of this paper, we isolated data from 15 interviews to focus on those self-identifying as women. Ten of these women identified as queer, and five identified as straight. As such, these findings are not representative of all hook-up app users, but offer a selection of the varied and rich perspectives on dating app use. All 15 participants were current or previous users of Tinder, Bumble, OkCupid or Her, among other less popular and widespread apps. Data were analysed via inductive, thematic analysis in the following sequence: (1) immersion in the data; (2) line-by-line coding; (3) integrating codes into broader themes; (4) refining and concretely defining themes and supplementing with extracted quotations. Although a variety of themes of interest were identified, we focus in this paper on findings that suggest ways intimacy is made public. We focus on habitual uses of hook-up apps; risk, privacy and safety; self-esteem and confidence; digital versus physical intimacy; sex and intimacy; social and public uses of hook-up apps; and friendship and community.

Findings

Habitual uses of hook-up apps

Many interviewees expressed that their daily use of hook-up apps was habitual. When media becomes habitual, it becomes a routine and it becomes intimate. The mundane and habitual process of opening up Tinder or Bumble and swiping left and right helps embed the intimate relations produced by dating apps within our users everyday lives. As Megan explains:

> When I was using them constantly, it was constant. It'd be in class in university, and messaging, or I would wake up in the morning and I would message. Even if you're out at the bar, when you go to the washroom, I'd pull it out just to see.

While all of the interviewees who spoke of their habitual app use spoke of their attempts to manage their time on the app, which often meant turning push notifications off or deleting the apps from their phone for a period of time, some time management strategies were not always in the service of a larger goal to find a better digital-physical life balance. Marnie spoke of her tendency to 'swipe until there's nobody left,' at which point she would not open the app up for a few days, but that was only to 'repopulate' possible matches for her to continue to swipe on.

Risk, privacy, and safety

Many participants discussed questions of risk, and often framed this in terms of their own personal safety and well-being, as opposed to through epidemiological concerns about the transmission of STIs and HIV. This supports Albury and Byron's (2016) findings about the negotiation of risk for queer hook-up app users, and also provides further evidence that straight hook-up app users understand risk in similar terms. Many participants would ask their potential dates enough personal questions to find them online and verify their identities via other social networks. Michelle, one of our straight participants, said:

> I would always tell someone, at least a friend or my mom or something, where I was going just in case. So I'm going on a date with this guy, we're going to this restaurant, just because. But I would do background research myself, try and find them on social media or look them up on Google or LinkedIn or something, just to corroborate what they were saying.

They would also meet their date in public and tell a friend or family member where they were going and who they were meeting as a further layer of security, establishing an intimate network of support around them.

Discussions of risk and safety were obviously gendered, with women taking more precautions meeting men than when they would meet women. However, this is more a question of degree than it is completely binary, as this exchange between a member of our research team and Sonia demonstrates:

> Interviewer: Going back to what you mentioned earlier about sort of the nervousness about meeting men, like they might be scary or different risks that are involved, can you tell me about a time where you didn't sort of have to navigate that because you wanted to meet somebody?

> Sonia: Yeah. I don't know if I can think of any specific times but I usually try to sort of manage that by picking a specific time and place to meet and then I feel sort of safer about that where I'm going somewhere where I know and I have been there and I'm going to meet him there and I know where to get the bus to go home and that sort of thing, but some guys will be like we should go out, I'll come pick you up and we will just go somewhere and I don't really want to do that with a total stranger from the internet.
>
> Interviewer: So, how is it different when you want to meet women?
>
> Sonia: I still do the same sort of thing like I still probably wouldn't want to just get in a stranger's car immediately, but I guess I worry about it a little less. Maybe partially because I get more messages from guys who seem creepy whereas women I'm sure can also be creepy but in different ways like I don't get as many rude messages from them or anything.

Queer participants were also more likely to frame their discussion of risk as taking a chance. While many hook-up app users usually spend quite some time talking on the app before meeting in person, Sophia noted that she would prefer to meet someone for coffee relatively quickly. When her friends would caution her against it, she would respond 'What is stopping me from doing it? It's a public place. They're grabbing their own coffee, I'm grabbing mine. I'm just meeting somebody. And that's what I wanted to do, just meet people and I have nothing to lose.' Jasmine noted that online anonymity provided her the comfort and safety to take more risks and talk with people she might not normally approach in person: 'I feel safer, I think [...] because you have nothing to lose and you can also just disappear.' This articulation of risk as chance underscores the complex considerations for meeting other users of hook-up apps in public.

Self-esteem and confidence

When curating their profile, many participants noted that they would choose photos that were particularly flattering and where they felt good about themselves. This, in turn, would elicit more likes and swipes from other users that would help affirm their confidence and self-esteem. Marnie said, 'To get people liking you or whatever [...] it's like good for your self image'. This was not consistent across all participants, and Rachel instead noted that hook-up app use has had a negative effect on her self-esteem:

> And I think my self-esteem is going down. Because it's really physical. I look at my body differently, so I, in the pictures where I thought I looked really good, I'd put it on Bumble, and I'm like, 'Ooh, maybe I don't look so good in that.' Or, 'I'm not as hot as this girl. So they're probably not going to like me.' And I find myself questioning a lot of things. Where I was super confident before, and I still think I'm confident, but I question a lot of things that I do now, or post. And I was never like that.

For Rachel, her lowered self-esteem is perhaps more a result of her own perception of herself than others; it was not the fact that people were rejecting her or not responding to her that lowered her self-esteem, but the act of constantly judging and curating your own profile that became the source of her lowered self-esteem. Indeed, in Michelle's experience, not getting a response from someone else on a hook-up app can have both positive and negative effects on self-confidence. She said,

> I think I'm more self-assured now and ... I said that, even on Bumble, a lot of people just didn't respond. If anything it was a hit to the confidence. But even that is kind of empowering, it's kind of like, 'All right, reject me, I don't care.'

For many of our participants, the relationships between their interactions with other users and the effects of their self-esteem can be ambiguous. Depending on the context, an interaction could be both positive and negative or neither. This suggests that not only do hook-up apps have more complex effects on our health and well-being, but that users are also aware of these complex and sometimes contradictory effects.

Distinction between digital and physical intimacy

All participants made a distinction between their time spent online using hook-up apps and their time not using the apps. For some participants this meant they had a strict 'no hook-up app use' policy when out with friends or in public, and they would place a higher value on connecting with their friends and family in person than with new people on hook-up apps. Many too would lament how hook-up apps have made it more difficult to meet people without the use of the app. As Michelle, one of our straight participants, explains:

> I've gone out with friends before, especially guys where I'll be sitting right across the table from them and they're sitting down looking at their phones trying to find someone nearby. It's just really sad. There are tons of beautiful women in this bar that you're at, yet you find it easier to look at your phone and swipe and talk to someone that way then actually get up and go start a conversation.

This lament for the 'old-fashioned' connection, as Michelle later describes it, is a nostalgia for a perceived time when technology did not mediate connection and intimacy. Rachel explained this saying,

> They're too scared to go out of their comfort zone in person. So they do it all through text, and all behind the phone, or behind a computer, me included. So I think it's hindered that personal connection. And so now it's hard for me to, or for anybody, I think, to make that personal connection quickly.

Many participants saw this technologically mediated intimacy as generational, and perceived that Millennials and Gen Y depended more on hook-up apps to find dates, relationships, and hook-ups than Gen X or Boomers. However, our data is unclear on whether or not this generational distinction is actually the case.

Sex and intimacy

There were divergent views on how much hook-up apps facilitated sex and intimacy. Rachel, one of our straight participants, found that after using hook-up apps she had more casual sex/hook-ups than she had previously. But many other women were using these apps explicitly to find, as Laura puts it, 'a bit more than that,' and wanted dates and the possibility of a relationship. Marnie, one of our queer participants, perceived these as a distinction of largely orientation, with straight women and men using hook-up apps for hook-ups, while queer women were using it for relationships and friendships. She said,

> I don't know I mean I feel like it's kind of a stereotype like guys who you see more a hookup. Well I feel like maybe straight people in general are more to just like hookup. In my experience a lot of the people that I've met are like using it to actually meet people just because it's easier.

However, many of our straight participants refuted this view, and reported using hook-up apps to seek out relationships and dates.

For Rachel, sex did not always equate with intimacy. She notes that hook-up apps have made her feel profoundly lonely. While it was easy for her to find hook-ups on hook-up apps, it was more difficult to find partners who were willing to cuddle and share other, non-sexual intimate moments. She said, 'I guess if I hook up with them after a date, I will leave right after we hook up. I won't sit and watch the rest of the movie or cuddle with them. It's just like, "Okay, see you later."'

This distinction between sex and intimacy that Rachel describes was also discussed by other participants, but within the framework of hooking-up versus finding relationships. Many participants would indicate that they would delete or swipe left on matches who were explicitly looking for sex, or would speak dismissively of those who were using hook-up apps just for sex. Sophia noted that she had difficulty finding other queer women who were looking for relationships when she used the apps:

> I would say maybe less than one percent if I'm being generous were looking for relationships. A lot of them was fun and games and just even probably either cybersex or probably one-night stands if it comes down to it. None of the people pretty much were looking anything close to a relationship which I was looking for.

The fact that those in relationships usually do have sex is elided by participants. But this distinction between sex and relationships suggests our participants saw relationships as a more valuable type of intimacy than casual sex.

Using hook-up apps socially or in public

A significant place of divergence between queer women's and straight women's experiences using hook-up apps were in the norms around using these apps in public and/or in social settings. As we noted above, many participants placed more value in in-person and non-digitally mediated forms of contact and intimacy and would establish rules around when it was appropriate to use hook-up apps in public. None of our queer participants said they would use the app in a social setting or in a public space like a bar unless they were alone and bored. Straight women, however, regularly will use the app together and in public and otherwise social settings. Erica says,

> You turn it on at a bar just to see who's there, around, or who you could meet up with. Even a bunch of girls would get together, and you'd swipe to see who you're talking to, and stuff like that. It's so funny when you're like, 'Look at this guy,' and someone's like 'Yeah, he was talking to me too.'

Megan notes that the act of swiping on Tinder together was a group was a game at a bachelorette party she attended, and also noted that she has used the app together with her family. She said, 'We were in Paris on New Year's Eve, we had brought this cable that we could connect the tablet to the TV. We are Tindering in Paris, and my whole family was there.' Straight women often gamified their interactions on hook-up apps in ways their queer peers did not.

Friendship and community

Another significant point of diversion between queer and straight women's experiences was the role friendship and community played in their app use. While queer women do use hook-up apps to find dates, relationships, and hook-ups, many of them also use them to find friends and a like-minded community. These communities are a quintessential intimate public. Some participants worked in fields with few other out queer women, and so hook-up apps became important sites for them not only to meet dates, but to find friends. As Sam puts it,

> As much as these apps are for the purpose of dating, moving into the next step in the relationship, it also did open up doors for people as just, 'Hey you know what? I don't like you that way, but I'm down to being friends'.

For Sophia, hook-up apps were important sites to build community because there were few people in physical queer spaces that she felt she had much in common with. She said

> I tried meeting people organically when I deleted the app briefly, I started going out to more queer events. But that lasted for a very short period of time, because a lot of these queer events weren't in the age that I was looking for they were much, much older. Some of them were much younger like teens, and I was like, oh my God, where am I going to meet somebody who I have something in common? And a lot of the times even when I went to gay bars, I started talking to women and they're like, well, I'm straight. And I'm like, what are you doing here then?

Straight women rarely used hook-up apps to make friends and build communities, though some of them would use hook-up apps to reconnect with friends and former crushes from high school. It was more common for straight participants to discuss how their friends would turn them on to hook-up apps, and subsequently help them curate their profile. Rachel said,

> I kind of got made fun of for the pictures that I posted, particularly for Bumble and Tinder. It was very much like, 'What are you thinking? You're not going to get people on Tinder and Bumble to like you when you look like that. You look like you are a strong, independent woman.' And apparently that's not what people want on Bumble and Tinder. Yeah. So it was more peer pressure and friend influence, who kind of knew a little bit more about it than I did.

By using hook-up apps together, either in groups or even with just one other friend, straight women were creating intimate publics where they could have conversations about sex or the kinds of intimacies hook-up apps could provide.

Discussion

Our findings suggest that the field of intimate publics available to women users of hook-up apps is broader than those afforded by in-app interactions; there is an entire network of intimacy and publicity that forms around hook-up apps. Even when our participants spoke about risks to their physical, mental or emotional health, they spoke of reaching out to other women and to their networks for support. These networks exceed the relationships formed in-app. While some of our participants were concerned about the role hook-up apps play in reorganising our intimate relationships with other users, others found them to be crucial mediators and catalysts for the formation of community and the production of intimate publics. Of course, these communities and intimacies are influenced by the unique economic contexts for creating dating apps for (queer) women (Murray & Ankerson, 2016), which none of our participants discussed in our interviews. Nevertheless, the intimacies afforded by these publics are broader than those of sex – community, sociality, and friendship are all part of the sphere of intimacy created by women users of hook-up apps.

While there were significant similarities and shared experiences for our participants that cut across sexuality, social class, and racial identity – including the habitual use of hook-up apps, negative and positive effects on self-esteem, and concerns over how hook-up apps digitally mediated intimacy – queer women and straight women had markedly different experiences and perceptions of using hook-up apps in public. Straight women would often use Tinder with friends and in public, and consistent with Tinder's founding ethos (Duguay, 2017) would gamify their use of the app. Queer women, on the other hand, were more reticent about using hook-up apps in public or in social settings. The difference can be attributed to the epistemology of the closet (Sedgwick, 1990), which structures queer life within discourses of (dis)closure and confession (Foucault, 1990). Using hook-up apps in public, even by oneself, is a public display of intimacy, and such displays have a long history of being regulated and of being a catalyst for abuse for queer people.

Using a hook-up app in public remains fraught for queer women, and points toward deeper questions about the role of shame within the formation of queer communities and identities (Sedgwick, 1993). For the queer women we spoke to, there is more shame around using the apps and they tend to use them more in private spaces than in public. This distinction is, of course, indicative of broader patterns within the intimate public sphere wherein only particular forms of heteronormative intimacy are permitted within the realm of public life (Berlant & Warner, 1998). The straight women in our study felt little shame over using hook-up apps in public; where they did feel shame, tellingly, was if they would have to reveal to their families that they met their partner through a hook-up app. But rather than see heterosexual women's app use as a feminist reclamation of the public sphere as a site of sexual sociality, the ease with which heterosexual women are able to integrate Tinder into public life compared to queer women only seems to support Berlant and Warner's (1998) thesis that the public sphere reproduces and supports heteronormative forms of intimacy and belonging. Indeed, the fact that both queer and straight participants placed more value on finding relationships, as opposed to hook-ups, suggests that heteronormative imperative toward monogamy still structures the types of intimate relationships these women seek out.

This points toward larger questions about the roles hook-up apps can play in women's health and women's abilities to live full and meaningful lives. For straight women, hook-up apps help further solidify their claim to public life, building a stronger support network of women to discuss questions of sex and dating openly, and to co-create strong senses of self. For queer women, hook-up apps can connect them with other queer women not just for sex and dating, but also to make friends and build community. Meeting physically without the use of apps is not a privilege afforded to many queer women, as there are few spaces devoted exclusively to queer women, and what spaces there are often attract heterosexual women and tend to skew younger, leaving many of the older queer Millennials we interviewed without physical spaces to meet other queer women of their generation.

Conclusion and areas for further research

We also noted in our interviews with queer women an underlying intimacy between interviewee and interviewer (Taylor, 2011). Because we matched the gender and sexuality of our interviewer with our participants, this opened up the possibility for sexual and other intimate relations between our queer interviewers and participants. Our queer women participants were more likely to ask their interviewer questions about their life and their own experience, as if they were on a date. At the end of numerous interviews with queer women, both women would often agree to turn the recorder off and keep talking. That privacy, that closing off their connection from the rest of the research team, signals a particular kind of intimacy produced between researcher and subject mediated by these apps. Further research needs to be done in how interviewing hook-up app users mimics the codes and conventions of dating and produces its own intimacies.

This research has a number of ramifications for health practitioners and app developers. For health practitioners, our research further supports the findings of Albury and Byron (2016) and suggests that the range of health-related effects of dating apps is broader than the transmission of STIs and HIV. While users continue to have concerns about the effects of dating apps on their mental and emotional health, health practitioners and scholars should also think more carefully about how hook-up apps can facilitate access to communities and networks of support. Dating apps have a wide variety of uses and as such their health effects cannot be determined in advance. For app developers and corporations, the wide variety of uses – including not only sex and relationships, but also friendships – should not be read as evidence for the production of new apps or new features that attempt to produce separate spheres where friendships can be built, while leaving other apps and features solely for those finding sex. Users are adept at navigating the interfaces and have developed norms and rules for app use that help them use them to find what they want. The ways intimacies develop is surprising and unpredictable; many of the women we spoke to downloaded these apps to find relationships and sex, but instead developed lasting friendships. The inability of many hook-up apps to allow users to easily, consistently, and reliably define the parameters of people they see and match with on the apps by type of intimacy sought – by friendship, casual sex, relationship, and so on – should not be seen as a bug that needs fixing. Rather, the inability to reliably narrow the scope of matches to a single sort of intimate relation is a key feature that allows these apps to produce intimate public spheres.

There are a wide array of intimate practices available to women who use or have used hook-up apps beyond their perceived normative uses around sex and dating. When used in social and public settings, hook-up apps can produce intimate publics and strengthen or develop the bonds of friendship and community. Despite the potential negative effects hook-up apps can have on mental and emotional health, they are also important mediators of bonds between women. These bonds created and mediated by hook-up apps are central to women's health and well-being, and their ability to live life fully.

Note

1. We define 'woman' as anyone who self-identifies as a woman. We use 'queer women' as an umbrella term for women who self-identified as bisexual, pansexual, gay, lesbian, or any other non-heterosexual sexuality.

Acknowledgements

We would like to thank Mary Grace Lao as well as our two anonymous reviewers for their perceptive and thoughtful comments on earlier drafts of this manuscript.

Disclosure statement

No potential conflict of interest was reported by the author(s).

Funding

This research was supported by the Social Sciences and Humanities Research Council of Canada.

ORCID

Jonathan Petrychyn http://orcid.org/0000-0003-3058-9226

References

Ahlm, J. (2017). Respectable promiscuity: Digital cruising in an era of queer liberalism. *Sexualities*, *20*(3), 364–379. doi:10.1177/1363460716665783

Albury, K., Burgess, J., Light, B., Race, K., & Wilken, R. (2017). Data cultures of mobile dating and hook-up apps: Emerging issues for critical social science research. *Big Data & Society*, 4, 1–11.

Albury, K., & Byron, P. (2016). Safe on my phone? Same-sex attracted young people's negotiations of intimacy, visibility, and risk on digital hook-up apps. *Social Media + Society*, *2*(4), 1–10.

Baum, F., Newman, L., & Biedrzycki, K. (2014). Vicious cycles: Digital technologies and determinants of health in Australia. *Health Promotion International*, *29*(2), 349–360. doi:10.1093/heapro/das062

Berlant, L. (1997). *The queen of America goes to Washington city: Essays on sex and citizenship*. Durham: Duke University Press.

Berlant, L. (1998). Intimacy: A special issue. *Critical Inquiry*, *24*(2), 281–288.

Berlant, L., & Warner, M. (1998). Sex in public. *Critical Inquiry*, *24*(2), 547–566.

boyd, d. (2010). Social network sites as networked publics: Affordances, dynamics, and implications. In Z. Papacharissi (Ed.), *A networked self: Identity, community, and culture on social network sites* (pp. 39–58). New York: Routledge.

Chun, W. H. K. (2016). *Updating to remain the same: Habitual new media*. Cambridge, MA: MIT Press.

Costa, L., & Matzner, A. (2007). *Male bodies women's souls: Personal narratives of Thailand's transgendered youth*. Binghamton, NY: Hawthorne Press.

Cousineau, L., Oakes, H., & Johnson, C. W. (2018). Appnography: Digital ethnography for app-based culture. In D. C. Parry, C. W. Johnson, & S. Fullagar (Eds.), *Digital dilemmas: Transforming gender identities and power relations in everyday life* (pp. 95–118). Cham, Switzerland: Palgrave.

David, G., & Cambre, C. (2016). Screened Intimacies: Tinder and the swipe logic. *Social Media + Society*, 2, 1–11.

Dean, J. (2010). Affective networks. *MediaTropes*, *2*(2), 19–44.

Duguay, S. (2017). Dressing up Tinderella: Interrogating authenticity claims on the mobile dating app Tinder. *Information, Communication & Society*, *20*(3), 351–367. doi:10.1080/1369118X.2016.1168471

Duguay, S., Burgess, J., & Light, B. (2017). Mobile dating and hookup app culture. In P. Messaris, & L. Humphreys (Eds.), *Digital media: Transformations in human communication* (pp. 213–221). New York: Peter Lang.

Foucault, M. (1990). *The history of sexuality: An introduction*. New York: Vintage Books.

Hobbs, M., Owen, S., & Gerber, L. (2017). Liquid love? Dating apps, sex, relationships and the digital transformation of intimacy. *Journal of Sociology*, *53*(2), 271–284. doi:10.1177/1440783316662718

Ito, M. (2008). Introduction. In K. Varnelis (Ed.), *Networked publics* (pp. 1–14). Cambridge, MA: MIT Press.

Jamieson, L. (2011). Intimacy as a concept: Explaining social change in the context of globalisation or another form of ethnocentricism? *Sociological Research Online*, *16*, 151–163.

Johnson, C. W., Petrychyn, J., & Parry, D. C. (2020). New methodologies for appnography. Manuscript in preparation.

Landovitz, R. J., Tseng, C.-H., Weissman, M., Haymer, M., Mendenhall, B., Rogers, K., … Shoptaw, S. (2013). Epidemiology, sexual risk behavior, and HIV prevention practices of men who have sex with men using GRINDR in Los Angeles, California. *Journal of Urban Health*, *90*(4), 729–739. doi:10.1007/s11524-012-9766-7

Lupton, D. (2014). Critical perspectives on digital health technologies. *Sociology Compass*, *8*(12), 1344–1359. doi:10.1111/soc4.12226

Lutz, C., & Ranzini, G. (2017). Where dating meets data: Investigating social and institutional privacy concerns on Tinder. *Social Media + Society*, *3*, 1–2.

Macapagal, K., Moskowitz, D., Li, D. H., Carrion, A., Bettin, E., Fisher, C. B., & Mustanski, B. (2018). Hookup app use, sexual behavior, and sexual health among adolescent men who have sex with men in the United States. *Journal of Adolescent Health*, *62*(6), 708–715. doi:10.1016/j.jadohealth.2018.01.001

Morris, J. W., & Murray, S. (Eds.). (2018). *Appified: Culture in the age of apps*. Ann Arbor: University of Michigan Press.

Møller, K., & Petersen, M. N. (2018). Bleeding boundaries: Domesticating gay hook-up apps. In R. Andreassen, M. N. Petersen, K. Harrison, & T. Raun (Eds.), *Mediated intimacies: Connectivities, relationalities and proximities* (pp. 208–223). New York: Routledge.

Murray, S., & Ankerson, M. S. (2016). Lez takes time: Designing lesbian contact in geosocial networking apps. *Critical Studies in Media Communication*, *33*(1), 53–69. doi:10.1080/15295036.2015.1133921

Papacharissi, Z. (2016). Affective publics and structures of storytelling: Sentiment, events and mediality. *Information, Communication & Society*, *19*(3), 307–324. doi:10.1080/1369118X.2015.1109697

Parry, D. C., Glover, T. D., & Mulcahy, C. M. (2013). From 'stroller-Stalker' to 'momancer': Courting friends through a social networking site for mothers. *Journal of Leisure Research*, *45*(1), 23–46. doi:10.18666/jlr-2013-v45-i1-2941

Parry, D. C., & Light, T. P. (2014). Fifty shades of complexity. *Journal of Leisure Research*, *46*(1), 38–57. doi:10.1080/00222216.2014.11950312

Phoenix, A. (2008). Analyzing narrative contexts. In M. Andrews, C. Squire, & M. Tamboukou (Eds.), *Doing narrative research* (pp. 64–77). London: SAGE.

Plummer, K. (2003). *Intimate citizenship: Private decisions and public dialogues*. Seattle: University of Washington Press.

Sedgwick, E. K. (1990). *Epistemology of the closet: Updated with a new preface*. Berkeley, CA: University of California Press.

Sedgwick, E. K. (1993). Queer performativity: Henry James's the art of the novel. *GLQ: A Journal of Lesbian and Gay Studies*, *1*(1), 1–16. doi:10.1215/10642684-1-1-1

Squire, C. (2008). Experience-centered and culturally-oriented approaches to narrative. In M. Andrews, C. Squire, & M. Tamboukou (Eds.), *Doing narrative research* (pp. 41–63). London: SAGE.

Taylor, J. (2011). The intimate insider: Negotiating the ethics of friendship when doing insider research. *Qualitative Research*, *11*(1), 3–22. doi:10.1177/1468794110384447

Tziallas, E. (2015). Gamified eroticism: Gay male "social networking" Applications and self-pornography. *Sexuality & Culture*, *19*(4), 759–775. doi:10.1007/s12119-015-9288-z

van Dijck, J. (2012). Facebook as a tool for producing sociality and connectivity. *Television & New Media*, *13*(2), 160–176. doi:10.1177/1527476411415291

Weltevrede, E., & Jansen, F. (2019). Infrastructures of intimate data: Mapping the inbound and outbound data flows of dating apps. *Computational Culture*, *7*. http://computationalculture.net/infrastructures-of-intimate-data-mapping-the-inbound-and-outbound-data-flows-of-dating-apps/.

'It's like getting an Uber for sex': social networking apps as spaces of risk and opportunity in the Philippines among men who have sex with men

Brooke Maria Hollingshead, Gary W. Dowsett and Adam Bourne

The HIV epidemic in the Philippines has been expanding rapidly, with most newly diagnosed cases occurring among 'men who have sex with men' (MSM). New social contexts of HIV are evident in the evolving phenomenon of more MSM seeking partners online via social networking applications ('apps'). This study examines findings from a virtual ethnography of app use among MSM, focus group discussions with community-based healthcare workers, and key informant interviews with healthcare workers, policymakers and researchers in Metro Manila. We argue that participants viewed the expanding epidemic and apps as intimately linked, regarding the apps as 'risky spaces' for 'risky behaviour'. However, such narratives neglected the agentive capabilities of the apps and how they have transformed sexual practice, creating new ways of being as sexual subjects, while perpetuating old imaginaries among healthcare workers of 'hard-to-reach' populations. Such narratives of 'risk' have led to new interventions by healthcare workers on the apps, viewing these technologies as opportunities to reach more MSM for health promotion. However, the interventions have created new complexities by reconfiguring boundaries with target populations. By conducting community-based outreach through encouraging behaviour change in one-to-one interactions with app users, the potential impact of these interventions is limited.

Introduction

The HIV epidemic in the Philippines has been changing rapidly. The past decade has witnessed dramatic increases in new diagnoses and a shift in the modes of transmission so that most new infections are now occurring among 'men who have sex with men' (MSM) (Gangcuangco, 2019; Ross et al., 2015). In 2019 there were 12,778 newly diagnosed cases of HIV, of whom 95% were men, making it the fastest growing epidemic in the Asia Pacific region, more than doubling in size between 2010 and 2016 (Department of Health, 2019; UNAIDS, 2017). However, the social changes that have produced this epidemiological shift remain underexamined, as are the appropriateness of the responses in this new phase of the epidemic.

The article will identify narratives that were used by participants to explain the rising number of diagnosed cases among MSM in the Philippines. It will explore how some participants viewed social networking applications used for sexual purposes (commonly termed 'apps') as spaces of 'risk' in themselves and a direct driver of the epidemic, attributing metonymically to these online spaces actual risk, not just as contributors to, or facilitators of sexual risk-taking. Others viewed the technologies agnostically, with any 'blame' or responsibility for HIV transmission determined by how individuals used these technologies. These perceptions and understandings are important to explore as they provide insight into how healthcare workers respond to the HIV epidemic.

We will argue that social and sexual networking has also been *reconfigured* by the rise of online technologies. The part played by these technologies in sexual experiences will be explored, as the agentive capacity of the apps transforms the operation of sexual desire and practice. They provide new affordances that enhance sexual connectedness and the possibility to shift depictions of the self and create new ways of being for MSM, while perpetuating old imaginaries of 'hard-to-reach' populations among healthcare workers. While some of this work bears relation to research on gay communities dealing with sexual health in high-income contexts (Albury, 2018; Bryant et al., 2018; Race, 2015a), there are many things about the Philippines that require a different frame of reference, and one of the major lessons from this pandemic has been finding ways to investigate sexuality without imposing visions of the West. One example of this is the APCOM Foundation (Asia-Pacific Coalition in Men's Sexual Health), whose work in the region including the Philippines involved partnerships with local organisations and international agencies such as the Global Fund fighting AIDS, Tuberculosis and Malaria, the Australian Federation of AIDS Organisations, aidsfond (the Netherlands) and many others, to share ideas, adapt strategies and develop locally appropriate interventions (see apcom.org).

The broader implications of these findings for the HIV response in the Philippines will then be discussed by exploring how such narratives of risk and blame have been used to justify new interventions. The healthcare workers who had been conducting their outreach work in bars now find themselves often working online, communicating via these apps to reach their target clients. Many healthcare workers are MSM themselves and personal app users too. While providing for valuable peer insight, this interweaving of the personal and the professional is a dynamic that can complicate community-based peer education (Dowsett, Wain, & Keys, 2005). Such interventions also re-install a biomedical focus on individuals as rational independent agents who, given appropriate information, will change their behaviours.

Most apps are centred on individual 'profiles' wherein users provide their age, height, weight, body type, relationship status, and preferred sexual positions (or these can be kept blank). Many of these fields are pre-populated with options to select from drop-down menus. Users can describe whom and what they are looking for and where and when they are available to meet. Profiles become visible to others based on location and proximity. When an image is clicked, the profile of that person expands and an option is given to send a message or pictures or the user's own location. The importance of such features lies in their ability to frame sexual desire and provide new affordances that enhance sexual connectedness.

Methodology

This research was conducted in Metro Manila from July 2018 to April 2019 and comprised three stages. The results and themes identified from each stage produced findings that informed the next.

First, a virtual ethnography of the apps was conducted by the first author acting as a passive observer. This documented how the apps functioned, the language used for sexual identities, and how the safety of sex was negotiated. These findings were used to develop questions for focus group discussions (FGDs) held with 17 healthcare workers from three community-based HIV organisations. Preliminary understandings of sexual identities and practices from the ethnography were tested, and the FGDs explored how participants believed their organisations understood online sexual networking and risk negotiation, and how it influenced service provision and health promotion initiatives to reach communities. The FGD participants were selected purposively in order to gain understandings from a range of perspectives and populations. Their professions included community healthcare workers for MSM or transgender women, support staff for people living with HIV, nurses, doctors and office managers.

An initial analysis identified themes on the risk and opportunities afforded in online sexual networking and how these linked to epidemiological change. These informed the interview schedule for the final stage of the research, in which 20 key-informant (KI) interviews were conducted with healthcare workers, researchers, and policymakers to explore the social contexts of HIV. Initial KIs were selected purposively for their experience working in the field and heterogeneity in the sample was sought to gain diversity in perspectives. Other KI participants were referred to the project from initial KIs and FGD participants. Each KI interview was semi-structured, lasting for between 60 and 90 min, and conducted at a location of the KI's choosing. The interviews and FGDs were digitally recorded and transcribed verbatim. Transcripts were subjected to an inductive thematic analysis (Braun & Clarke, 2006).

The study received ethics clearance from the La Trobe University Human Ethics Committee (HEC18132 and S17-171).

Findings

'Risky' online technologies

The apps used for sexual purposes were understood to be shaping risk-taking behaviour by increasing the availability and convenience of sex, with one FGD participant arguing now that everyone had a smartphone, '[i]t's so much easier. It's like getting an Uber for sex' (FGD 1, member 1, gay male, doctor). This was elaborated upon by KIs who compared the accessibility of sex now with earlier times:

> I've experienced that time when social media was not yet common, so when you wanted to hook-up you just go to cruising areas, hot spots, a bar. But right now, at the convenience of their homes, you can just have sex there and meet anyone. (KI 16, gay male, community-based healthcare worker)

However, participants reported that these technologies could be used for networking as well as sex, and a proliferation of 'Clans' (online text message-based chat groups) had arisen that were used to connect people and organise offline meetings. During one FGD with the community organisations, the participants talked excitedly about the Clans they were a part of (and, with sadness, about those they were not). Clans were also divided into factions depending on sexual preferences or common interests (e.g. groups for gym bunnies, pageant lovers, or orgies). Some Clans had strict criteria for who could join, with a negative HIV result being required (with FGD participants noting the relevance of the window period was obviously not considered). Consequently, the administrative ability of these technologies to bring together large groups of people conjured an assumed vision of a mass of participants searching for sexual partners. KI 2 (bisexual female, human rights worker) argued that such chat groups were therefore 'a recipe for infection, especially if in orgies', perpetuating a perception that these were spaces of high-risk.

Some participants reported that it was not just apps being used for sex seeking; other platforms intended purely for social networking were also becoming sexualised as an avenue to meet people:

> Back in 2008 there were all these sex dating apps and networking sites, but now, you don't have to be in those forums, you can just be on Facebook … you can just be on Twitter, and these are platforms that were not created for that, but they have become utilised for that, so it's actually very easy to access sex online. (KI 2, bisexual female, human rights worker)

KI 11 (gay male, community-based healthcare worker, living with HIV) regarded the HIV epidemic as being driven by online sexual networking, as partner selection was often determined by the willingness to engage in what were termed 'high-risk behaviours' such as anal sex generally and anal sex without condoms specifically:

> When I was still young, the common practice is just vaginal sex, penis and vagina, or oral sex. If you are a gay or MSM, during my time, the practice is more on oral, mutual masturbation. But now it's different. It's like, aside from oral, you should also practise anal sex. Sometimes, if you just met someone online, social media, and you are talking with these people, bargaining for possible meetups—sometimes if you don't agree with them to have anal sex, they just ignore you. And I believe that many people are trying to practise that high-risk activity. And the problem will come in if you don't have any knowledge about condom use and protection. So, that is a big problem now. Many MSM are practising high-risk behaviour, [having] anal sex unprotected.

In the global HIV response, the concept of what is considered 'risky' sex is rapidly evolving. The availability of Pre-Exposure Prophylaxis (or PrEP, where an HIV-negative individual takes daily antiretroviral medication to prevent acquiring HIV) and the increase in undetectable viral loads among people living with HIV taking similar medication (when HIV cannot be detected by standard viral load tests and becomes unable to be transmitted, termed 'treatment as prevention' or TasP) have contributed to this reframing of 'risk'. In situations where these medications are widely available and used, it has become possible for penetrative sex without condoms to be engaged in with, effectively, no risk of HIV transmission, and therefore these biomedical technologies have reframed the concept of risk. However, both biomedical tools currently have limited availability in the Philippines. Where available, people living with HIV are often lost to follow-up and not linked effectively to antiretroviral treatment and, therefore, widespread supressed community viral load is far from being realised. PrEP has had limited roll-out (a demonstration project and few current providers) and, therefore, it is hard to access, expensive if available, and still a highly charged political issue as to whether it should be offered at all due to the current problems facing treatment access. Some discussions of risk as they are framed in the Global North are therefore not as pertinent to the current Philippines context where the predominant understanding of risk still refers to sex without condoms.

App use was also associated with exposing men to potentially new risks, as FGD participants mentioned widespread references in app users' profiles to drug-related activities. One participant (FGD 1, member 1, gay male, doctor) highlighted how '[i]t's very much commonplace. Grindr. You get invites to PNP [Party and play]'. KI 4 (queer male, activist, living with HIV) added that this had contributed to a 'normalisation of drug use in the gay community in the Philippines, particularly in the urban setting, [which] has also contributed to more sexual activity as well'. Such arguments are challenging to explore further due to the difficulty in discussing such issues amid concerted efforts by the police and other law enforcement agencies, sanctioned and promoted by President Duterte, to persecute those who use drugs. Hence, community healthcare workers' understandings of the actual contribution of drug use to the HIV epidemic among MSM in the Philippines is unclear.

Other FGD participants raised concerns that these online sexual networks were developing 'under the radar' and outside the purview of public health authorities, arguing that some individuals would not have received safe sex messaging. In such narratives, participants tied changes in the epidemic to changes in sexual culture, which were seen to emerge with the new social contexts of sex as apps reshaped risk-taking behaviour.

Online technologies as innocent vessels for risky behaviour

Some KI participants regarded this technology as neutral or innocent and saw the 'problem' as lying with the individuals who decided to use apps to facilitate risky sex. Such narratives recognised the benefits and limitations posed by the technologies but viewed them critically, as argued by KI 16 (gay male, community-based healthcare worker):

> I'm not blaming the app. I'm not blaming technology, because I believe technology is a double-edged sword. It could be used for the good or for the downfall ... but then a lot of people [don't] recognise that technology's just like, a vessel.

In such narratives, online technologies appear not to be awarded a value, as participants attempted to take an agnostic position with the intention of assigning responsibility instead to individuals who used these technologies for determining their own behaviour. However, 'double-edged sword' is a heavily laden, common-placed trope, and this participant clearly had some misgivings even as other participants were clearly trying to be seen as staying away from anything that might appear to their peers as holding a moralistic or value-laden opinion. In such narratives, participants were determined that blame or risk cannot be constituted in the apps but in how individuals use them to make friends and build networks, whilst others used them for 'bad behaviour'. Following this logic, risky sex is seen to occur because of poor decisions by undisciplined and out-of-control individuals (Bryant et al., 2018). Given the fact that some of these KI and FGD participants were also personal app users, there appeared to be a few possible motivations underlying these ways of representing the apps and their use. However, no participant raised this possibility as such, but we note it here given the literature on this issue cited earlier in this paper.

HIV risk and blame

These narratives grappling with concepts of risk and blame drew on a wider discourse. The tendency to identify *the* problem and who is to blame for it has been prominent since the beginning of the epidemic. In speaking of risk and blame, the healthcare workers were reaching for these old motifs that have been part of a longstanding discursive manoeuvre in literature on HIV to locate cause and blame in gay men or other MSM. Discussions of 'bad behaviour' and 'riskiness' within the apps revealed that this story was still operating in the Philippines, perpetuated by the healthcare workers themselves.

In these continuing narratives of risk in Manila, either the apps or their users were construed as *the* problem driving the HIV epidemic. Each was represented as either facilitating or performing sex that occurred in 'the shadows', under the noses of health professionals everywhere, yet somehow out of reach from healthcare initiatives. The apps were understood to shape risk-taking through facilitating opportunities to practise what was regarded as bad behaviour. As KI 18 (heterosexual female, government worker) argued, 'If you have the social apps, for example, you have Grindr, you have Tinder, you have Blued, whatever, it means you're practising very risky behaviour. But if you don't have, you're practising safe sex'.

Of course, risky sex can happen without the assistance of apps, so these narratives mistakenly confine risk to the apps and those who use them, and echo the panic and warnings from public health officials and in popular commentary ever since people began seeking sex on the Internet (Lehmiller & Ioerger, 2014). In an article published by the *Wall Street Journal* entitled 'HIV Cases Soar in the Philippines as Dating Apps Spread' (Rana, 2019), the journalist drew a clear connection between the expanding epidemic and the increasing use of apps:

> The internet opened an avenue for the gay community to meet and experiment ... but infections skyrocketed a few years later as cheap smartphones flooded Filipino homes. By 2012, AIDS had claimed the lives of many friends.

In this way, the journalist drew a confronting picture by speaking in the same breath of the growing presence of digital technologies and of the death of people from AIDS-related illnesses, thereby suggesting that one caused the other in an attempt to create panic and raise awareness of activities occurring within the apps.

In academic research, such popular warnings have been validated by studies that demonstrated increased risk of HIV transmission was associated with seeking sex online. These studies found men who sought sex online were more likely to report having had unprotected anal intercourse (Landovitz et al., 2013), a recent sexually transmissible infection (Patel, Masyukova, Sutton, & Horvath, 2016), more sex partners (Bien et al., 2015), or having engaged in drug use (Sun, Reboussin, Mann, Garcia, & Rhodes, 2016). Davis (2008) argued that much of this panic about apps was focussed on 'barebacking', i.e. having 'intentionally unprotected anal intercourse in circumstances in which risk has not been ruled out' (Carballo-Diéguez et al., 2006, p. 476). Barebacking has long been regarded as the motivation of much online sex seeking and of particular concern to health professionals since it was regarded as contrary to public health advice. However, various researchers have also long argued that this conceptualisation may not be the most useful way to understand unprotected sex (Carballo-Dieguez et al., 2009; Kippax, Crawford, Davis, Rodden, & Dowsett, 1993), and such concerns are largely moot in many contexts in the era of PrEP and TasP.

However, apps can also be seen as a vehicle to reach people and for health promotion and the riskiness of apps has not always demonstrated in research. The internet, and more recently social media, began to be used for HIV/AIDS health education in the late 1990s (Taggart, Grewe, Conserve, Gliwa, & Roman Isler, 2015), and gay men's HIV/AIDS prevention was among the first to use these technologies (Johnson, Hedges, & Diaz, 2003). Various studies since have documented the value of such technologies, e.g. Grindr users being more open to using PrEP (Hoenigl et al., 2019), and increased safe sex practices (Race, 2015a), higher levels of testing (Goedel, Halkitis, Greene, Hickson, & Duncan, 2016) and better knowledge of PrEP (Rice et al., 2012) has been found among gay male social media users. There is, however, minimal research on this in the Philippines.

The agentive capacity of apps in reconfiguring sexual practice

Human agency is central to the framing of narratives of risk and blame, and participants regarded the apps as passive stages on which the activities of individuals took place. This has led to interventions by the participants' organisations being directed at the individual level to change behaviours and educate, which will be discussed later. Yet, such narratives disregarded the agency of the apps themselves and how online technologies have actively contributed to the ongoing reconfiguration of sex. As such, these narratives also neglected the broader determinants of behaviour and vulnerability influencing individuals. This is an issue discussed in many contexts in relation to ongoing risk-taking and continuing HIV epidemics. For example, arguments have been made in relation to technology use for sexual networking in high-income countries that risk practices are now occurring as an individualised and embodied response to the material conditions shaped by neoliberalism. It is argued that 'chemsex' or sexual networking provides a 'collectivity' moment that obviates a growing existential dilemma (Hakim, 2019). That may be true for high-income contexts; however, such a frame of reference cannot be readily applied to the Philippines, where the effects of neoliberalism are not anywhere near as strong, particularly among the majority of Filipinos where extended family living and shared subsistence work outside late-capitalist market-driven relations are common. Therefore, a different frame of reference is required in the search for whatever motivates any desire for collectivity among MSM using these apps.

The agentive potential of the apps to provide new affordances by changing understandings of sexual practice, perceptions of gay space, and to provide new ways of being for MSM were apparent in the narratives of participants. The capacity for app users to specify their identities and desires created the opportunity to plan sexual encounters ahead of time by sharing details of their upcoming travel plans, thereby constituting desire through suspense and expectation, sexual speculation and fantasy construction (Race, 2015b). KI 19 (gay male, researcher) argued that this ability to preplan sex had produced new gay communities in tourist spots:

> I hear the party scenes in places like Boracay [an island in the Philippines known for its beaches, resorts and parties] also do a gay scene, and this is because of Planet Romeo and other apps, as they do provide for, 'Let's meet up somewhere', or 'I'm going to Boracay' and you can prepare beforehand so you know what the scene is like in a city.

This example highlighted the agentive capacity of the apps to transform and create experiences; however, it was also evident in how they provided active ways to shift depictions of the self and of what was regarded as gay space.

Creating new forms of being: the 'discreet' and 'hard to reach'

Online sex-seeking via these technologies have also produced new ways of being and new forms of sexual subjectivity as the apps provided active ways to shift depictions of the self. This was most evident in the notion of 'discreet', a term that FGD participants argued has been taken up by many MSM to describe a sexual sense of self. The term discreet was linked in profiles to other terms such as being 'straight-acting', or to men exhibiting 'no trace' of being gay (alluding to being covert, unmarked, unrecognisable and hidden). Discreet could be used to hide sexual activities by using such language as a protective barrier, signalling to a broader fear of stigma in operation. However, FGD and KI participants outlined how it was also used to represent the app user as more masculine and, therefore, more desirable and marketable. These were supported visually by the many masked faces and grids of faceless bodies of men who wished to be anonymous.

This sense of hiddenness seems more similar to the struggles of homosexual people to emerge from the stigmatised margins in pre-gay-liberationist times in the West than to any neoliberal, individualist and existential dilemma today. This limits the direct applicability to the Philippines of analyses of app use and changing sexual cultures among gay men in the Global North where new forms of sexual community and new sexual publics have been documented (Race, 2015b). The longstanding, very public, gay communities of the Global North provide a locus of their changing sexual cultures, e.g. in the way the Sydney Gay and Lesbian Mardi Gras provides a collective symbol under which more prosaic sexual lives are lived and pursued in Sydney. Visible gay communities in the Philippines are very small, mostly comprising middle- and upper-class, well-educated people often with considerable exposure to the Global North. Most sex between Filipino men does not happen under the discursive framing of 'gay' sexual culture or community, and common understandings of being gay or what gay men do and are cannot be taken for granted. What is occurring on these apps in the Philippines is certainly producing new sexual possibilities and cultures as has been noted in the Global North, but these are emerging from a different base or starting point. This emergence is akin more to the 'unregulated' improvisation among young queer people reported by Byron and Albury (2018) than to transforming existing community. It is yet to be seen whether the confluence of these technologies, globalising sexuality discourses such as 'gay', and the increasing spaces created by the new possibilities for sex that involve such technologies will shift men with sexual interests in other men from discreet and masked lives into the kinds of shared cultures, collectives and communities.

The anonymity suggested by these masked faces and pixelated profile pictures was linked to understandings of risk conveyed by many FGD and KI participants in intimations that any potential partners found via the apps – by their clients or by themselves personally – may be hiding something, thereby reinforcing the understanding that such activity was occurring in 'the shadows'. This idea of anonymity and shadowy sexual agents was discomforting to many healthcare workers, as they were regarded as endangering public health. What emerged was an understanding and imagination of the sexual subjects using these online technologies to find sex who, when describing themselves as 'discreet', were rendered 'closeted' individuals seeking anonymous sex online.

> These people could be 'discreet', they could be closeted individuals. And these are the most hard-to-reach individuals, because their stigma, their fear, is very much ingrained. They're paranoid when people see them going near to a testing centre. (KI 16, gay male, community-based healthcare worker)

> It is precisely your discreet males who are shadow populations. (KI 19, gay male, researcher)

These narratives from healthcare workers reinforced this idea of 'hard-to-reach' 'shadow' populations who must be diligently tracked down by community healthcare workers for their 'bad behaviour' on 'bad apps'. It was evident in the narratives noted above in which sexual networking via these apps was viewed as dangerous due to its occurrence beyond the purview of public health, amid consensus among healthcare workers that 'discreet' MSM were unlikely to be aware of the need to use condoms or practise safe sex. It was also evident when healthcare workers accused MSM of deception and presenting 'false' selves in their profiles, even though this practice has long been regarded as commonplace in online sexual networking technologies (Plummer, 2001).

Understandings of space and time have also been transformed by the agentive capacity of the apps, with the centrality of location promoting an orientation towards immediacy and a prioritisation of spatial proximity as vital for sexual encounters. The convenience of securing sex through the apps compared with traditional methods was evident in the narratives of both FGD and KI participants. However, as Brubaker, Ananny, and Crawford (2016) argued, the geolocation functionality of apps is not only about finding someone but also about positioning oneself in places where one can readily be found by others. Location awareness therefore reconfigures sexual activity by providing a way for potential partners to be filtered by spatial and temporal attributes to provide opportunity for a steady stream of potential sex partners. Such sex-seeking via apps was embedded in everyday activities of their users. As KI 4 (queer male, activist, living with HIV) reported: 'I think it's fair to say that, for many people, their approach to Grindr is [that] it passes the time, it helps address boredom, waiting while travelling like two hours to and from work every day'.

The apps have transformed the conceptualisation of gay space, once bounded by distinct physical places such as cruising areas or bars that required insider knowledge. Metro Manila is a large conurbation comprising many contiguous cities, with great distances to travel. Gay venues have traditionally concentrated in just a few inner-city neighbourhoods, rendering them difficult to reach for many MSM, particularly those of more limited means. For those who could go to such places, these venues were and are known to provide small refuges of safety and acceptance for men seeking sex with other men; they are shielded by their boundaries.

These technologies have contributed to an expansion of social worlds in which sex between men is available, possible and facilitated. Beyond the large distances to be travelled to gay venues in Manila, KI 10 (heterosexual male, community-based healthcare worker, living with HIV) noted that increased access to online technologies has also connected men to others with same-sex interests when previously they did not have the financial means to go to bars and other venues:

> They don't go anymore to the mall ... 'Cause these young people, they don't have money, so they can't afford to go to bars.

Implications

Online technologies as an opportunity to reach MSM

In response to the changing epidemic and the blame and risk attributed to online technologies, healthcare interventions have emerged, led by healthcare workers from community-based organisations and local government units, which have sought to meet MSM where they were, i.e. online. This was being done by healthcare workers creating profiles on various apps to raise awareness about HIV and offer free testing, viewing the technologies as a vehicle to reach more people. Certainly, there has been an increase in testing programs in the Philippines (Department of Health, 2017), thereby increasing access for MSM and other populations. Yet, the extent to which the rising incidence is a consequence of increased detection or an increase in risk behaviour (as has been explored in other contexts, see Dougan et al., 2007) has not been determined. The problem that was explained to justify these interventions by participants was one of access and a hidden epidemic; efforts to encourage HIV testing were regarded as the solution. This was formulated through references to greater access to testing, especially for the 'hard-to-reach'.

The effectiveness of interventions delivered via social networking apps has been examined in other contexts. A systematic review by Cao et al. (2017) found that HIV-testing uptake increased after implementation of social media interventions. However, the authors noted that few online interventions had occurred in low- and middle-income countries. Another study assessing the effectiveness of using Grindr to increase HIV self-testing among Black and Latino MSM in Los Angeles found online interventions resulted in more linkage to testing than offline outreach, and a greater likelihood to reach untested high-risk populations (Maloney, Bratcher, Wilkerson, & Sullivan, 2020). Yet, it was found that such interventions were also limited to individual behaviour change by only encouraging testing and education, resulting in an absence of interventions addressing linkage to and retention in care, or adherence. Such online interventions have increased in the time of COVID-19, in the Philippines as well as in high-income contexts, as traditional ways of having sex have become difficult during lockdowns. Health promotion and outreach initiatives have used technologies to promote ways risk can ameliorated, moderated and negated online (Love Yourself, 2020).

New complexities for healthcare workers

There has been a reconfiguration of the relationships and boundaries between target populations and healthcare professionals, as healthcare workers operate in online spaces when conducting outreach. Community-based workers reported difficulties when MSM denied their offers of testing and, instead, pursued the workers themselves for sex – sometimes successfully. This was most obvious when KI 12 (gay male, community-based healthcare worker, living with HIV) stated:

> I have advertisements on social dating apps about CBS [community-based screening] and HIV tests. There are a few who offer sex, but I first decline them, because I am there for the HIV test. But if they insist then I tell them that it is OK if we have sex, but we must be protected, that's what I insist, use condoms.

Such experiences revealed how many of these community-based workers were embedded in these populations, which was a strength of their peer education and testing programmes but also a weakness whenever tensions arose as these workers navigated balancing their professional and personal interests and boundaries. Their embeddedness was also evident when healthcare workers struggled to separate their professional experiences of these apps from their personal use:

> The idea of going to a bar, it's not that common anymore. I mean going to bar and hook-up there? Not common … Wherein my experience, I still use my apps if I go to the bar. I get my hook-ups using the apps, and not only my talking to someone. (KI 16, gay male, community-based healthcare worker)

The assumptions underlying each narrative of risk, opportunity and blame have shaped how the participants and their organisations have responded to the epidemic and the tools they have used to control it. Each of these narratives was informed by an individualised perspective that prioritised the behaviour change of clients in adopting safe sexual practices and coming forward for testing. This individualisation of HIV risk is clear in the framing of online sexual networking as inherently risky, with the onus of responsibility, or blame, lying with the individual. Bryant et al. (2018) argue that these narratives remove risk from its context, ignoring the ways that men protect themselves and each other when having sex. Consequently, each outreach initiative occurred on a one-to-one basis by messaging individual app users. Such initiatives re-installed a biomedical focus on individuals as rational independent agents who, given appropriate information by the healthcare worker, would change their behaviour. In doing so, the healthcare workers lay the blame of being unreachable on these 'hard-to-reach' individuals rather than recognising the broader influences on why people do not engage with healthcare programmes, or how such conceptualisations may further stigmatise same-sex attracted men and hinder much-needed HIV programming (Moen, Aggleton, Leshabari, & Middelthon, 2012).

This kind of initiative also perpetuated a focus on surveillance and control, which has long been the model upon which the government and community response to HIV has been based. Writing on an earlier time in the Philippines' epidemic occurring among female sex workers, Tan (2000) referred to this focus on surveillance and control as *utak pulis*, or 'police brains', with the role of healthcare workers being to track down and provide HIV testing to target populations. He argued that this need for control often manifested itself through a fixation on HIV testing, used as a tool for surveillance and punishment. Central to the process of social control was the creation of the 'other' or 'high-risk groups', or a construction of the 'deviant', seen anew among this current study's participants in the 'hard-to-reach' and 'discreet' subjects of digital health technologies. The new opportunities for surveillance offered by working in the sexualised spaces of the apps, and their ability to identify and regulate what was seen as 'bad behaviour', functioned as an extension of this surveillance and control.

Conclusion

The changing HIV epidemic in the Philippines was regarded by a number of healthcare workers participating in this study as largely due to the rise in online technology use, as these have created a readily available and convenient means of obtaining what was regarded as 'risky' sex. Other participants viewed any 'blame' as determined by how apps were used for 'good' or 'bad' behaviour. Consequently, healthcare workers have reinforced this idea of a 'hard-to-reach' group of men, or 'shadow' populations who must be diligently tracked down. Such reasoning disregarded the agentive capabilities of the apps as transforming sexual practices, delimiting gay space and the ability to shift depictions of the self. Such narratives have led to interventions being diversified, from traditional physical events and place-based outreach at beauty pageants, gay bars and sex-on-premises venues to conducting online health promotion via the apps. However, these online interventions have perpetuated an individualised approach to outreach in prioritising one-to-one interactions and a focus on individual behaviour change. Furthermore, they have reconfigured boundaries between healthcare workers and target populations, as the apps provided a window on to what were viewed as risky individuals practising 'bad behaviour'. In order to understand the complex relational dynamics in which individuals vulnerable to HIV are embedded, a deeper understanding of the social contexts from which MSM are engaging with healthcare is needed, one that engages with the complex and rapidly changing sexual cultures emerging as a result of new technologies.

Given the seriousness of the growing HIV epidemic in the Philippines among MSM, and in the context of an unpredictable political climate and precarious socioeconomic situation, getting the HIV prevention response right for the Philippines is a challenge. Major epidemics elsewhere among MSM occurred largely in recognisable visible gay communities and did so early in the pandemic; the Philippines in experiencing a unique, late emergence of its MSM epidemic in a very different era, one which prevention responses now have a long history, treatments are available (but not accessible to many), and new technologies are changing the face of sexual life. Innovative responses are needed that reflect the particular situation of the Philippines, its old and new sexualities, and its engagement with, not duplication of, the Global North and the global HIV response.

Acknowledgements

Thank you to all who provided support and guidance, with special mention to Professor Michael Tan (former Chancellor of University of the Philippines Diliman), Dr Mikee Inton-Campbell (University De La Salle), and Dr Gundo Weiler and Leila Coppens (WHO Philippines Office).

Disclosure statement

No potential conflict of interest was reported by the author(s).

ORCID

Gary W. Dowsett http://orcid.org/0000-0002-0841-3964

References

Albury, K. (2018). Young people, digital media research and counterpublic sexual health. *Sexualities*, *21*(8), 1331–1336. doi:10.1177/1363460718771338

Bien, C. H., Best, J. M., Muessig, K. E., Wei, C., Han, L., & Tucker, J. D. (2015). Gay apps for seeking sex partners in China: Implications for MSM sexual health. *AIDS and Behavior*, *19* (6), 941–946. doi:10.1007/s10461-014-0994-6

Braun, V., & Clarke, V. (2006). Using thematic analysis in psychology. *Qualitative Research in Psychology*, *3*(2), 77–101.

Brubaker, J. R., Ananny, M., & Crawford, K. (2016). Departing glances: A sociotechnical account of 'leaving' Grindr. *New Media & Society*, *18*(3), 373–390. doi:10.1177/1461444814542311

Bryant, J., Hopwood, M., Dowsett, G. W., Aggleton, P., Holt, M., Lea, T., Drysdale, K., & Treloar, C. (2018). The rush to risk when interrogating the relationship between methamphetamine use and sexual practice among gay and bisexual men. *International Journal of Drug Policy*, *55*, 242–248. doi:10.1016/j.drugpo.2017.12.010

Byron, P., & Albury, K. (2018). 'There are literally no rules when it comes to these things': Ethical practice and the use of dating/hook-up apps. In A. S. Dobson, B. Robards, & N. Carah (Eds.), *Digital intimate publics and social media* (pp. 213–229). Cham, Switzerland: Palgrave Macmillan. doi:10.1007/978-3-319-97607-5_13

Cao, B., Gupta, S., Wang, J., Hightow-Weidman, L. B., Muessig, K. E., Tang, W., Pan, S., Pendse, R., & Tucker, J. D. (2017). Social media interventions to promote HIV testing, linkage, adherence, and retention: Systematic review and meta-analysis. *Journal of Medical Internet Research*, *19*(11), e394. doi:10.2196/jmir.7997

Carballo-Dieguez, A., Ventuneac, A., Bauermeister, J., Dowsett, G. W., Dolezal, C., Remien, R., Balan, I., & Rowe, M. (2009). Is 'bareback' a useful construct in primary HIV-prevention? Definitions, identity and research. *Culture, Health & Sexuality*, *11*(1), 51–65.

Carballo-Diéguez, A., Dowsett, G. W., Ventuneac, A., Remien, R. H., Balan, I., Dolezal, C., Luciano, O., & Lin, P. (2006). Cybercartography of popular internet sites used by New York City men who have sex with men interested in bareback sex. *AIDS Education and Prevention*, *18*(8), 475–489.

Davis, M. (2008). *Sex, technology and public health*. Basingstoke: Palgrave Macmillan.

Department of Health. (2017). Philippines addresses rising trend in new HIV infections [Press release]. Department of Health: Retrieved from https://www.doh.gov.ph/node/10649

Department of Health. (2019). *HIV/AIDS & ART Registry of the Philippines – October-December 2019*. Manila: Department of Health, Epidemiology Bureau.

Dougan, S., Elford, J., Chadborn, T. R., Brown, A. E., Roy, K., Murphy, G., Gill, O. N., & Dukers, N. H. T. M. (2007). Does the recent increase in HIV diagnoses among men who have sex with men in the UK reflect a rise in HIV incidence or increased uptake of HIV testing? *Sexually Transmitted Infections*, *83*(2), 120–125. doi:10.1136/sti.2006.021428

Dowsett, G. W., Wain, D., & Keys, D. (2005). Good gay men don't get "messy": Injecting drug use and gay community. *Sexuality Research and Social Policy*, *2*(1), 22–36.

Gangcuangco, L. M. A. (2019). HIV crisis in the Philippines: Urgent actions needed. *The Lancet Public Health*, *4*(2), e84. doi:10.1016/S2468-2667(18)30265-2

Goedel, W. C., Halkitis, P. N., Greene, R. E., Hickson, D. A., & Duncan, D. T. (2016). HIV risk behaviors, perceptions, and testing and preexposure prophylaxis (PrEP) awareness/use in

Grindr-using Men Who have sex with men in Atlanta, Georgia. *Journal of the Association of Nurses in AIDS Care, 27*(2), 133–142. doi:10.1016/j.jana.2015.11.005

Hakim, J. (2019). The rise of chemsex: Queering collective intimacy in neoliberal London. *Cultural Studies, 33*(2), 249–275. doi:10.1080/09502386.2018.1435702

Hoenigl, M., Little, S., Stockman, J., Skaathun, B., Grelotti, D., Weibel, N., & Smith, D. (2019). Grindr™ on Screen activity on iPhones Correlates with HIV risk and Substance Use in Men Who have Sex with Men, San Diego. *Open Forum Infectious Diseases, 6*(2), S63–S64.

Johnson, W. D., Hedges, L. V., & Diaz, R. M. (2003). Interventions to modify sexual risk behaviors for preventing HIV infection in men who have sex with men. *Cochrane Database of Systematic Reviews,* (1), CD001230. doi:10.1002/14651858.CD001230

Kippax, S., Crawford, J., Davis, M., Rodden, P., & Dowsett, G. (1993). Sustaining safe sex: A longitudinal study of a sample of homosexual men. *AIDS, 7*, 257–264.

Landovitz, R. J., Tseng, C.-H., Weissman, M., Haymer, M., Mendenhall, B., Rogers, K., Veniegas, R., Gorbach, P. M., Reback, C. J., & Shoptaw, S. (2013). Epidemiology, sexual risk behavior, and HIV prevention practices of men who have sex with men using GRINDR in Los Angeles, California. *Journal of Urban Health: Bulletin of the New York Academy of Medicine, 90*(4), 729–739. doi:10.1007/s11524-012-9766-7

Lehmiller, J. J., & Ioerger, M. (2014). Social networking smartphone applications and sexual health outcomes among Men who have sex with men. *PLoS ONE, 9*(1), e86603. doi:10.1371/journal.pone.0086603

Love Yourself. (2020). Giving virtual consultations (Part 2 of 3). *Innovating in times of crisis.* Retrieved from http://www.loveyourself.ph/2020/06/innovating-in-times-of-crisis_1.html

Maloney, K. M., Bratcher, A., Wilkerson, R., & Sullivan, P. S. (2020). Electronic and other new media technology interventions for HIV care and prevention: A systematic review. *Journal of the International AIDS Society, 23*(1), e25439. doi:10.1002/jia2.25439

Moen, K., Aggleton, P., Leshabari, M. T., & Middelthon, A.-L. (2012). Not at all so hard-to-reach: Same-sex attracted men in Dar es Salaam. *Culture, Health & Sexuality, 14*(2), 195–208. doi:10.1080/13691058.2011.632825

Patel, V. V., Masyukova, M., Sutton, D., & Horvath, K. J. (2016). Social media use and HIV-related risk behaviors in young black and Latino gay and bi men and transgender individuals in New York City: implications for online interventions. *Journal of Urban Health, 93*(2), 388–399. doi:10.1007/s11524-016-0025-1

Plummer, K. (2001). *Documents of life 2: An invitation to critical humanism* (K. Plummer Ed.). London: SAGE Publications.

Race, K. (2015a). 'Party and play': Online hook-up devices and the emergence of PNP practices among gay men. *Sexualities, 18*(3), 253–275. doi:10.1177/1363460714550913

Race, K. (2015b). Speculative pragmatism and intimate arrangements: Online hook-up devices in gay life. *Culture, Health & Sexuality, 17*(4), 496–511. doi:10.1080/13691058.2014.930181

Rana, P. (2019, October 3). HIV Cases Soar in the Philippines, as Dating Apps Spread. *Wall Street Journal.* Retrieved from https://www.wsj.com/articles/hiv-cases-soar-in-the-philippines-as-dating-apps-spread-11570095003

Rice, E., Holloway, I., Winetrobe, H., Rhoades, H., Barman-Adhikari, A., Gibbs, J., & Dunlap, S. (2012). Sex risk among young men who have sex with men who use Grindr, a smartphone geosocial networking application. *Journal of AIDS and Clinical Research,* S4. doi:10.4172/2155-6113.S4-005

Ross, A. G., Ditangco, R. A., Belimac, J. G., Olveda, R. M., Mercado, E. S., Chau, T. N., & Crowe, S. M. (2015). The dire sexual health crisis among MSM in the Philippines: An exploding HIV epidemic in the absence of essential health services. *International Journal of Infectious Diseases, 37*, 6–8. doi:10.1016/j.ijid.2015.06.001

Sun, C. J., Reboussin, B. A., Mann, L., Garcia, M., & Rhodes, S. D. (2016). The HIV risk profiles of Latino sexual minorities and transgender persons who use websites or apps designed for social and sexual networking. *Health Education & Behavior, 43*(1), 86–93. doi:10.1177/1090198115596735

Taggart, T., Grewe, M. E., Conserve, D. F., Gliwa, C., & Roman Isler, M. (2015). Social media and HIV: A systematic review of uses of social media in HIV communication. *Journal of Medical Internet Research*, *17*(11), e248. doi:10.2196/jmir.4387

Tan, M. L. (2000). AIDS, medicine and moral panic in the Philippines. In R. Parker, R. M. Barbosa, & P. Aggleton (Eds.), *Framing the sexual subject* (pp. 143–164). London: University of California Press.

UNAIDS. (2017, August 1). UNAIDS report indicates new HIV infections in the Philippines have doubled in the past 6 years [Press release]. Retrieved from https://unaids-ap.org/2017/08/01/press-statement-unaids-report-indicates-new-hiv-infections-in-the-philippines-have-doubled-in-the-past-6-years/

Data-driven intimacy: emerging technologies in the (re)making of sexual subjects and 'healthy' sexuality

Jacinthe Flore and Kiran Pienaar

ABSTRACT

Wireless sex toys are new technologies that enable sexual partners to connect remotely across long distances. Promoted as enhancing intimacy and pleasure as part of a healthy sex life, these devices buttress a 'sex for health' discourse which relies on the collection of intimate data purportedly used to improve current and subsequent teledildonics models. This article draws on two case studies of sex toys developed by leading sex-tech/teledildonic companies Lovense® and Kiiroo® to examine how the relationship between data and sexual subjectivity is being transformed through these emerging technologies. Applying concepts from new materialism, and extending the work of Faustino [(2018). Rebooting an old script by new means: Teledildonics–the technological return to the 'coital imperative'. *Sexuality & Culture*, 22, 243–257]', we explore how sexual practices, intimacy and pleasure become 'datafied' through these sensory technologies. Inspired by the concept of the 'sexuality-assemblage', we pose teledildonic-enhanced sex as a 'sexuotechnical-assemblage', a term that highlights the uniquely technological dimensions of sex in the age of teledildonics. Approaching these devices as sexuotechnical-assemblages highlights the generative role of data as lubricants of long-distance intimacy, and central actors in the (re)making of sexual subjects, and by extension, 'healthy' sexuality.

Introduction

Smart devices are becoming ubiquitous in everyday life, as part of a broader shift in human–computer interactions enabled by advances in voice-activated technology, artificial intelligence, proprietary algorithms, Wi-Fi and Bluetooth. These advances, combined with aesthetically pleasing designs, are converging into an ever smarter and automated Internet of Things (IoT). The convergence of sex and technology has contributed to these innovations: from online pornography to sex 'robots' and wireless sex toys, technology has permeated the domains of sexual desire and intimacy. This article focuses on wireless sex toys – known as 'teledildonics' – in the context of broader changes in sexual and gender norms that have emerged in contemporary, neoliberal societies. Viewed in light of these larger social transformations, the teledildonic is not an unprecedented phenomenon; rather it has evolved alongside other biomedical and biodigital technologies of sex and intimacy, including drugs such as Viagra® for men, and more recent 'sexuopharmaceuticals' targeting women such as Addyi® and Vyleesi® (Cacchioni, 2015; Flore, 2018).

Linking the contemporary neoliberal emphasis on health and wellness with the pursuit of a 'healthy sex life', these technologies contribute to a 'sex for health' imperative which uses 'medical and scientific data connecting regular sexual activity to quantifiable health benefits' (Gupta & Cacchioni, 2013, p. 450). The idea that one can improve health *through* sexual activity brings sex into the ambit of health and can be understood as part of the 'healthicisation' of sex. Connecting sex and sexual pleasure to health optimisation is presented as an uncontroversial health promotion strategy in popular and scientific discourses (Frith, 2015). Within this understanding of sexual pleasure as a prerequisite for good health, the wireless sex toy emerges as an agent of optimisation. It makes previously private, hard-to-access data – intimate practices and preferences – accessible to the broader neoliberal projects of the 'healthicisation' and commodification of sex.

Against this backdrop of the rise of biodigital technologies, the capabilities of teledildonics have been augmented in recent years through new media and data analytics (Bardzell & Bardzell, 2011). As the case studies we will discuss demonstrate, these toys are marketed as sensory devices that can enhance a healthy and active sex life. They aim to engage the whole body in its connections with technology, and they operate through haptic technology or kinaesthetic communication; that is, technology that communicates and responds to movement and touch. Wireless sex toys are typically paired with smartphone applications (apps), which transmit haptic data. In addition to facilitating sexual connections across long distances, some apps enable users to record personal preferences. Designed to personalise intimate experiences and maximise pleasure, teledildonics promise to increase sexual performance and pleasure through the algorithmic analysis of data. Such optimisations can only function through the collection of intimate data that are purportedly used to improve the design of current and subsequent models. Thus, data collection – and the willingness of users to submit their desires to technological optimisation – is central to how these devices work. This article draws on two case studies of sex toys developed by leading teledildonic companies, Lovense® and Kiiroo®, to examine how the relationship between data and sexual subjectivity is being transformed through the design and functionality of these emerging technologies. We focus on the company's flagship wireless sex toys for couples, Lovense's *Max2* (https://www.lovense.com/male-masturbators) and *Nora* (https://www.lovense.com/rabbit-vibrator), and Kiiroo's *Onyx+* (https://www.kiiroo.com/collections/for-him/products/onyx-plus) and *Pearl2* (https://www.kiiroo.com/collections/for-her/products/pearl2). Details of the design and functionality of the devices are provided in the analysis that follows.

Our analysis focuses on the promissory discourses used to market these new technologies and as such builds on research in the sociology of expectations. This body of scholarship has demonstrated that technological innovations involve cycles of hype and disappointment when the promises and predictions of new technologies fail to fully materialise (Brown, 2003; Petersen & Krisjansen, 2015). As Brown (2003, p. 3) observes, 'early hopes [of new technologies] are rarely proportionate to actual future results' but this does little to temper optimistic marketing claims about the promises and value of new technologies. Extending this work, economic sociologists and science and technology studies scholars have charted the role of promissory discourses in creating and maintaining markets (Butler, 2010; MacKenzie, Muniesa, & Siu, 2007; Petersen, 2018). In doing so, they have highlighted the *performativity* of marketing discourses: they help to produce that which they describe, although seldom in a predictable, straightforward manner. Indeed, the performative effects of a marketed product may differ dramatically from its promised outcomes since it is impossible to predict whether actual use by consumers will challenge or disrupt its intended applications.

With this in mind, our article focuses on the marketing discourses and design features of the selected teledildonics. Applying concepts from new materialist approaches, and extending the work of Faustino (2018) on teledildonics and the 'coital imperative', we explore how sex is 'datafied' through these sensory objects. Our analysis also elaborates the concept of the sexuality-assemblage (Fox & Alldred, 2013) by proposing that sex in the age of teledildonics is usefully understood as a 'sexuotechnical-assemblage', a term intended to capture the distinctly technological dimensions of teledildonic-enhanced sex and its implications for contemporary forms of intimacy. We argue that through wireless sex toys, data become the lubricant of long-distance intimacy, and central actors in the (re)making of sexual subjectivities, intimacies and 'healthy' sexuality. We conclude by reflecting on the implications of our analysis for the enactment of sexual desires, gendered bodies and norms of sexual health in relation to the promises and limits of teledildonic sex.

The dynamics of technology and sexuality

The intersections of technology and sexuality have long been a topic of critical social science analysis with scholars tracking the role of technology in transforming sexual practices. For example, studies have highlighted how digital technologies such as the internet, social media and smartphone apps have reshaped a range of sex-related phenomena, including sexual practices (Albury, Burgess, Light, Race, & Wilken, 2017), pornography (Ashton, McDonald, & Kirkman, 2019) and sex work (Jones, 2015). More recently, scholars have turned their attention to internet-enabled sex toys, analysing the history of these devices (Nixon, 2017) and how they shape ideas of intimacy, sexuality and gender (Liberati, 2017). Others have addressed questions of safety and privacy (Wynn et al., 2017) and the role of technology in enhancing pleasure (Bardzell & Bardzell, 2011).

Of particular relevance to this article is the growing body of social science research that examines how new technologies have been harnessed to record and purportedly improve sexual performance. This includes studies of apps that invite users to enter data on the number and duration of sexual encounters, and to record sound levels – taken as indicators of sexual enjoyment – and thrusts per minute (Lupton, 2015). Some of these apps analyse the data using algorithms and then generate graphic representations which users may share with partners to increase mutual enjoyment. Similarly, in some contemporary incarnations, the vibrator has been transformed into a sensory, digitally-connected technology capable of collecting and processing personal data to increase pleasure, and enhance intimacy and sexual wellbeing. Bringing sex into the purview of health through technology (the 'healthicisation of sex') is connected to the broader digitisation of health and the proliferation of apps, wearables and sensors that continually mine data and claim to improve individual wellbeing (Rich & Miah, 2017). Within this broader project of health optimisation, injunctions to monitor sexual activity and individual performance are framed as key aspects of a healthy sex life (Gupta, 2011). Together these studies demonstrate how the domains of sexuality and intimacy have become 'hacked' by the harnessing of data and the possibilities for algorithmic analysis generated through the sensory dimensions of wireless sex toys. Further, the dynamics of promise and optimism play out in promotional discourses that depict teledildonics as enhancing long-distance intimacy, supporting healthy sex lives and augmenting sexual pleasures. The circulation of these discourses, combined with the collection of intimate data, have the potential to transform sexual subjectivities. Individuals are increasingly encouraged to understand desires and sexual activity *through* data and algorithms. This data-driven approach to sex reinforces the prescience of recent calls for an approach to digital sex that sheds light on 'the performative dynamics or affective intents of digital exchange' (Race, 2018, p. 1327). As critical scholars have amply demonstrated, data-driven conceptions of sexual desire and sexuality are inextricably bound up with prevailing social norms and understandings of what constitutes 'sex' (Liberati, 2017; Nixon, 2017).

For example, in a recent analysis of technology-driven transformations to sexual intimacies, Faustino (2018) argues that the design and functionality of wireless sex toys extend the 'coital imperative'. The 'coital imperative' refers to the positioning of peno-vaginal intercourse as the central sex act, which naturalises the reproductive function of heterosexual sex, and valorises sexual practices directed towards achieving male orgasm. Drawing on a feminist discourse analysis of the marketing material of three teledildonics companies Lovense®, Kiiroo® and the now discontinued LovePalz®, Faustino argues that 'the physical interaction promoted by teledildonics devices strategically reduces the sensorial and bodily responses to the genital core' (2018, p. 249). Hence, the design of these devices reproduces legitimate areas of erotic pleasure (genitalia) that are fundamentally heteronormative in their emphasis on penetrative sex. This echoes Berlant and Warner's (1998, p. 562) point that heteronormative intimacy is supported in material ways by institutions, which, we would suggest, include teledildonics corporations. In the process, other desires and practices are relegated to the periphery, and rendered optional extras for the central sexual act. Reading this insight through Rubin's (1984) influential model of the sex hierarchy and the 'charmed circle' of sexual practices, we suggest that by positioning peno-vaginal intercourse as the central sex act, these devices implicitly relegate other, non-heteronormative sexual practices to Rubin's outer circle, constituting them as, at best optional precursors to the 'fundamental' peno-vaginal sex act and, at worst non-normative and deviant. Hence, the design of these devices contributes to reinforcing, rather than challenging the sex hierarchy, suggesting that the model of sexual practices elaborated by Rubin almost three decades ago remains relevant to understanding contemporary sexual norms. To return to Faustino's account of teledildonics and the coital imperative, she notes that they present 'a strong resonance of the reproductive model' (2018, p. 256), a model that remains focused on penetration, with other practices considered optional or merely *en route* to intercourse. Faustino's account powerfully illuminates the heteronormative imperatives underpinning the design and marketing of wireless sex toys. For example, the toys for men are suction devices designed to simulate the act of penetration, while those targeting women are shaped to mimic the penis and include functions to stimulate the clitoris – we discuss these aspects of teledildonics design in more detail below. By examining a key aspect of the sensory experience of teledildonics in action, *data-driven intimacy,* we aim to extend Faustino's analysis. As we go on to argue, in the design and functionality of teledildonics, data are themselves sensory and agentic: they are shaped by and active in shaping the collection and transmission of intimate data.

This raises questions of what kinds of data are being collected and processed by sex-tech companies. Both Lovense® and Kiiroo® emphasise the stringency of their encryption systems. Lovense®, which was the centre of a class action lawsuit related to privacy breaches (Carman, 2017), notes:

> [e]very byte of your data that passes through our servers, including your text, picture, and voice messages, are fully encrypted … All video calls are peer-to-peer with end-to-end encryption and never pass through our servers … none of your data is ever kept on our servers longer than seven days. (Lovense, 2020a)

Meanwhile, Kiiroo's app developer, Feel Technology (2018), notes that it

> collects and stores information like (i) IP address, (ii) Bluetooth MAC address and device type of a device connected to the website and/or app upon 'sharing rooms' within the app and (iii) on- and offline times of devices when connected to an online service. Feel Robotics also collects, but does not store … various sensor values of touch sensors on any and all devices connected to the website and/or app.

Given their dependence on intimate practices, the companies aim to reassure users that sensitive data are not being stored and that any data collected are fully encrypted. Nonetheless, the Lovense case, which it claims was due to a 'minor bug' (Carman, 2017), highlights the slipperiness of data and privacy policies. As Duller and Rodriguez-Amat (2019, p. 230) note, the reliance on online connectivity 'means that the use of those devices involves giving up anonymity and privacy' and the devices produce 'data and metadata that will be stored in computing clouds – that is, on someone else's computer'.

We suggest that these concerns about data privacy, surveillance and algorithmic measurement are heightened in relation to the collection and commercial use of intimate data. Cognisant of the significant implications of teledildonics for new forms of intimate surveillance, our analysis builds on the work of Wilson-Barnao and Collie (2018, p. 741) who argue that teledildonics are indicative of 'refined, distributed, and autonomous forms of an intimate surveillance assemblage'. In line with this interest in intimate surveillance, a growing body of research has identified governance, privacy and control as pressing issues in the context of emerging sexual technologies (Duller & Rodriguez-Amat, 2019). Extending this research, our analysis explores how digital sex technologies are creating novel forms of data- and object-optimised intimacy with significant implications for sexual subjectivity and norms of 'healthy sexuality'. We aim to illuminate the assumptions surrounding sexuality, gender and sexual health that are built into the design of wireless sex technologies, and the ways in which these work to constitute sexual subjects. Doing so involves a shift in focus from epistemological questions – such as what the objects 'represent'– to ontological questions about the kinds of realities that they help to materialise or enact (Mol, 1999). Implicit in the concept of 'enactment' is a recognition of ontological instability and contingency: the idea that phenomena (or 'objects') are not fixed, but rather contingent on their relations with particular human and non-human practices. We elaborate on these ideas next as they relate to our approach to theorising the dynamics of sex toys, data-driven intimacy and sexuality.

Approach: (de)coding technology in the sexuality-assemblage

Queer and post-structuralist approaches to sexuality have long problematised essentialist views and destabilised hetero- and gender-normativity (e.g. Berlant & Warner, 1998; Halberstam, 2005). Scholars drawing on queer theory conceptualise sexuality and gender as dynamic phenomena mediated by historical and social forces, rather than as fixed identities (Berlant, 1998; Butler, 1990). Building on these ideas while affirming the centrality of matter, new materialist approaches have emerged as a 'new metaphysics' within the ontological turn and its efforts to rethink the nature of 'matter' in relation to discourse, power and the body (Dolphijn & van der Tuin, 2012). For example, feminist philosopher Rosi Braidotti has drawn on feminist and new materialist scholarship to theorise sexuality as a 'complex, multi-layered force that produces encounters, resonances and relations of all sorts' (2011, p. 148). Her account challenges the dominant view of sexuality as defined by an enduring pattern of sexual attraction to individuals of a particular gender.

In line with these processual accounts of 'sex' and 'sexuality', Fox and Alldred (2013), apply Deleuze's influential concept of the 'assemblage' to the domain of sexuality, coining the term 'sexuality-assemblage'. Intended to query the status of the human as the sole progenitor of agency and sexual desire, the notion of the 'sexuality-assemblage' explores the affective dynamics of human and non-human actors that jointly produce sex and sexuality. A focus on affective relations does not dispense with the discursive production of sexual norms; instead, it considers discourse as one of the many constitutive dimensions of the sexuality-assemblage. On this understanding, sexuality is not reducible to an effect of matter or discourse, but is a thoroughly *material-discursive* phenomenon (Barad, 2007). Recognising the multiple and distributed nature of sexuality, the concept of the 'sexuality-assemblage' invites close attention to how sexuality is relationally produced through the bio-physical, social, discursive, material, and we would add, technological enactment of bodies. The concept has since been productively applied to analyse sexual harassment in secondary schools (Renold & Ringrose, 2017a), teenagers' use of social media (Renold & Ringrose, 2017b), and young people's sexual practices (Fox & Bale, 2018). Applied to our work, the notion of 'sexuality-assemblage' invites us to approach the wireless sex toy not as fixed object that 'reflects' sexual norms, but as an emergent phenomenon that is both shaped by and active in shaping sexual norms, practices and subjects. Here *all* matter, including the wireless sex toy, the associated app and user data, is relational and agentic in the production of sexual subjectivities.

Treating teledildonics as inextricable from the entanglements of bodies and data extends to how 'biological' data are collected and enacted through sexual practices. We refer here to both the sensory functions embedded in wireless sex toys and the embodied experience of the toy itself. In their encounters with human and non-human actors, sensors can offer 'insights into the interiorities of our bodies and subjectivities' (Smith, 2016, p. 115). As scholars have observed, a life 'optimised' by data and the IoT poses complex ethical and social questions. While these require careful consideration and have been explored in related research (Duller & Rodriguez-Amat, 2019; Lupton, 2016), our concern in this article is to explore how the teledildonic as an emergent technology is (re)shaping sexual subjectivities, with important implications for experiences of intimacy and conceptions of 'healthy sexuality'. Applying the concept of the 'sexuality-assemblage' to the domain of teledildonics, we argue that sex in the age of teledildonics can be referred to as a *sexuotechnical-assemblage*: a term that points to the range of actors and relations imbricated in teledildonic sex, including human bodies and desires, sexual practices, technological devices, internet connections, intimate data, and neoliberal understandings of sexual health.

Methods

Building on Faustino's (2018) analysis of the sexual norms underpinning popular teledildonics, we selected two well-known international companies commercialising teledildonics, Lovense® and Kiiroo®. While both companies offer a range of products, this article focuses on the latest generation of wireless sex toys that are synchronised between remote partners. Our analysis draws on publicly accessible data on the relevant products from Lovense's (*Max 2* and *Nora*) and Kiiroo's (*Onyx+* and *Pearl2*) websites. Importing screenshots into MS Word, we collected and analysed the content published between December 2019 and January 2020, including all previous publications still available online. We also accessed the devices' user manuals and other guidelines on the websites as additional data for our analysis. The data were coded using an iterative inductive approach in which a preliminary list of codes was drawn up based on our overarching interest in the sociosexual and subjectification effects of teledildonics and the relevant social science literatures on sex technologies. The preliminary list of codes related to discourses of sexual pleasure, intimacy and enhancement; the datafication of sexuality; and sex and health (or the 'healthicisation' of sex). These were collaboratively refined and supplementary codes were added across the dataset to capture a wider range of themes derived from the empirical material (Dicks, 2012). Based on the coding, we identified three overarching themes evident in the data: (1) augmented intimacy, (2) detachable body parts and techno-pleasures, and (3) intimate data and the commodification of sex. These themes guided the analysis in terms of the promissory discourses used to market the products, and their relationship to the broader project of enhancing sexual health and wellbeing.

Analysis

Augmented intimacy through teledildonics

Founded in 2010 and based in Hong Kong, Lovense® explicitly brands itself as a teledildonics company with its homepage featuring a banner titled 'Sex tech for every bedroom: Use teledildonics to improve your sex life!' (Lovense, 2020b). While Lovense® offers a range of internet-connected devices, their 'flagship' devices aimed at couples are *Max 2* and *Nora*, with the former targeting men and the latter designed for women. Launched in 2013, Kiiroo® is based in Amsterdam and like its competitor, offers products for 'him', 'her' and 'couples'. Its 'couples sets' comprise several generations of products including *Onyx* + and *Pearl2*, with their sequential names signalling Kiiroo's ongoing quest for innovation 'to keep people satisfied' (Kiiroo, 2020d).[1] In this respect, Kiiroo® collaborates extensively with the Amsterdam-based FeelRobotics, a company that aims to improve how IoT devices communicate. Kiiroo® presents its aim as enabling sexual partners to 'feel [their] lover from anywhere in the world'. Echoing their emphasis on facilitating distance-agnostic intimacy, the 'couples' product page features a large banner claiming that 'Kiiroo® was created to close the gap between long-distance relationships' as '[m]issing your lover hurts less when you can still feel every movement they make' (Kiiroo, 2020a). Implicit here is the role of the devices' internet-connected functionality, sensors and use of personal data in facilitating remote, synchronous sexual connections.

Indeed, both websites' central marketing hook is that the devices are designed to be synched and respond to the movements of remotely located partners. As noted above, they rely on digital connectivity, which in turn enables the collection and transmission of personal, intimate data. We argue that this process constitutes a 'datafication' of sex: a process by which intimate desires and practices are coded as data packets that can travel long distances to a partner. In doing so, data act as lubricants of long-distance intimacy, enabling users to engage in technologically 'augmented' sexual encounters through the exchange and processing of data, or they can relinquish control and allow data sent from a partner's app to program their teledildonic-enhanced pleasures. From a new materialist perspective, the potential of data to act as a lubricant of intimacy raises the question of 'what the body can do to other bodies in assemblages of quantification' (Rich & Miah, 2017, p. 89). Here, data – as an inextricable component of the sexuotechnical-assemblage – enable desires and pleasures to flow through remotely connected teledildonics, while also enacting sexual and affective relations between human and non-human actors. The performativity of data as a lubricant of intimacy is further reflected in how Lovense® and Kiiroo® market the devices as strengthening *coupled* relationships. The potential for three or more people to use the devices simultaneously is not mentioned as a possibility, thus affirming norms of dyadic (heterosexual) monogamy. Further reinforcing dominant sexual and aesthetic norms, the website images used to promote the products suggest that the target demographic is a white, slim and able-bodied heterosexual couple. Kiiroo® in particular features models with athletic and purportedly 'healthy' bodies (Kiiroo, 2020a), which we suggest serves to reproduce an idealised form of 'healthy sexuality' as part of the broader move to bring sex into the purview of health.

Detachable parts for techno-pleasures

Turning to each company's teledildonics products, Lovense's *Max 2* is a suction device with an adjustable air vent, designed to stimulate the penis when it is inserted. For an additional cost, *Max 2* can be fitted with a 'Vagina Sleeve', a pink-cream coloured sleeve, the shape of which is designed to imitate the labia and the interior walls of the vagina. The sleeve's colour is presumably intended to emulate that of flesh racially coded as 'white'. This design choice, along with the images of exclusively white heterosexual couples on Lovense's website, suggests they are the imagined users of these devices, which serves to reinforce a heteronormative, racialised ideal common to the design of many new technologies (Atanasoski & Vora, 2019). The sleeve, comprising one component in a techno-machinery of detachable body parts, claims to offer the user an enhanced sensory experience of vaginal penetration (Lovense, 2020c). For the female partner engaged in long-distance heterosex, *Nora*'s design features aim to stimulate the clitoris and 'optimise' penile penetration. The 'shaft' of the toy purports to 'easily stimulate your G-spot' by rotating and vibrating, and is 'designed to gently stimulate the right places during thrusting' (Lovense, 2020d). Noteworthy here is the heteronormative, phallocentric language: 'shaft' evokes a penis and, coupled with the toy's phallic design, suggests that it is intended to simulate a penis – a point that echoes Faustino's (2018) observation that popular teledildonics rely on and reinforce a heteronormative 'coital imperative'.

Kiiroo's *Onyx+* and *Pearl2* couples sets operate in similar ways to *Max 2* and *Nora. Pearl2* and *Onyx+* are connected via Bluetooth and the FeelConnect app. The 'interactive' male masturbator *Onyx+* is equipped with '10 contracting rings that [simulate] intercourse' (Kiiroo, 2020b). Capable of up to '140 strokes per minute', their pulsations are designed to mimic the vaginal contractions of a partner using *Pearl2*, which offers 'intense vibrations' to users. Much like *Nora, Pearl2* is marketed as the 'world's most technologically advanced G-spot vibrator, designed to fulfil your most intimate needs' (Kiiroo, 2020c). Importantly, as these quotes demonstrate, references to 'the G-spot' feature prominently in the marketing of *Pearl2* and *Nora*. Not only do such references reify the 'G-spot' as a discrete, physiologically homogenous entity that can be targeted in the functionality of the sex toy, they also reiterate the primacy of vaginal over clitoral orgasms. This emphasis ignores the extensive body of feminist research contesting the existence of the G-spot and emphasising that people with vaginas do not only experience orgasms through vaginal penetration (Cacchioni, 2015). Such work has revealed how the notion of the 'G-spot' reinforces the dominant view of the female orgasm as a fundamentally physiological phenomenon, the result of penetrative stimulation of a purportedly highly erogenous area of the vagina. We suggest that the companies' unreflexive emphasis on the G-spot is connected to the 'body work' involved in the healthicisation of sex, which includes the embodied monitoring of sexual responses to maximise pleasures (Gupta, 2011, p. 140). In this regard, it is also worth noting that connections between female orgasms, the G-spot and sexual health are often made in popular media (Frith, 2015). In line with feminist and queer critiques, we suggest that the enactment of the 'G-spot' as a highly erogenous zone erases the specificities of female sexuality and reduces the experience of sexual pleasure to physiological arousal, thus ignoring the affective, erotic and sensual dimensions of pleasure. Despite these reductive assumptions, claims about stimulating the G-spot and vaginal orgasms are not only prominent marketing tools in the Lovense® and Kiiroo® discourses, but depicted as markers of a healthy, pleasurable and increasingly datafied sex life.

In her analysis of *Max2, Nora, Onyx2* and *Pearl2*, Faustino (2018, p. 253) argues that these toys buttress the 'coital imperative' where 'the ubiquity of penetration is left unchallenged' even as the companies claim that their toys are suitable for non-heterosexual couples. We do not dispute this critique of wireless sex toys and indeed, as noted above, our analysis strongly resonates with Faustino's argument. However, in work inspired by feminist and queer theories, the dildo is positioned as a tool that simultaneously valorises peno-vaginal penetration *and* enhances 'fluidity by allowing sexual partners to assume different roles' (Das, 2014, p. 698). This argument reflects the multiple and contradictory positions of sex toys more broadly. Further, the combination of technology, toys designed for men and women, and long-distance partners provokes complex questions pertaining to the entanglement of data, sensors, bodies and subjectivities. We suggest that new materialist perspectives can extend these insights by shedding light on the specificities of these human-technological entanglements. The argument that these devices strengthen the 'coital imperative' focuses on what a particular toy is ostensibly designed to do, that is, its primary and programmed function. However, new materialist approaches consider all matter relational and contingent, made and changed in its encounters with myriad practices, relations and human and non-human phenomena.

Tracing these entanglements illuminates the teledildonic as an object-in-the-making, its materiality contingent and emergent rather than fixed and technologically determined. In other words, rather than treating the teledildonic in conventional terms, as an ontologically bounded object that pre-exists sexual relations and subjects, we treat it as a co-constituted phenomenon, made in its enfolding with other phenomena including human bodies, desires, relationships and modes of intimacy, as well as a host of 'non-human' phenomena such as data connectivity, charged batteries, Virtual Reality equipment, lubricant and sensors. In other words, we approach the teledildonic as 'slippery' matter, unable to be fully contained by its design and programming. Likewise, 'sex' or 'intimacy' in the age of the teledildonic cannot be limited to the 'coital imperative' or other practices more directly associated with sex, such as masturbation using the toy. Rather, sex materialises through a sexuotechnical-assemblage which involves multiple human and non-human actors, agencies and affective relations. With its functionality reliant on the seamless intra-actions of various human and non-human phenomena, the teledildonic exposes sexuality, desire and pleasure as complex achievements, rather than naturally given functions of the human body – a point that echoes the observations of many queer theorists (e.g. Berlant, 1998; Berlant & Warner, 1998), albeit framed here in more explicitly posthumanist terms.

Data as a lubricant: the commodification of sex

In the context of teledildonics, we suggest that data must work as a lubricant; they hold together the sexuotechnical-assemblage and ensure the various human and non-human phenomena intra-act smoothly to facilitate a sexual encounter. A real-time, long-distance intimate encounter requires, for example, an uninterrupted Bluetooth connection, a functioning and recently updated app, and properly charged toys. Reaching for one's smartphone, swiping through to locate the app, loading the app and connecting to a partner's device while ensuring that one's device is functioning, and a partner is doing the same across distance, are all practices – among others – that co-produce a the sexuotechnical-assemblage. Such material and affective flows enact a sexual subjectivity from which data are always inextricable. In addition, personal and intimate data are harnessed and processed for the improvement of future generations of teledildonics. Lovense®, for example, promotes the *Nora* vibrator in terms that highlight this emphasis on data-driven improvement: '*Nora* is the result of years of development and is designed to live up to your needs and expectations. By working with our users, both the hardware and software has been continually perfected to live up to meet your needs' (Lovense, 2020e). The improved versions of the toys and their sensors mean that ever more finely calibrated personal data can be harvested for commercial purposes.

In this way, an individual's intimate data are transformed into valuable assets for commercial purposes and private gains, i.e. to inform targeted marketing and optimisation of current and future teledildonics products. Extending the insights of Campbell and Carlson (2002) on online surveillance and the commodification of privacy, we suggest that the collection and analysis of personal, sexual data can be understood as a 'commodification of techno-intimacy'. This is central to a 'bioeconomy' (Lupton, 2016, p. 93) where bodies, health and intimate pleasures are exploited for commercial purposes. In the case of Lovense® and Kiiroo®, this is not accomplished by 'duping' users into giving information but rather by mobilising the language of physiology and optimisation (e.g. the references to the G-spot), and appealing to the agency of consumers to make informed choices in pursuit of their preferred techno-pleasures. The commodification of techno-intimacy is further reflected in the supplementary products that can be purchased online, supporting a form of bespoke marketing that is tailored to highly individualised desires. For example, *Onyx+* and *Pearl2* offer the option of accessing 'augmented' Virtual Reality (VR) pornographic videos and interactive content (via FeelMe.com) when paired with a compatible VR headset sold separately from the teledildonics. While these devices are primarily marketed as facilitating remote intimacy for couples, some of the toys designed for men (e.g. Kiiroo's *Onyx+* and *Titan* and Lovense's *Max*) are also promoted as enhancing solo sex by integrating virtual porn stars and other VR-porn into the experience of masturbation. Whether the VR features are marketed in terms of their potential to enhance partnered or solo sex, they operate as part of the sexuotechnical-assemblage to further commodify sex and increase the profits of teledildonics' companies and the sex industry more generally.

To draw these threads together, the wireless sex toys we have analysed materialise through networks of human and non-human actors. Central to these networks are sensors that transform physiological responses into data for algorithmic analysis and technological optimisation. In other words, while teledildonics are promoted in ostensibly benign terms as devices for enhancing sexual pleasure and a 'healthy sex life', they rely on the commodification of users' intimate data. The commercial use of these data is legitimated through recourse to discourses of 'health and wellbeing' in which sex is implicitly drawn into the purview of health. Kiiroo®, for example, has a blog that includes articles on the health benefits of masturbation using vibrators and teledildonics (Kiiroo, 2020e). It also has a page listing media reviews of their products that feature comments on the value of teledildonics for sexual wellbeing (Kiiroo, 2020f). Importantly, the healthicisation of sex through technology cannot be viewed as a 'top down' tool of surveillance or control over bodies. Instead, it operates more subtly as a distributed process made possible by the commodification of intimate data, and the willingness of sexual subjects to submit these data for algorithmic optimisation. This process contributes to the operation of the sexuotechnical-assemblage where teledildonic sex, desires, individual bodies and sexual health norms converge to generate sexual subjects defined in part by the commodification of their intimate data.

Importantly, the sexuotechnical-assemblage is characterised by ontological multiplicity and contingency: it varies in relation to the specificities of the Kiiroo® and Lovense® products (among a host of other factors). In this respect, it is worth highlighting a key difference between the features of each company's couples sets: Lovense® offers an 'intelligent playback feature' that Kiiroo's teledildonics does not feature. The website presents 'intelligent playback' as popular among military couples who are often apart (Lovense, 2020d). This particular function demonstrates the *capaciousness and agency of data*: beyond simply enabling the devices to be optimised, the collection of data can then be harnessed to 'play back' users' preferences, allowing users to re-enact intimate moments (whether alone or together). It seems particularly apposite, when speaking of the agency of data, to reflect on Barad's comment that '[m]atter, feels, converses, suffers, desires, years and remembers' (cited in Dolphijn & van der Tuin, 2012, p. 59). Data here are agents *of* and *with* memory: the algorithms enable the teledildonics to reference (or 'remember') users' preferences in order to reproduce intimate encounters. In this way, desires and sexual practices, specifically those leading to simulated peno-vaginal penetration (the coital imperative) are repeated and reinforced.

Conclusion

In this paper, we have applied concepts from new materialist scholarship to theorise digitally-connected sex toys as objects-in-the-making, their materiality contingent and emergent, rather than fixed and technologically determined. Doing so has enabled us to trace the network of human and non-human forces that intra-actively constitute sex in the age of teledildonics. Within this network (or what we refer to as the 'sexuotechnical-assemblage'), intimate data play a key role: physiological responses are not simply data mined to improve performance, data here are themselves sensory and act as lubricants of intimacy. The data generated through users' engagement with sex technologies actively participate in the sexuotechnical-assemblage. We have also highlighted the ontological instability of the teledildonic, tracing the ways in which it materialises through its entanglement with human bodies, sexual practices, data flows and algorithmic analysis. Or to put this in terms of the sexual encounter, the wireless sex toy is a 'slippery' object, both in the sense of acting as a lubricant of intimacy and in the more fundamental sense of being mercurial, open-ended and shape-shifting.

Teledildonics' potential to generate pleasure, combined with sensors and continual communication with apps, has material implications for how these devices enact sexual subjects, desire and intimacy. Further, the experiences of pleasure or intimacy are simultaneously corporeal *and* embedded in socio-sexual (and gendered) norms. The devices, then, can be understood as generating new forms of algorithmic intimacy and bio-technical sexual subjectivities from which the collection, processing and circulation of data are inextricable. Users submit their intimate data for algorithm-driven optimisation, which is marketed as enabling product improvements, but the underlying imperative remains commercial. The commodification of intimate data has implications for the sexual norms underpinning these emerging technologies. In this respect, the reproduction of narrow, heteronormative assumptions about sexuality is significant as it contributes to enacting an increasingly globalised, commercialised and monolithic form of sexuality partly defined through the digital transmission of intimate, personal data.

To return to the concept of the 'sexuality-assemblage' that inspired this analysis, it encompasses all the relations that materialise sex, including human desires and intimate practices, and non-human actors such as smartphones, sex toys and data. To capture the technological dimension of teledildonics we have elaborated the notion of the sexuality-assemblage, coining the term 'sexuotechnical-assemblage'. We have also sought to extend Faustino's (2018) analysis beyond the coital imperative by tracing how the sexuotechnical-assemblage enacts 'datafied' forms of subjectivity, sexuality and sexual health. Rather than a static, stable subject that pre-exists the sexuotechnical-assemblage, the subject materialises as, and through, *networked* sexual subjectivity, produced through specific sexual practices in their encounters with teledildonics, associated apps and the processing of intimate data. On this view, data cannot be considered exterior to sexual subjectivity. Instead the data generated through teledildonics literally and figuratively penetrate the interiority of bodies, desires and subjectivities, in the process enabling intimate encounters to be commodified in the service of 'optimising' current and future sex products. This, we suggest, may have an impact on how teledildonics are used and how they are helping to (re)make sexual subjects in the digital age. While beyond the scope of this article, these issues point to important avenues for future research that could include ethnographies and interviews with users of teledildonics. Such work has the potential to shed much-needed light on the affective and embodied transformations wrought by the sexuotechnical-assemblage of teledildonics.

Note

1. The companies' respective marketing strategies emphasise their quest for continual technological improvement. This is evident in the fact that during the course of drafting this article, Kiiroo® launched a new version of *Onyx*, the *Onyx+*. The functionalities remain largely similarly to *Onyx2*, but it is marketed as quieter and more effective at 'simulating intercourse' (Kiiroo, 2020b).

Disclosure statement

No potential conflict of interest was reported by the author(s).

ORCID

Jacinthe Flore http://orcid.org/0000-0002-3136-9236
Kiran Pienaar http://orcid.org/0000-0003-4770-7882

References

Albury, K., Burgess, J., Light, B., Race, K., & Wilken, R. (2017). Data cultures of mobile dating and hookup apps: Emerging issues for critical social science research. *Big Data & Society*, *4*(2), 1–11.

Ashton, S., McDonald, K., & Kirkman, M. (2019). What does 'pornography' mean in the digital age? Revisiting a definition for social science researchers. *Porn Studies*, *6*(2), 144–168.

Atanasoski, N., & Vora, K. (2019). *Surrogate humanity: Race, robots, and the politics of technological futures*. Durham: Duke University Press.

Barad, K. (2007). *Meeting the universe halfway: Quantum physics and the entanglement of matter and meaning*. Duke University Press.

Bardzell, J., & Bardzell, S. (2011, May). 'Pleasure is your birthright': Digitally enabled designer sex toys as a case of third-wave HCI. In G. Fitzpatrick et al. (Ed.), *CHI '11 proceedings of the SIGCHI conference on Human Factors in Computing Systems* (pp. 257–266). ACM SIGCHI Conference on Human Factors in Computing Systems.

Berlant, L. (1998). Intimacy: A special issue. *Critical Inquiry*, *24*(2), 281–288.

Berlant, L., & Warner, M. (1998). Sex in public. *Critical Inquiry*, *24*(2), 547–566.

Braidotti, R. (2011). *Nomadic theory*. New York: Columbia University Press.

Brown, N. (2003). Hope against hype: Accountability in biopasts, presents and futures. *Science Studies*, *16*(2), 3–21.

Butler, J. (1990). *Gender trouble: Feminism and the subversion of identity*. New York: Routledge.

Butler, J. (2010). Performative agency. *Journal of Cultural Economy*, *3*(2), 147–161.

Cacchioni, T. (2015). *Big pharma, women and the labour of love*. Toronto: University of Toronto Press.

Campbell, J. E., & Carlson, M. (2002). Panopticon.com: Online surveillance and the commodification of privacy. *Journal of Broadcasting & Electronic Media*, *46*(4), 586–606.

Carman, A. (2017). Sex toy company admits to recording users' remote sex sessions, calls it a 'minor bug' [webpage]. Retrieved from https://www.theverge.com/2017/11/10/16634442/lovense-sex-toy-spy-surveillance.

Das, A. (2014). The dildo as a political transformative tool: Feminist and queer perspectives. *Sexuality & Culture, 18*, 688–703.

Dicks, B. (2012). *Digital qualitative methods. Volume 3: Data analysis*. London: SAGE Publications.

Dolphijn, R., & van der Tuin, I. (Eds.). (2012). *New materialism: Interviews & cartographies* (pp. 48–70). Ann Arbor: Open Humanities Press.

Duller, N., & Rodriguez-Amat, J. R. (2019). Sex machines as mediatized sexualities: Ethical and social implications. In T. Eberwein, M. Karmasin, F. Krotz, & M. Rath (Eds.), *Responsibility and resistance: Ethics in mediatized worlds* (pp. 221–239). Wiesbaden: Springer.

Faustino, M. J. (2018). Rebooting an old script by new means: Teledildonics–the technological return to the 'coital imperative'. *Sexuality & Culture, 22*, 243–257.

Feel Technology. (2018). Privacy [webpage]. Retrieved from https://feeltechnology.com/privacy.php.

Flore, J. (2018). Pharmaceutical intimacy: Managing female sexuality through Addyi. *Sexualities, 21* (4), 569–586.

Fox, N. J., & Alldred, P. (2013). The sexuality-assemblage: Desire, affect and anti-humanism. *The Sociological Review, 61*, 769–789.

Fox, N. J., & Bale, C. (2018). Bodies, pornography and the circumscription of sexuality: A new materialist study of young people's sexual practices. *Sexualities, 21*(3), 393–409.

Frith, H. (2015). Sexercising to orgasm: Embodied pedagogy and sexual labour in women's magazines. *Sexualities, 18*(3), 310–328.

Gupta, K. (2011). 'Screw health': Representations of sex as a health-promoting activity in medical and popular literature. *Journal of Medical Humanities, 32*, 127–140.

Gupta, K., & Cacchioni, T. (2013). Sexual improvement as if your health depends on it: An analysis of contemporary sex manuals. *Feminism & Psychology, 23*(4), 442–458.

Halberstam, J. (2005). *In a queer time and place: Transgender bodies, subcultural lives*. New York: NYU Press.

Jones, A. (2015). Sex work in a digital era. *Sociology Compass, 9*(7), 558–570.

Kiiroo. (2020a). For couples [webpage]. Retrieved from https://www.kiiroo.com/collections/for-couples#product-details.

Kiiroo. (2020b). KIIROO® Onyx+™ Interactive Male Masturbator [webpage]. Retrieved from https://www.kiiroo.com/products/onyx-plus.

Kiiroo. (2020c). KIIROO® Pearl2™ G-Spot Vibrator [webpage]. Retrieved from https://www.kiiroo.com/products/pearl2.

Kiiroo. (2020d). KIIROO® Our Story [webpage]. Retrieved from https://www.kiiroo.com/pages/about.

Kiiroo. (2020e). KIIROO® Articles [webpage]. Retrieved from https://www.kiiroo.com/search?q=health.

Kiiroo. (2020f). KIIROO® Welcome to our press kit! [webpage]. Retrieved from https://www.kiiroo.com/a/press-kit.

Liberati, N. (2017). Teledildonics and new ways of 'being in touch': A phenomenological analysis of the use of haptic devices for intimate relations. *Science Engineering Ethics, 23*, 801–823.

Lovense. (2020a). Privacy [webpage]. Retrieved from https://www.lovense.com/faq/Privacy.

Lovense. (2020b). Sex tech for every bedroom: Use teledildonics to improve your sex life! [webpage]. Retrieved from https://www.lovense.com/.

Lovense. (2020c). Max2: Revolutionizing male masturbators [webpage]. Retrieved from https://www.lovense.com/male-masturbators.

Lovense. (2020d). Nora: The original Bluetooth vibrator [webpage]. Retrieved from https://www.lovense.com/rabbit-vibrator.

Lovense. (2020e). Our long-distance sex toys are the best way to stay intimate! [webpage] Retrieved from https://www.lovense.com/long-distance-sex-toys.

Lupton, D. (2015). Quantified sex: A critical analysis of sexual and reproductive self-tracking using apps. *Culture, Health & Sexuality, 17*(4), 440–453.

Lupton, D. (2016). Digital health technologies and digital data: New ways of monitoring, measuring and commodifying human bodies. In F. X. Olleros, & M. Zhegu (Eds.), *Research handbook in digital transformations* (pp. 85–102). Cheltenham: Edward Elgar Publishing.

MacKenzie, D. A., Muniesa, F., & Siu, L. (Eds.). (2007). *Do economists make markets? On the performativity of economics*. Princeton: Princeton University Press.

Mol, A. (1999). Ontological politics. A word and some questions. *The Sociological Review, 47*(S1), 74–89.

Nixon, P. G. (2017). Hell yes!!!!! Playing away, teledildonics and the future of sex. In P. G. Nixon, & I. Düsterhöft (Eds.), *Sex in the digital age* (pp. 201–212). London: Routledge.

Petersen, A. (2018). Capitalism on ageing anxieties: Promissory discourses and the creation of an 'anti-ageing treatment' market. *Journal of Sociology, 54*(2), 191–202.

Petersen, A., & Krisjansen, I. (2015). Assembling 'the bioeconomy': Exploiting the power of the promissory life sciences. *Journal of Sociology, 51*(1), 28–46.

Race, K. (2018). Towards a pragmatics of sexual media/networking devices. *Sexualities, 21*(8), 1325–1330.

Renold, E., & Ringrose, J. (2017a). Pin-balling and boners: The posthuman phallus and intra-activist sexuality assemblages in secondary school. In L. Allen, & M. Rasmussen (Eds.), *The Palgrave handbook of sexuality education* (pp. 631–635). London: Palgrave Macmillan.

Renold, E., & Ringrose, J. (2017b). Selfies, relfies and phallic tagging: Posthuman part-icipations in teen digital sexuality assemblages. *Educational Philosophy and Theory, 49*(11), 1066–1079.

Rich, E., & Miah, A. (2017). Mobile, wearable and ingestible health technologies: Towards a critical research agenda. *Health Sociology Review, 26*(1), 84–97.

Rubin, G. S. (1984). Thinking sex: Notes for a radical theory of the politics of sexuality. In G. S. Rubin (Ed.), *Deviations: A Gayle Rubin reader* (pp. 137–181). Durham: Duke University Press.

Smith, G. J. D. (2016). Surveillance, data and embodiment: On the work of being watched. *Body & Society, 22*(2), 108–139.

Wilson-Barnao, C., & Collie, N. (2018). The droning of intimacy: Bodies, data, and sensory devices. *Continuum: Journal of Media & Cultural Studies, 32*(6), 733–744.

Wynn, M., Tillotson, K., Kao, R., Calderon, A., Murillo, A., Camargo, J., … Rueda, S. (2017, November). Sexual intimacy in the age of smart devices: Are we practicing safe IoT? In T. Benson, & S. Sundaresan (Eds.), *IoTS&P'17 Proceedings of the 2017 Workshop on Internet of Things Security and Privacy* (pp. 25–30). ACM Conference on Computer and Communications Security.

Conceptualising the continuum of female genital fashioning practices

Alexandra James, Jennifer Power and Andrea Waling

ABSTRACT

Genital fashioning practices, such as Brazilian waxing and female genital cosmetic surgery, have become increasingly prevalent within contemporary western societies. This paper explores the role of genital fashioning in the construction of contemporary femininity. It uses in-depth interviews and focus groups with Australian women aged 18–30 to investigate female genitalia as a site of alteration. Drawing on broader understandings of the body as socially mediated, this paper contends that multiple modification practices are employed to produce genital appearance. It departs from previous investigations which consider genital fashioning practices in isolation. In identifying the scope of genital fashioning, this research reveals a continuum of genital fashioning practices, both physically and discursively mobilised by women to negotiate their identity, sexuality, and femininity.

Introduction

Female genitalia have held cultural significance throughout history in art, culture, and folklore. Recently, however, they have become a site for modern beauty regimens. With increased popularity of pubic hair removal since the 1980s (Labre, 2002), female genitalia receive greater scrutiny than in the past and have become a more visible part of feminine presentation and performance. The new ideal genital appearance is characterised by a 'clean slit'; hairless, pale in colour, with a hidden labia minora (McDougall, 2013). A large range of genital fashioning options have emerged as routine components of pursuing this ideal – from hair removal to surgery – with a marked increase in demand for these practices over recent decades (Braun, Ticklebank, & Clarke, 2013; McDougall, 2013; Tiggemann & Hodgson, 2008; WHV, 2013).

Options for pubic hair fashioning are extensive, ranging from trimming and styling to a full 'Brazilian', involving removal of all hair from the genital and anal regions (Labre, 2002). Australian and international research has shown a majority of young women remove substantial or total amounts of their pubic hair (Braun et al., 2013; Li & Braun, 2017; Tiggemann & Hodgson, 2008). Other forms of temporary genital modification include vajazzling, in which diamantes or sequins are glued to a hairless mons pubis (Turney, 2016), vaginal or anal bleaching, or use of genital deodorising products (wipes, powders, douches) (Herbenick et al., 2012). Women have also begun to adopt permanent modifications, including genital (labia or clitoral) piercing, pubic tattooing (Armstrong, Caliendo, & Roberts, 2006; Davis, 2002), and genital cosmetic surgery (FGCS). FGCS takes genital fashioning practices far outside beauty clinics, tattoo parlours or do-it-yourself forms of modification. Labiaplasty or vulvoplasty are expensive surgical procedures with costs varying between AUD$3,500-$9,000 (Nurka, 2019). Yet surveys have shown increasing demand for FGCS within Australia, the U.S. and U.K. (Braun, 2010; WHV, 2013).

There is an observable continuum between Brazilian waxing and more extreme forms of genital fashioning. Although labiaplasty and other surgical procedures are relatively rare compared to hair removal, some researchers suggest women who remove public hair may be more likely to adopt further practices of genital modification (DeMaria & Berenson, 2013). Tiefer (2008, p. 467) identifies the hairless vulval norm as having made female genitalia 'more visible and exacerbated pre-existing negative genital perceptions', thus contributing to demand for FGCS.

Trends in genital fashioning

Female genitalia have long attracted specific 'pudendal disgust' (Tiefer, 2008), with trends in genital modification reoccurring throughout history. Surgical intervention began with practices of labiaplasty recorded during the Greco-Roman period (Nurka, 2019). Similarly, pubic hair removal has a long history; ancient Egyptians reported to have removed all of their body hair, including pubic hair. However, in this period, bodily depilation was a normative practice for men and women (Hope, 1982). It has been suggested that contemporary preferences for labial size have their origins in racist, colonial disdain for the Hottentot apron; the supposed elongated labia of south-west African women serving to distinguish them from European counterparts as less human *and* less feminine (Jones, 2017; Nurka, 2019). Hope (1982) documents more recent trends in female public hair depilation, with the U.S. advertising industry instrumental in establishing norms of underarm and leg hair removal during the period 1915–1945. Normative notions of the hairless female body culminated in full pubic hair removal trends in the late 1980s. In 1994, the J-Sisters Salon in New York brought the 'Playboy bikini wax' to the public – later to become the Brazilian wax (Labre, 2002). Likewise, contemporary trends of labiaplasty emerged in the early 1980s (Braun, 2010) and became more commercial in the 1990s with the promotion of the 'designer vagina' (Tiefer, 2008). Analysis of medical marketing or surgical discourses found the promotion of an idealised designer vagina described as 'neat', symmetrical, with unprotrusive labia minora (Braun, 2010; McDougall, 2013).

There are various explanations for increased attention on genital aesthetics. Some argue the trend occurred as a result of the feminist push to destigmatise and demystify the vagina (Holliday, 2018). However, with only some exceptions (Holliday, 2018; Nurka, 2019), it is often attributed to widespread accessibility of internet-based pornography in tandem with expanded commercial services in hair removal and enhanced popularity of cosmetic surgery (Braun, 2010; Braun et al., 2013; Green, 2005; McDougall, 2013). Cosmetic surgery is also increasingly normalised and publicised through various media (Labre, 2002), via reality television and celebrities (e.g. Schott, 2016), with genitals joining the list of standard sites for procedures. Genital fashioning operates in a context where media and the body are entangled in a symbiotic relationship; media images represent the body, and the body is surgically altered to conform to media imagery (Jones, 2017).

Feminist scholars have observed an inherent contradiction between presentations of genital modification in advertising, often framed in discourses of sexual agency and empowerment, and the practices themselves, which entrench greater restriction on women's bodily agency (Li & Braun, 2017). The once ignored aesthetics of the vagina are increasingly subject to scrutiny, surveillance and judgment. Greater availability and awareness of FGCS reinforces normative aesthetics by the implication that anything other than the ideal 'vulval slit' can, or should, be 'fixed' (McDougall, 2013). The 'problem' of an imperfect vagina has been created by the existence of a (commercial) surgical 'solution' (Braun, 2010). Likewise, the development and advertisement of hygiene products also contribute to a cultural disdain for genitalia. These narratives position natural, unmodified female genitalia as deficient (Braun & Kitzinger, 2001) and form a component of the cultural lexicon in which women's genitalia are considered 'smelly' (Braun & Wilkinson, 2001) and in need of remediation through the purchase of products.

The culmination of contemporary trends toward fashioning of genitalia have resulted in the vagina being publicly scrutinised. Genitalia are now a locus of cultural tension in which women inscribe meaning upon their body through modification. Women make decisions about how to mark their bodies as appropriately feminine, risking social judgement and stigma if they fail to meet normative standards. As with other beauty ideals, standards for genital appearance can constitute a source of anxiety for women, with negative self-perceptions potentially impacting adversely on sexual health, self-esteem and sexual enjoyment (WHV, 2013). Dissatisfaction with genital appearance can prompt women to seek surgical intervention, and is a rising concern in some countries including the U.K., U.S. and Netherlands (Zwier, 2014). In an Australian study, a 'sizeable percentage' of women sampled (17%) expressed interest in undergoing labiaplasty (Sharp, Tiggemann, & Mattiske, 2015) and, in a study by Simonis, Manocha, and Ong (2016), almost all surveyed Australian general practitioners reported having been asked about the normality of genital appearance by patients.

Choice, agency, and engagement in genital refashioning

Women's engagement with beauty practices has come under much scrutiny in feminist literature. Early works positioned beauty practices as oppressive, designed to keep women as decorative objects for men's pleasure (e.g. Wolf, 1990). Bartky's (2002) work includes similar themes regarding thinness, highlighting that if women remain focused on their weight, they have limited capacity to engage in areas of social life traditionally reserved for men. Women's use of beauty modification practices, such as surgery, has been positioned as a form of oppression, whereby women are compelled to engage in bodily transformations to appease a heterosexist male gaze (Bartky, 1997).

Contemporary scholars, such as McGladrey (2015), Davis (1995) and Gill (2007a), have sought to build on feminist narratives by analysing women's agency in their choices to use beauty products or modify their bodies, and how that functions within structures of oppression. For instance, Davis (1995) calls for an appreciation of cosmetic surgery, arguing it should be seen as oppressive *and* liberating. Cosmetic surgery, for Davis (1995), is undertaken in the context of oppressive social structures, but is generally a rational and considered choice about its value (relative to the risks). It is seen as something that can enhance individual value and power. McGladrey (2015) argues that investigation of how young women engage in beauty practices needs to consider how practices can be simultaneously pleasurable and problematic. Women receive some intrinsic pleasure from the process, even if they are in some ways 'complicit' in oppressive norms.

Gill (2007a) presents a nuanced perspective on choice and agency that accounts for contradictions and complexities. Gill (2007a) critiques contemporary post-feminist ideology, wherein traditional modes of femininity have been replaced by the celebration of consumerist values, encapsulated by assertiveness, materialism, and individualism. Scholars have observed that women are subject to intensified expectations around bodily production via beauty practices (Gill, 2007a). Post-feminist ideology recasts such practices as empowering or liberating, as a practice of self-care, rather than a source of oppression (Gill, 2007b). Advertising for cosmetic surgery frames it as 'the best or most effective means of attaining satisfaction, chosen by the most active, self-reliant subjects' (Fraser, 2003, p. 39). Such ideas are observable in FGCS discourses (Braun, 2010) as well as those underpinning the promotion of other genital fashioning practices, such as vajazzling (Turney, 2016) and Brazilian waxing. Gill argues that post-feminist assumptions of beauty practices as empowering obscure the social and commercial forces which produce and police choices. She also argues that women often have a detailed and complex understanding of their social environment which needs acknowledgement alongside feminist critique of beauty practices. Jones (2017) similarly argues that labiaplasty represents a method for managing how others view the body and, whilst individuals are unable to control meanings that others project onto them, labiaplasty provides the opportunity to reflexively negotiate cultural scripts and self-display.

Despite creating (often unachievable) beauty standards for women, genital fashioning is also part of the complex ways in which women negotiate feelings of inadequacy or enhance self-confidence. For example, genital piercings have been associated with enhanced sexual experience, expression and positive self-perception (Armstrong et al., 2006). Likewise, pubic depilation has been found to be pleasurable and shape sexual expression and confidence (Herbenick et al., 2012; Tiggemann & Hodgson, 2008). However, others (Labre, 2002) have suggested that women may experience bodily satisfaction as a result of adhering to feminine norms of hairlessness.

When situated within contemporary makeover cultures and self-display norms (Widdows, 2018), post-feminism (Gill, 2007a), and women's reclaiming of a more visual or raunchy sexuality (Gill, 2007b), there are opportunities to critically consider how women engage in genital fashioning. In this paper, we aim to better understand how Australian women engage with genital fashioning practices. We examine women's attitudes toward the range of options for genital fashioning, how they view such practices, and the ways women make sense of their choices to adopt, or reject them.

Methodology and methods

Methodology

This research is underpinned by a feminist, post-structural methodology in which the body is positioned as socially produced rather than a biological given. In exploring tensions between women's decisions to engage with genital fashioning, and the structural imperatives to maintain idealised standards of appearance, we draw on Gill's concept of contextualised choice whereby 'women make choices ... but they do not do so in conditions of their own making' (2007a, p. 72). Following Davis (1995), we contend that research participants are knowledgeable actors, who are aware of cultural limitations but make decisions in accordance with their needs and desires. Considering the embodied subject as situated within context, not 'statically determined by it' (Davis, 1995, p. 169), we acknowledge that participant choices about genital modification operate within the confines of femininity, but can also shape this culture. Genital fashioning presents a tension, whereby women are not free from patriarchal influence and beauty cultures, but are not necessarily without capacity to consider their decisions within these framings (Gill, 2007a). In this research, we attend closely to *how* participants make sense of their choices.

This approach is in keeping with Gill's (2007a) proposal of 'critical respect' as a way to make sense of how women engage with practices of body modification, whilst seeking to 'interrogate the structures of everyday life' (Gannon & Davies, 2012, p. 73) and make visible the social pressures which inform engagement with beauty practices. Gill's (2007a) concept of critical respect is utilised as a framework to prioritise women's perspectives whilst critically situating these within a cultural context.

Terminology

Feminist writers have noted the problems and uncertainties associated with terms to describe female genitalia (Braun & Kitzinger, 2001). Anatomically, the vagina refers to the birth canal, 'the "passage" between a woman's external genitals and her cervix' (Braun & Wilkinson, 2001). However, whilst 'vagina' may be popularly misappropriated within lay talk and surgical advertising, neither vagina nor vulva accurately describes the entirety of female genitalia (Frueh, 2003). The complexity of terminological reference to female genitalia has resulted in numerous feminist attempts to reclaim terms laden with culturally symbolic meanings, such as 'vagina' and 'cunt' (Braun & Wilkinson, 2001; Rees, 2013). To contribute to this process of reclamation and reflect the ordinary usage of terms with which women are comfortable (Braun & Wilkinson, 2001), the term vagina is adopted in this paper.

Methods

Young women's understandings of genital fashioning were investigated through in-depth qualitative interviews and focus groups with Australian women aged 18–30. The age range was selected on the basis of literature showing greater popularity of genital alteration among young women (DeMaria & Berenson, 2013), and the lead author's own 'insider' status within this cohort, aiding in access to the research population (Corbin Dwyer & Buckle, 2009).

Qualitative research was used to explore the nuance in young women's choices about genital fashioning. Focus groups generate rich responses through group interaction (Lewis in Wilkinson, 1998) and are guided by participants (Wilkinson, 1998), in keeping with the aim to prioritise participant perspectives. However, the sensitive nature of the topic required offering options of single person interviews for participants uncomfortable discussing the topic in a group setting.

There was no requirement that study participants had experience in any form of genital fashioning as the aim was to explore attitudes, not direct experience. The study, project number CF14/3999–2014002045, was approved by Monash University Research Ethics Committee.

Recruitment

Participant recruitment was conducted via a combination of advertising and word-of-mouth promotion. Research flyers were displayed in women's bathrooms on university campuses. To increase participant numbers, word-of-mouth promotion was undertaken via the researcher's university network. Contacts were provided with a copy of the recruitment flyer that could be forwarded to potentially interested parties. In all cases, participation was self-selected.

Data collection – focus groups

In 2014/2015, 11 focus groups were conducted and audio recorded with a total of 28 women participating. Each group lasted 30–50 min and was conducted in safe, public venues such as library meeting rooms. Focus groups were guided by a series of open questions (Appendix 1) about participants' understanding of genital fashioning and the social context associated with the uptake of such practices; however, participants were free to guide discussion.

Data collection – interviews

Following the focus groups, in-depth one-on-one audio-recorded interviews were conducted with 10 women, of which four had also participated in a focus group. Interviews lasted 20–40 min and were semi-structured. Topics included: norms of genital appearance, the role of media in informing women of genital ideals, the influence of sexual partners, and the 'right' or 'wrong' reasons to engage in genital fashioning. Interview participants were asked to comment on an extract about genital fashioning from Cosmopolitan magazine to elicit thoughts on media representation of these practices (Appendix 2). The open nature of the interview questions allowed participants scope to discuss ideas to the extent with which they felt comfortable. This resulted in the wide variation of interview session lengths.

Participant characteristics

As this was a small self-selected sample largely recruited from a university campus, the majority of participants had, or were undertaking, higher education. A small number were not students and had not previously obtained tertiary degrees. Those participants with higher education ranged widely in their level and discipline of degree.

Participants were asked about their relationship with feminism. The majority described themselves as feminists, ranging from liberal to radical feminists, or indicated support of the feminist movement. Only two regarded themselves not to be feminists. Feminism in Australia has been noted to have an increasingly broad influence on the lives of young women (Garden & Toffoletti, 2017), with visibility in public discourse on issues such as sexual objectification, sexual and domestic violence, and mothering. It is also important to note that studies on gender and sexuality, such as this one, are more likely to attract participants involved in, or cognisant of, social movements such as feminism (Strassberg & Lowe, 1995).

Demographic questions around ethnic identity, sexuality, social background, or area of residence were not asked. However, during discussion, participants indicated they were from a range of social backgrounds and the sample included people from rural, outer suburban and inner-city locations.

Data analysis

The method of thematic analysis applied is drawn from Braun and Clarke (2006) who outline processes for inductive coding of qualitative data in which data are coded according to broad themes and refined into sub-themes through further identification of patterns, trends, emphasis, tensions or discord within the data.

Findings

Whether physically enacted or discursively mobilised, genital fashioning locates the vagina as a site through which normative femininity is negotiated. Below, we discuss the ways in which women discussed genital fashioning as differentially normative, subversive, or commercialised.

Pubic depilation – a normative, hygienic, and expected practice

The majority of interview and focus group participants discussed pubic depilation as a normative and routine practice among women, particularly for younger generations:

> I would say most ladies in Australia under the age of 40 don't have hair [on their pubic area]. (Ally, IP)

> These days it is more normal to get a Brazilian or just go out and get a wax or just go out and completely be bald. And I think a lot of people have sort of grown up with that and … having pubic hair is no longer normal. (Dianne, IP)

Despite agreement that full pubic hair removal was normal for young women, participants reflected on it being enforced on younger women through pressure from peers, media or partners. Young women were seen as more vulnerable to this pressure than older women due lessened capacity to resist, or critically assess, the practice:

> I really felt the pressure [to wax] when I was younger, for sure. (Ling, FGP)

> Yeah. Up until the age of 17, 18, I used to do pretty much what was standard, what most young women do. Shaving everything basically. (Nelle, FGP)

The topic of hygiene arose in various contexts throughout the participant discussion. The extent to which a practice is considered hygienic became part of young women's critical appraisal of the practice, its social implications and, in some cases their narratives for depilation. Participants associated pubic depilation with *feelings and perceptions* of hygiene, generally agreeing that social messages led women *and* men to regard a hairless genital region as more hygienic:

> I definitely think there is a really common theme about people thinking its unhygienic not to shave. I definitely think that the really common perspective is that you're unhygienic [if you're unshaved]. (Willow, FGP)

Participants were aware that narratives about hygiene impacted how women viewed their body by positioning the unwaxed vagina as unclean or improper for women:

> About the waxing, some women say that it's cleaner. Like hair is something dirty. [The] Vagina smells because of the hair … People make us think that women's bodies are dirty and you have to try to clean most as you can, like with all your hair gone. (Phoebe, FGP)

However, being aware of the social impact of waxing practices did not necessarily empower women to challenge them. Many participants were unsure whether the hygiene narrative was based on fact or not, but it influenced how they felt about waxing. Removing hair helped them to feel clean:

> I mean, it's nature, so probably just, if you leave it that's perfectly fine … But I think it feels, sometimes it feels like, my friends wax, and I might have a quick shave every now and then, it just feels cleaner. But I think there's a difference between feeling clean, and actually being more hygienic, if you know what I mean? (Andy, FGP)

Participants were similarly critical of vaginal hygiene products. However, they were more likely to regard the need for these products as artificially promoted through marketing campaigns that drew on broader discourses positioning female genitalia as unclean or odorous:

> I know that there's a lot of marketing around having a clean smelling vagina, and how bullshit that is really for health. … And also washing vaginas and stuff, cause there's, you know, a lot of marketing around dirty vaginas and therefore you must wash. 'Femfresh' bullshit. (Nelle, FGP)

Likewise, the commercial promotion of bleaching products was discussed as mobilising women's insecurities about genital appearance:

> I guess media plays in a way to just hurt them into what they actually want to sell … Right now, if whitening is in then I'm going to sell it to you to say that a white vagina is nice. (Alexis, IP)

Alexis' comment reveals how colonial imaginations continue to shape ideals of beauty and hygiene – dark vaginas are considered less nice and less hygienic (LaForteza, 2016; Nurka, 2019). In this way, social powers and hierarchies of race are perpetuated through body altering practices which reinforce stigma associated with darkness (LaForteza, 2016) – be it anal bleaching or genital lightening washes – in each case, whiteness is insidiously preferenced.

The normalisation of pubic depilation, compared to use of hygiene products or bleaching, meant participants were more likely to hold ambivalence about hygiene arguments – they understood that the hygiene argument was not factual and had negative implications for how women's bodies were perceived, but were comfortable accepting that they 'felt' cleaner with a waxed vagina. The use of hygiene or bleaching products, however, was viewed critically as something being 'sold' to women. A similar narrative about the commercialisation of waxing or shaving was not evident.

Female genital cosmetic surgery – achieving normality

As with depilation, participants' attitudes toward FGCS wavered between critical awareness of social pressure and empathy, or experiential understanding, of why women might pursue surgery. Participants were aware FGCS was both a product, and a cause, of an ever-narrowing view of what is considered a 'normal' vagina:

> I think there are a lot of norms that, like a lot of women think that oh this is normal, is my vulva and vagina supposed to look like this, which encourages that type of behaviour like waxing and labiaplasty. (Monica, IP)

> I think stuff like labiaplasty is, you know, my labia don't look normal. I want to look normal. Not even about looking sexy, I think it's genuinely about being normal. (Willow, IP)

Participants were empathetic about people's desires to have their body look 'normal', Sookie said:

> I mean, I can understand if people wanted to get surgery you know, to fix lengths or things like that. I mean, my stepsister had that done which, I mean, I don't think it makes much of a difference but like, visually I think it bugs people, you know, those kind of things. (Sookie, FGP)

Even if they adopted a critical stance on normality as a concept, participants generally did not rule out surgery as an option they might pursue in particular circumstances. Summer explained, she would probably undertake surgery if she were unhappy with her body, even though she recognised that surgery may not provide a resolution to this:

> If I was definitely very unhappy and felt that I wasn't sexually confident … I would probably get surgery. But at the same time … I'd have to recognise that it would probably be my own problem, and if I could overcome it in a way that wasn't surgery then I think that would be beneficial. (Summer, FGP)

Similarly, Carol explained the availability of surgery with an option to manage the negative emotional impact of these pressures and insecurities, even if it did not address the cause:

> I guess they don't feel comfortable with themselves. I don't want to generalise, but a lot of plastic surgery seems to be 'cause they're not feeling comfortable with their bodies so they want to alter it. (Carol, FGP)

Genital piercings and tattooing – subverting norms

In contrast to pubic depilation or FGCS, which were done in the interests of achieving an ideal genital appearance, genital piercings and tattoos were seen as non-normative and resisting this ideal. They were associated with empowerment and linked to greater personal choice:

> It depends on, like, their relationship with their body and, um, like, I think definitely genital piercing and all of that would be a choice, but probably not hair removal. (Carol, FGP)

> Those people who do tattoos and piercings, I don't think they're very influenced by the society but they actually, they like to express themselves. (Phoebe, FGP)

By their cultural association with an enhanced sense of agency and resistance to normative practices, piercing and tattoos were seen to be means of marking individuality in a way practices like waxing were not:

> I think maybe if, it was like a piercing or tattoo, maybe they might draw more identity, same as if you had like a regular tattoo somewhere else or a piercing on your face or something, um, it might have to do with your identity. But waxing nor surgery I don't, I see it more just as like a practice that you do, whereas tattoos or piercings then you might get I don't know, more identity related reasons, or things like that. (Sookie, FGP)

Although participants considered genital piercings as practices associated with enhanced agency, and occasionally discussed them as a means of reclaiming the body, participant conversation also revealed stigmatising perceptions of piercings and tattoos:

> Well even my tattoo. I first of all got it as a yeah, I own my body, this is my thing. As a bit of a joke too, like, 'cause a bit of trauma's attached to that area, but it was kind of like you need to remember to laugh, like you came through and you need to laugh. You know what I mean? This is your body and you own it. But at the same time I remember reading an article that was like, oh well girls who get stuff down there are, that's kind of a bit more out of the norm, that kind of points to that they're really messed up. And that messed me up for a few months. I kind of sat there and go, well, well, am I? (Faith, FGP)

Genital tattoos and piercings were discussed as physical markers of the 'other', related to subversive and alternative cultures, but also associated with perceptions of sexually deviant behaviour:

> Like you see, you know, the pierced girl, and you know, oh she's probably got one down there, she's a bit you know, weird. And she'll be into the freaky stuff. (Ebony, IP)

The stigma associated with tattoos and piercings reinforces its status as a non-normative, empowering practice; undertaken by women actively seeking to differentiate their embodied femininity from conventional appearance norms. The transgressive nature of bodily modifications such as intimate piercings may therefore challenge normative gendered bodies and identities. Practices of genital piercings and tattooing can be understood within the context of other modification options that enact 'an identity shifting performance which "destabilize[s] many of our preconceived notions about beauty, identity, and the female body"' (Pitts-Taylor, 1998, p. 80).

Vajazzling – a commercialised practice

In contrast to piercings and tattoos, vajazzling was viewed as a frivolous practice. Unlike other forms of genital fashioning, which were considered legitimate options for bodily modification – be it to normalise or reclaim the body – vajazzling was generally positioned as a commercially driven and media promoted practice that was not worth the cost:

> I just think ugh how ridiculous, what a waste of time. I guess you've got nothing better to do. I mean you would have to have a lot of time and a lot of cash, I'm just too much of a cheapskate. I'd sooner have I don't know my eyebrows or my lashes tinted or something else, that's so far down on the list, I think it's a bit ridiculous. (Andy, FGP)

Laughter frequently accompanied discussion of vajazzling which was regarded a comical practice, a parody of femininity. The participants' mocking and scorn of vajazzling served to distinguish their own position of correctly embodied femininity from women who go too far:

> We started talking about vajazzling, like putting diamantes, because apparently Jennifer Love Hewitt started that whole thing. I feel like that's really silly. We laughed about it. We actually sat around and laughed at it. 'Cause I was like, what do you do, get your hot glue gun and stick on diamonites? (Patty, FGP)

The vajazzled body reveals the artifice of femininity and, in altering the vagina in an obvious manner, the practice destabilises notions of femininity as natural (Jones, 2008). In participant discussion, vajazzling serves to distinguish the Other, those that engage in genital fashioning to a level deemed too extreme, and, in so doing, solidifies notions of normal and acceptable embodiment as achievable through practices of pubic depilation or FGCS.

Discussion

The study's findings reveal there is no form of genital presentation free from scrutiny or judgment – even the unmodified 'natural' vagina has a social meaning and value attached to it. For the women in this study, perceptions of genital modification were framed by negotiation of what it means to be feminine *and* feminist, whereby different genital fashioning practices contained varying meanings associated with choice, agency, and bodily normality.

Previous research has identified women's reluctance to identify their own depilatory practices as influenced by social pressure (Tiggemann & Lewis, 2004). Our research builds on this, showing how descriptions of genital modification contain multiple, sometimes contradictory, narratives that enable women to feel comfortable to engage in genital modification while acknowledging these practices are products of social pressures on women to look 'normal'. The participants reproduced feminist understandings of the natural body as a 'feminist body' (Holliday, 2018). Participants recognised that vaginal modification was linked to social pressure and bodily insecurity, especially for young women, and it was implicit in participant narratives that the 'natural', unmodified vagina was more aligned with feminist values (Holliday, 2018). However, there were also multiple references to the 'normal' vagina. Depilated genitalia were described by several participants as 'normal', especially younger women. 'Normal' was not the same as 'natural'. If anything, an unwaxed, natural vagina was considered abnormal because it was less common for women not to wax. There is a tension that emerges here, whereby women are negotiating notions of the 'natural' and the 'normal' vagina, as articulated by competing discourses of feminism (the natural) and medical and beauty industries (normal). 'Achieving normality' was the core basis on which most participants explained their own genital modification and empathised with others who undertook more extreme modification, such as labiaplasty, to normalise their vaginal appearance.

The women were aware, and critically engaged, with social pressures to appear 'normal'. However, this also resulted in participants' awareness and ability to articulate the impact of not adhering to normative feminine standards. As such, the women did not view the choice to wax, or modify their vagina in other ways, as undermining their feminism or values. A possible interpretation could locate this as a function of social pressure and the commericalisation of beauty regimes – as practices are normalised, they become less visible and subject to critique. However, this does not account for participant's social critique of vaginal modification. Participants located their critique in practices with which they did not engage or which were not seen as part of normal practice. Waxing was described as normal, and less subject to critique, but labiaplasty was seen as extreme or invasive, and vajazzling or use of hygiene wipes was seen as overly commercial and tacky. By distancing themselves from these practices, participants held a critical lens to genital modification practices in general. However, by normalising their own practices, they avoided judging themselves – or their own choices – under this same lens.

Norms of genital appearance exert control over options for female embodiment, but at the same time the women in this study were using genital fashioning practices to actively negotiate their relationship to their identity and social position. Some theorists have argued that women are positioned as lacking agency or insight if they engage in any form of beauty practice or body modification (for example Jeffreys, 2005), positioning the 'natural' unmodified body as a form of agency – a choice to not modify. This, of course, is problematic given that all forms of bodily presentation hold cultural meaning (Fraser, 2003; Jones, 2008; Pitts-Taylor, 2009). There is no 'natural' body that exists outside of gendered cultural norms. Women are continually required to navigate the cultural meanings ascribed to their body and bodily practices, both in terms of how they feel about themselves and how they are 'read' by others. Real or imagined, this viewer serves as the panoptic disciplinarian as women reflexively negotiate their identity in response to perceived cultural expectations and repercussions.

The extent to which women are subject to this ongoing scrutiny remains more extreme, with more severe consequences attached to failure, than it does for their cisgender male counterparts. While men have long since become subject to bodily appearance standards (Bordo, 1999), including for their genital presentation (Braun et al., 2013), they are generally afforded access to a wider array of embodiment options as well as options for cultural power that are not reliant on appearance alone. This is dependent on where men are situated culturally, economically, socially, and politically. For example, gay and bisexual men are more likely to experience bodily surveillance and appearance expectations than straight men (Duncan, 2010). However, for women, their access to power is continually located in their appearance, and the often-extreme measures they are expected to engage to achieve this (i.e. dieting, surgery, fitness regimes) which has economic, political, and social impacts (Bartky, 2002). As noted by previous feminist scholars (Bartky, 1997; Widdows, 2018; Wolf, 1990), this cycle risks further limiting women's power as they remain focused on achieving impossible appearance standards that take up time, energy, mental and physical capacity, and financial resources.

Women in this study were aware of beauty standards imposed on women, young women in particular, and spoke about this in relation to genital modification practices. However, they did not necessarily apply this lens to their own practice or describe their personal genital fashioning as disempowering. These findings problematise traditional approaches to understanding women's engagement with beauty practices and present new opportunities for conceptualising the complexities and tensions between experience, identity, and practice that pay attention to both experiences of oppressive gendered power relations, and engagements with body modification practices.

For the women in this study, the function of genital modification in shaping identity was dependent on both the discursive and physical mobilisation of bodily alteration practices. The way women described these practices was just as important as the physical act. Narratives around tattoos and genital piercing as subversive had potential to imbue an individual with a greater sense of agency as such narratives align with subversion of oppressive feminine ideals and 'reclaiming' the body (Pitts-Taylor, 2003). Similarly, narratives describing waxing as 'normal' enabled participants to construct an experience of waxing that was uncomplicated – it was just something that all women do rather than something they are pressured to do. For researchers, attending to the narratives to describe body modification practices can reveal how women navigate social pressure, stigma and judgment in accordance with their own sense of what it means to have agency or be a feminist. Our findings show that participants were keen to hold onto their critique of genital modification practices while also describing their practices in ways that recognised their choice as well as their lack of choice.

Conclusion

In examining the full range of genital fashioning practices, it is possible to examine the ways women consider genital fashioning and make sense of these practices in relation to each other. Genital fashioning practices work together to construct normative ideals – women produce their identity by partaking in some practices and not in others. Understandings of genital fashioning as a disciplinary practice influenced by cultural norms for women are not limited to academic dialogue; perhaps as a result of a broad uptake of (post)feminist ideology and strong media literacy. This was evident among women in this study. They were keenly aware of the social sanctions and circumstances within which they operate – but did not consider it a viable option to abstain from genital fashioning without risking social sanction. Instead, they constructed their own state of being and identity through discursive processes – the way they spoke about genital fashioning practices.

Female genitalia are an important site in the contemporary construction of feminine embodiment; it is a site at which women negotiate complex and often contradictory ideas about their identity, sexuality, femininity, agency and feminism. Genital fashioning practices inscribe meaning on the body, even in instances when women do not engage with them – the presence of pubic hair acquiring as much cultural meaning as the absence. As such, there is no body which remains free from cultural inscription. Exploring women's attitudes to a continuum of genital fashioning and modification practices enabled us to unpack women's narratives regarding their engagement in genital fashioning in a unique way. Women's feelings and descriptions of their own practices were often described in relation to awareness of the range of genital fashioning practices, not just those they had personally adopted.

Different practices of genital fashioning have differing social implications, but all exist on a continuum. The continuum of genital fashioning is both physically and discursively used by women to navigate the cultural and social context of beauty practices. Contemporary western culture is characterised by an intensification of requirements for the physical inscription of femininity on the body (Gill, 2007a), whilst, at the same time, there is a more visible presence of feminist discourse and ideology. In this study, the narratives constructed around genital fashioning enabled young women to maintain their critical, feminist stance toward social expectations for female embodiment, yet also partake in practices to avoid the sanctions of which they were acutely aware.

Acknowledgements

This research was conducted as component of a Ph.D. at Monash University, supervised by Professor Jo Lindsay and Professor JaneMaree Maher. It was made possible by the generous contributions of research participants. Thanks to The Australian Sociological Association Families and Relationships Mentoring Program and mentor Dr Emma Kirby for support in producing this paper.

Disclosure statement

No potential conflict of interest was reported by the author(s).

Funding

This project was supported during PhD candidature through the Australian Postgraduate Award.

ORCID

Jennifer Power http://orcid.org/0000-0002-6566-3214
Andrea Waling http://orcid.org/0000-0003-1370-5600

References

Armstrong, M. L., Caliendo, C., & Roberts, A. E. (2006). Genital piercings: What is known and what people with genital piercings tell us. *Urologic Nursing*, *26*(3), 173–179.

Bartky, S. (1997). Foucault, femininity, and the modernization of patriarchal power. In D. T. Meyers (Ed.), *Feminist social thought: A reader* (pp. 129–154). New York, NY: Routledge.

Bartky, S. (2002). *'Sympathy and solidarity' and other essays*. Lanham, MD: Rowman & Littlefield.

Bordo, S. (1999). *The male body*. New York, NY: Farrar, Straus and Giroux.

Braun, V. (2010). Female genital cosmetic surgery: A critical review of current knowledge and contemporary debates. *Journal of Women's Health*, *19*(7), 1393–1407.

Braun, V., & Clarke, V. (2006). Using thematic analysis in psychology. *Qualitative Research in Psychology*, *3*(2), 77–101.

Braun, V., & Kitzinger, C. (2001). The perfectible vagina: Size matters. *Culture, Health & Sexuality: An International Journal for Research Intervention and Care*, *3*(3), 263–277.

Braun, V., Ticklebank, G., & Clarke, V. (2013). 'It shouldn't stick out from your bikini at the beach': Meaning, gender, and the hairy/hairless body. *Psychology of Women Quarterly*, *37*(4), 478–493.

Braun, V., & Wilkinson, S. (2001). Socio-cultural representations of the vagina. *Journal of Reproductive and Infant Psychology*, *19*(1), 17–32.

Corbin Dwyer, S., & Buckle, J. L. (2009). The space between: On being an insider-outsider in qualitative research. *International Journal of Qualitative Methods*, *8*(1), 55–63.

Davis, K. (1995). *Reshaping the female body: The dilemma of cosmetic surgery*. New York, NY: Routledge.

Davis, S. W. (2002). Loose lips sink ships. *Feminist Studies*, *28*(1), 7–35.

DeMaria, A. L., & Berenson, A. B. (2013). Prevalence and correlates of pubic hair grooming among low-income Hispanic, black, and white women. *Body Image*, *10*(2), 226–231.

Duncan, D. (2010). Embodying the gay self: Body image, reflexivity and embodied identity. *Health Sociology Review, 19*(4), 437–450.

Fraser, S. (2003). The agent within: Agencies repertoires in medical discourse on cosmetic surgery. *Australian Feminist Studies, 18*(40), 27–44.

Frueh, J. (2003). Vaginal aesthetics. *Hypatia, 18*(4), 137–158.

Gannon, S., & Davies, B. (2012). Postmodern, post-structural and critical theories. In S. N. Hesse-Biber (Ed.), *Handbook of feminist research: Theory and praxis* (2nd ed., pp. 65–91). Thousand Oaks, CA: Sage.

Garden, H., & Toffoletti, K. (2017). Feminism, celebrity and lifestyle in the Australian digital news site Mamamia. *Outskirts, 36*, 1–20.

Gill, R. C. (2007a). Critical respect: The difficulties and dilemmas of agency and 'choice' for feminism. *European Journal of Women's Studies, 14*(1), 69–80. Retrieved from http://peer.ccsd.cnrs.fr/docs/00/57/12/97/PDF/PEER_stage2_10.1177%252F1350506807072318.pdf

Gill, R. C. (2007b). Postfeminist media culture: Elements of a sensibility. *European Journal of Cultural Studies, 10*(2), 147–166.

Green, F. J. (2005). From clitoridectomies to 'designer vaginas': The medical construction of heteronormative female bodies and sexuality through female genital cutting. *Sexualities, Evolution and Gender, 7*(2), 153–187.

Herbenick, D., Hensel, D., Smith, N., Schick, V., Reece, M., Sanders, S. A., & Fortenberry, J. D. (2012). Pubic hair removal and sexual behavior: Findings from a prospective diary study of sexually active women in the United States. *The Journal of Sexual Medicine, 10*(3), 678–685.

Holliday, R. (2018). Vagina dialogues: Theorizing the 'designer vagina'. In G. Griffin & M. Jordal (Eds.), *Body, migration, re/constructive surgeries* (pp. 192–208). Oxon: Routledge.

Hope, C. (1982). Caucasian female body hair and American culture. *Journal of American Culture, 5* (1), 93–99.

Jeffreys, S. (2005). *Beauty and misogyny*. New York, NY: Routledge.

Jones, M. (2008). *Skintight*. Oxford: Berg.

Jones, M. (2017). Expressive surfaces: The case of the designer vagina. *Theory, Culture & Society, 34* (7–8), 29–50.

Labre, M. P. (2002). The Brazilian wax: New hairless norm for women? *Journal of Communication Inquiry, 26*(2), 113–132.

LaForteza, E. (2016). *The somatechnics of whiteness and race*. London: Taylor and Francis.

Li, A. Y., & Braun, V. (2017). Pubic hair and its removal: A practice beyond the personal. *Feminism & Psychology, 27*(3), 336–356.

McDougall, L. J. (2013). Towards a clean slit: How medicine and notions of normality are shaping female genital aesthetics. *Culture, Health & Sexuality, 15*(7), 774–787.

McGladrey, M. (2015). Lolita is in the eye of the beholder: Amplifying preadolescent girls voices in coversations about sexualization, objectification and performativity. *Feminist Formations, 27*(2), 165–190.

Nurka, C. (2019). *Female genital cosmetic surgery*. Cham: Palgrave Macmillian.

Pitts-Taylor, V. L. (1998). 'Reclaiming' the female body: Embodied identity work, resistance and the Grotesque. *Body & Society, 4*(3), 67–84.

Pitts-Taylor, V. L. (2003). *In the flesh: The cultural politics of body modification*. New York, NY: Palgrave Macmillian.

Pitts-Taylor, V. L. (2009). Becoming/being a cosmetic surgery patient. *Studies in Gender and Sexuality, 10*(3), 119–128.

Rees, E. L. E. (2013). *The vagina*. New York, NY: Bloomsbury Academic.

Schott, J. (2016, April 12). Everything you wanted (or didn't want) to know about the $3,500, Kardashian-endorsed 'vaginal laser'. *Elle*. Retrieved from www.elle.com/beauty/news/a35562/kardashian-vaginal-laser/

Sharp, G., Tiggemann, M., & Mattiske, J. (2015). Predictors of consideration of labiaplasty: An extension of the tripartite influence model of beauty ideals. *Psychology of Women Quarterly, 39*(2), 182–193.

Simonis, M., Manocha, R., & Ong, J. J. (2016). Female genital cosmetic surgery: A cross-sectional survey exploring knowledge, attitude and practice of general practitioners. *BMJ Open*, *6*. doi:10.1136/bmjopen-2016-013010

Strassberg, D. S., & Lowe, K. (1995). Volunteer bias in sexuality research. *Archives of Sexual Behavior*, *24*, 369–382.

Tiefer, L. (2008). Female genital cosmetic surgery: Freakish or inevitable? Analysis from medical marketing, bioethics, and feminist theory. *Feminism & Psychology*, *18*(4), 466–479.

Tiggemann, M., & Hodgson, S. (2008). The hairless norm extended: Reasons for and predictors of women's body hair removal at different body sites. *Sex Roles*, *59*(11–12), 889–897.

Tiggemann, M., & Lewis, C. (2004). Attitudes toward women's body hair: Relationship with disgust sensitivity. *Psychology of Women Quarterly*, *28*(4), 381–387.

Turney, J. (2016). Vajazzled!!! Pursuits for the hirsute. *Clothing Cultures*, *3*(2), 143–153.

Widdows, H. (2018). *Perfect me*. Princeton, NJ: Princeton University Press.

Wilkinson, S. (1998). Focus groups in feminist research: Power interaction, and the co-construction of meaning. *Women's Studies International Forum*, *21*(1), 111–125.

Wolf, N. (1990). *The beauty myth*. London: Vintage.

Women's Health Victoria (2013). *Women and genital cosmetic surgery*. Author. Retrieved from http://whv.org.au/publications-resources/publications-resources-by-topic/post/women-and-genital-cosmetic-surgery-issues-paper/

Zwier, S. (2014). 'What motivates her': Motivations for considering labial reduction surgery as recounted on women's online communities and surgeons' websites. *Sexual Medicine*, *2*(1), 16–23.

Appendices

Appendix 1. Focus group discussion guide

- **What were your thoughts when you first heard about this project?**
- **Can you tell me what you would associate with the term genital fashioning or modification?**
  (Prompt: Any specific practices?)
- **What are your opinions and thoughts about genital modification practices?**
  (Prompts: Reasons? Associated benefits or drawbacks?)
- **Can you tell me about any recent media discussion, or discussions you may have had or overheard, about genital fashioning?**
  (Prompts: Media articles offering options or advice? Any discussion amongst friends?)
- **Can you share with me any experiences you or your friends may have had in relation to genital fashioning?**
  (Follow up: Were there any circumstances around this experience that stood out for you?)
- **Why do you think women might want to their genitalia?**
  (Prompt: Does modification or not have any bearing on a woman's identity? Does modification relate to hygiene? Is it a matter of choice?)
- **Are there any stories you may wish to share with me in relation to our discussion today?**
- **Can you tell me about your relationship to feminism?**

Appendix B. Extract from Cosmopolitan magazine

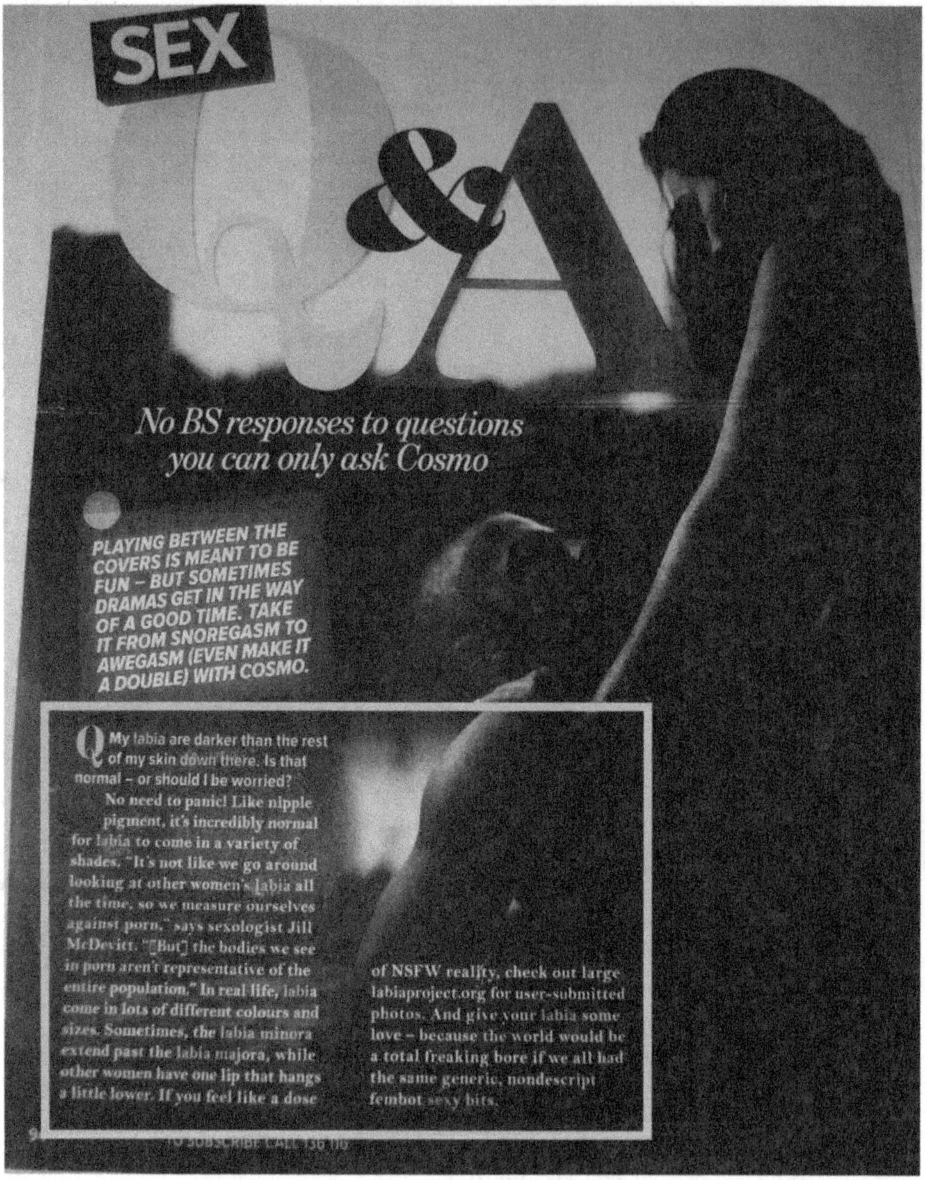

SEX

Q&A

No BS responses to questions you can only ask Cosmo

PLAYING BETWEEN THE COVERS IS MEANT TO BE FUN – BUT SOMETIMES DRAMAS GET IN THE WAY OF A GOOD TIME. TAKE IT FROM SNOREGASM TO AWEGASM (EVEN MAKE IT A DOUBLE) WITH COSMO.

Q My labia are darker than the rest of my skin down there. Is that normal – or should I be worried?

No need to panic! Like nipple pigment, it's incredibly normal for labia to come in a variety of shades. "It's not like we go around looking at other women's labia all the time, so we measure ourselves against porn," says sexologist Jill McDevitt. "[But] the bodies we see in porn aren't representative of the entire population." In real life, labia come in lots of different colours and sizes. Sometimes, the labia minora extend past the labia majora, while other women have one lip that hangs a little lower. If you feel like a dose of NSFW reality, check out largelabiaproject.org for user-submitted photos. And give your labia some love – because the world would be a total freaking bore if we all had the same generic, nondescript fembot sexy bits.

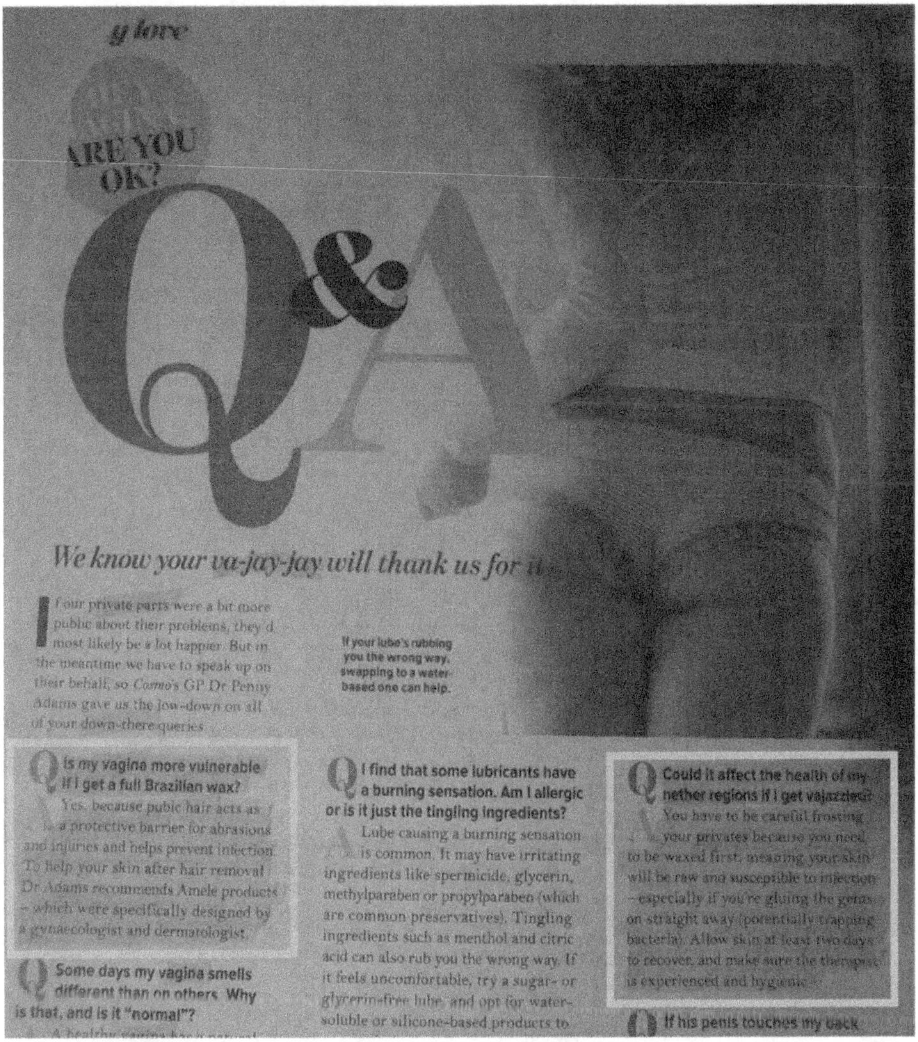

ARE YOU OK?

Q&A

We know your va-jay-jay will thank us for it

If our private parts were a bit more public about their problems, they'd most likely be a lot happier. But in the meantime we have to speak up on their behalf, so *Cosmo's* GP Dr Penny Adams gave us the low-down on all of your down-there queries.

Q Is my vagina more vulnerable if I get a full Brazilian wax?

A Yes, because pubic hair acts as a protective barrier for abrasions and injuries and helps prevent infection. To help your skin after hair removal Dr Adams recommends Amele products – which were specifically designed by a gynaecologist and dermatologist.

Q Some days my vagina smells different than on others. Why is that, and is it "normal"?

Q I find that some lubricants have a burning sensation. Am I allergic or is it just the tingling ingredients?

A Lube causing a burning sensation is common. It may have irritating ingredients like spermicide, glycerin, methylparaben or propylparaben (which are common preservatives). Tingling ingredients such as menthol and citric acid can also rub you the wrong way. If it feels uncomfortable, try a sugar- or glycerin-free lube, and opt for water-soluble or silicone-based products to

If your lube's rubbing you the wrong way, swapping to a water-based one can help.

Q Could it affect the health of my nether regions if I get vajazzled?

A You have to be careful frosting your privates because you need to be waxed first, meaning your skin will be raw and susceptible to infection – especially if you're gluing the gems on straight away (potentially trapping bacteria). Allow skin at least two days to recover, and make sure the therapist is experienced and hygienic.

Q If his penis touches my back

The age of LARC: making sexual citizens on the frontiers of technoscientific healthism

Jenny Dyck Brian, Patrick R. Grzanka and Emily S. Mann

ABSTRACT

Routinely positioned as the 'first-line option' for contraceptive choice-making, long-acting reversible contraception (LARC) promotion efforts have come under critical scrutiny by reproductive justice advocates for the extent to which public health actors' preference for LARC devices may override potential users' ability to freely (not) choose to use contraception among an array of options. We identify LARC promotion discourse as constituting 'The Age of LARC': multifarious strategies for producing responsible sexual citizens whose health behaviours are empowered via a LARC-*only* approach to contraceptive use. We suggest that immediate postpartum LARC insertion policies, which have proliferated in the U.S. since 2012, exemplify the new era of LARC hegemony, in which urgency, efficiency, cost-effectiveness, and outcomes dominate both health policy and clinical practice around these contraceptive technologies. By following these efforts to facilitate access to and use of immediate postpartum LARC, we find a discourse on sexual citizenship that paradoxically constructs sexual health freedom through the use of a single class of contraceptive technologies.

In 2012, South Carolina introduced a Medicaid guidance for immediate postpartum long-acting reversible contraception (LARC) insertion. LARC, which include intrauterine devices (IUD) and subcutaneous implants, are contraceptive technologies that are inserted in the body for the purpose of preventing pregnancy for up to 10 years. Policies like the South Carolina guidance provide physicians and hospitals with payment for IUD or implant insertion after a woman[1] on Medicaid has given birth and usually within a specified time period. Since 2012, 43 U.S. states and the District of Columbia have since adopted similar policies, effectively creating a nationwide policy regime of immediate postpartum LARC. These extra-juridical and extra-legislative policies are all created within the amorphous space of Medicaid rules and regulations, which are largely controlled by individual states' Medicaid offices (Walls et al., 2016). Proponents of the new policies argue that LARC is a safe, effective and affordable means of reducing unintended pregnancies (Rodriguez, Evans, & Espey, 2014).

South Carolina's policy was described as a novel way to deal with the enduring problem of reducing unintended pregnancies (e.g., Bingham, 2017). *The New York Times* detailed the perceived successes:

> The change seems to have done the unimaginable: connect large numbers of poor women with new methods of birth control that have the potential to give them a lot more say over when, and with whom, they have children. Since South Carolina started the policy in 2012, unplanned pregnancies have declined by 6 percent, and the state Medicaid office has saved $1.7 million. (Tavernise, 2016)[2]

LARC promotion, as constituted by public health campaigns, policy statements (e.g. American Academy of Pediatrics, 2014; CDC, 2015; WHO, 2012), advertisements, and clinical research, is expressly about health and empowerment, particularly among those at elevated risk for unplanned and short-interval pregnancies, including young and low-income women, who are disproportionately women of colour (Thomas & Karpilow, 2018).

While LARC promotion discourse is characterised by well-intentioned appeals to help women and families, LARC promotion efforts—especially immediate postpartum strategies—raise important questions about the state's role in regulating reproductive practices, particularly those of society's most marginalised: young, poor, racial-ethnic minority women. In response to the Medicaid policies and increased enthusiasm for LARC in public health, the National Women's Health Network and SisterSong (2016) released a joint statement:

> We reject efforts to direct women toward any particular method and caution providers and public health officials against making assumptions based on race, ethnicity, age, ability, economic status, sexual orientation, or gender identity and expression. People should be given complete information and be supported in making the best decisions for their health and other unique circumstances.

Reflecting key reproductive justice principles (Ross & Solinger, 2017), they underscore the importance of LARC as contraceptive options, while arguing that enthusiasm can quickly become coercion.

Our research interrogates LARC promotion discourse, which we argue both *reflects* normative ideas about sexuality and health and *produces* responsible sexual citizens. Following longstanding feminist and antiracist engagements with technoscience as objects and practices that can both expand and constrain the agency of marginalised subjects (Clarke, Shim, Mamo, Fosket, & Fishman, 2003), we analyse immediate postpartum LARC (hereafter IPLARC) promotion obliquely. Extending critical scholarship on LARC, our paper investigates IPLARC promotion via what we term a 'textual ethnography of a device' (Ahmed, 2006). Specifically, we trace these devices' travels through three discursive sites: state Medicaid policies, health policy, and clinical research on IPLARC. Our methods are informed by Clarke's (2005) situational analysis and Ahmed's ethnography of texts, which attend to silence in discourse and the shape of power/knowledge, i.e. not only the *content* but the *forms* in which discursive activity comes to matter or affect the empirical world. As feminist science and technology studies (STS) scholarship has demonstrated, policies are not neutral reflections of best medical practices and expertise, but instead produce particular meanings, and influence which technologies are preferred (Akrich, 1992). Ultimately, we conceptualise LARC promotion efforts both as a manifestation of reproductive governance (e.g. Waggoner, 2017) and, perhaps more importantly, as *sexual healthism* that functions to produce forms of sexual citizenship (Epstein & Mamo, 2017). More than just repressive or empowering, we argue that LARC promotion is ideologically productive. Illuminating the subtle distinction between repression and productivity exposes the hegemonic logic of contemporary LARC promotion in the U.S., which we term 'The Age of LARC.'

Mapping 'new' LARC promotion: soft sterilization in the twenty-first century?

IPLARC policies manifest in the context of widely circulating constructions of women who choose LARC as responsible and empowered subjects in control of their reproductive futures (Mann & Grzanka, 2018). The discourse on contemporary LARC promotion in the U.S. implicates overlapping transnational, historical discourses of LARC promotion, the invention and proliferation of sexual health, and sexual citizenship. Our work stitches these together.

Sexual health as the new normal

While research on LARC promotion globally illustrated mechanisms of reproductive governance (Takeshita, 2011), our concern is as much with the regulation of reproductive health as it is with how LARC promotion indexes normative ideas of sexual health. Arguably ubiquitous in public health discourse in the twenty-first century, Epstein and Mamo (2017) traced the genealogy of sexual health to the relatively recent past. We pick up here their concern with sexual health*ism*. Akin to governmentality, healthism denotes a kind of moralisation of health (Conrad, 1992; Crawford, 1980), whereby individual subjects are compelled to self-fashion and maximise their well-being, particularly in the context of the state's disinvestment from social welfare programs and public health care. Epstein and Mamo identify a curious omission in scholarship on healthism: the central role that sexuality has played in the deployment of healthism worldwide. They found that the diffusion of sexual health since the 1970s has resulted in multiple discourses rather than simply a dilution of the term. The diversification of sexual health 'niche' concerns (e.g. STI prevention, reproductive and sexual rights, population control, sexual dysfunction) means that sexual healthism*s* compel different goals through different—albeit sometimes overlapping—health practices. Notably, they observe how the coupling of reproduction with sexuality means that contemporary concerns with reproductive health appear inextricable from sexual health.

How might IPLARC represent another node of sexual healthism? Metzl and Kirkland's (2010) critique of health's moralising dimensions is especially helpful in connecting Medicaid policy to broader ideological currents. By rejecting public health recommendations as benevolent a priori, Metzl and Kirkland posit health as a *value* that reflects existing inequalities while imposing those values on the targets of health promotion. Their theorisation is germane insomuch as our concern is less with LARC technologies themselves, but the scripting of those technologies and the work they do in the world. Who does IPLARC help, and whose interests are advanced by such Medicaid policies?

Sex and the state

The extensive uptake of IPLARC Medicaid policies across the U.S. suggests sexual citizenship is central to LARC promotion discourse. Sexual citizenship broadly refers to normative configurations of personhood that are linked to national goals or ideals; to recognise the state as sexual and sexuality as central to the state exposes the powerfully consequential role that sexuality and nation play in making each other up (Puri, 2016). The state remains deeply invested in producing a normative model of sexual citizenship, predicated on a specific life course trajectory wherein one should first complete their educational goals, achieve economic self-sufficiency, *and then* get married and become a parent (Geronimus, 2003). However, unlike state-sanctioned forced sterilisation policies of the twentieth century, much of the contemporary discourse on sexual citizenship is neoliberal and emphasises individuals' roles in assuming responsibility for adherence to a normative model of sexual citizenship in order to prevent socially undesirable outcomes (Ezer, Jones, Fisher, & Power, 2019). Thus, the neoliberalization of sexual health promotion frames personal responsibilization as inherently empowering, even as its effects are punitive (Grzanka, Mann, & Elliott, 2016).

New LARC: sexual health meets technoscience

Sexual citizenship, healthism, and technoscience collide in LARC's fraught global trajectories. The history of IUDs in the U.S. is one of 'corporate greed and medical neglect' (Takeshita, 2011, p. 76). An early IUD device, the Dalkon Shield, caused the death of at least 15 women and thousands of others suffered life-threatening infections, miscarriages, and sterilisations in the U.S. (Ross & Solinger, 2017). After the Dalkon Shield was removed from the market in 1976, the IUD disappeared from the U.S. medical system until 2002. The implant also has its own problematic history. In the 1990s, policy proposals to financially incentivize or require Norplant use for women receiving public benefits proliferated. Further, while state Medicaid programs made Norplant free for poor women, requests for removal due to serious side effects were routinely denied or rendered inaccessible due to out-of-pocket costs of $150–500 (Roberts, 1997, p. 130).

But LARC advocates have identified new IUDs and implants as the ideal tools for eliminating teenage and unintended pregnancy and reducing associated health disparities, primarily because they are relatively cheap and essentially infallible (Gomez, Fuentes, & Allina, 2014). Nevertheless, rates of IUD use hovered between 2–12% between 2002 and 2012 (Kavanaugh & Jerman, 2018). In 2007, the Contraceptive CHOICE Project began offering young women any birth control of their choice for free, coupled with a tiered approach to contraceptive counselling that emphasised LARC as the best options due to their efficacy (Secura, Allsworth, Madden, Mullersman, & Peipert, 2010). Approximately 70% of the 10,000 women who participated selected an IUD or implant (McNicholas, Madden, Secura, & Peipert, 2014). This signalled that women were interested in LARC. In Colorado, a similar campaign was launched in 2012 to offer free IUDs to teenagers, which resulted in significant declines in teen pregnancy, birth, and abortion rates (Ricketts, Klingler, & Schwalberg, 2014). Almost immediately, articles declaring LARC's superior effectiveness (e.g. Rodriguez et al., 2014) began to pervade the U.S. public health imaginary (Gomez et al., 2014; Gubrium et al., 2016; Higgins, 2014).

Health campaigns and corporate advertising about new LARC foreground the kind of woman who chooses an IUD or an implant. They make good choices for their health and their future children, because while LARC is heavily promoted, sterilisation is not (Mann & Grzanka, 2018). Because LARC is 'hassle free,' the 'enlightened' user has the freedom to be more productive and consciously engaged in their life more broadly (Takeshita, 2011, p. 155). And while contraception is explicitly about sex, LARC promotion discourse remains particularly silent about sex itself, including what effects LARC has on sexual pleasure (Higgins, Ryder, Skarda, Koepsel, & Bennett, 2015). The targets of LARC promotion are implicitly cast as irresponsible; LARC promotion is a disciplinary instrument that promotes the exercise of sexual control while effacing the structural factors that constrain autonomy (Mann & Grzanka, 2018; Gomez & Wapman, 2017). This is a critical point: this single class of contraceptive technologies has become the vehicle through which young women and postpartum mothers achieve sexual health. LARC is not just a birth control but a technological life hack for health and happiness.

While LARC is deemed a commonsense tool for pregnancy prevention, only some young women are identified as especially in need of LARC because they cannot be trusted to manage their fertility in accordance with the normative model of sexual citizenship. This neoliberal discourse constructs the responsible and healthy subject in contrast with the irresponsible and unhealthy subject, which is racialized, classed, and gendered (Mann, 2018). Young women who focus on their education and careers, and delay childbearing until their thirties, are able to participate in the late capitalist economy as both unencumbered workers and consumers. By contrast, poor single mothers have long been racialized as Black and Latina—historically labelled 'welfare queens' (Bridges, 2011)—precisely because they are perceived to be lazy and irresponsible. While LARC promotion discourse assumes that all young women should *and will* be empowered to choose LARC to prevent pregnancy, the implicit focus on low-income young women of colour as especially in need of LARC forecloses a consideration of how such targeted LARC promotion invokes a long history of population control and the denial of agency for those with the fewest resources. The multidimensional targeting of society's most vulnerable women, including incarcerated women, for LARC use has prompted Winters and McLaughlin (2019) to ponder the extent to which LARC promotion may sometimes enact a power akin to 'soft sterilization:' a version of eugenics whereby the state does not have to blatantly infringe upon civil rights in order to achieve its aims. Instead, soft sterilisation is involuntarily, 'temporarily' *chosen*—eugenics *vis-à-vis* empowerment.

Method

Our work was driven by the following overarching research question: how does IPLARC discourse produce ideas about sexual health and sexual citizenship? Our work was informed by critical discourse analysis and feminist, constructivist qualitative research (Clarke, 2005). Inspired by and expanding upon Ahmed (2006), we conduct a textual ethnography to examine the subtle pedagogical moments wherein state public health policies and campaigns construct and instruct subjects. Our analysis focuses on three primary sites. We examined all state-level Medicaid policies on LARC reimbursement; publicly available policy statements by public health organisations; and published clinical literature on the IPLARC published as of December 2019. In contrast to a systematic review or meta-analysis, Ahmed describes textual ethnography as *following texts around.* Accordingly, rather than implement rigid inclusion/exclusion criteria, we individually and collectively engaged in a variety of data collection practices, including: tracing citation networks to see which documents received the most uptake, collected and coded Medicaid policies according to what they did (not) specify, and iteratively analysed policy statements and clinical literatures for their ideological investments. The primary investigators maintained a shared data archive supplemented by research assistants' targeted investigations of specific state-level policies that resulted in supplementary data points, such as training modules on LARC insertion for health care providers and presentations at health policy meetings. Some of these data collection procedures (e.g. policy analysis) overlapped with a larger multidisciplinary, mixed-methods study of LARC promotion (Mann & Grzanka, 2018 Grzanka & Schuch, 2020; Mann, White, Rogers, & Gomez, 2019). We maintained what Levitt, Motulsky, Wertz, Morrow, and Ponterotto (2017) call 'fidelity'—an intimate relationship between researchers and the researched (i.e. our data)—by engaging in ongoing memoing, group dialogue, and iterative reflection on our emerging ideas and developing argument.

Results

Proliferating clinical literature on LARC emphasises rates of LARC use, tiered contraceptive counselling, policy implementation, and maternal health outcomes (e.g. Madden, Mullersman, Omvig, Secura, & Peipert, 2013; Moniz et al., 2016; Tyler et al., 2012). LARC supplements a particular kind of reproductive health, while seemingly effacing concerns about sexuality and sexual health. In addition to the limited attention to any discussion about sexuality or sexual well-being in LARC promotion, users' experiences with LARC are largely overlooked in policies and clinical literature. Such omissions suggest researchers and policymakers tend to regard contraceptive use as a straightforward proposition and that when barriers to access are removed—whether financial or epistemic—women will choose to use LARC. In sum, clinical and policy-based enthusiasm for LARC signals the assumption that LARC is best among available contraceptive options. We observe four intersecting axes central to hegemonic LARC promotion, or the 'Age of LARC': *urgency, efficiency, cost-effectiveness*, and *outcomes.*

Urgency

The state's enthusiasm for LARC is based on an assumption that there is an urgent need to change behaviours. Unintended pregnancy is framed by public health actors as an economic, social, and health crisis that we desperately need to prevent (Rodriguez et al., 2014; Sonfield & Kost, 2015). The state's anxiety over unintended pregnancy is not new nor tied fundamentally to LARC. However, IPLARC promotion discourse yokes unintended pregnancy to reproductive technoscience by framing IPLARC as *the* solution to an otherwise intractable crisis. Statistical information disseminated by health agencies identifies IPLARC as historically urgent, as well as cost-effective (a theme we return to below); recall that South Carolina claimed unplanned pregnancies declined by 6 percent, and its Medicaid office saved $1.7 million through IPLARC (Tavernise, 2016). Additionally, unintended pregnancy is associated with short interpregnancy intervals (conceiving within 12–18 months of a previous live birth) and both are associated with adverse birth outcomes (Appareddy, Pryor, & Bailey, 2017); thus, preventing unintended and short interval pregnancies through LARC use is positioned as the best way to reduce adverse birth outcomes, which disproportionately occur among women of colour. These and other statistics are mobilised as evidence of an urgent, widespread exigency for implementing IPLARC across the state. Further, IPLARC exponents insist that the timing of the insertion is equally vital. Because half of Medicaid recipients do not return for a six-week postpartum checkup, the explicit motivation for IPLARC insertion is to leverage a time when a woman is in the health care system, most likely to have health insurance, and certain to not be pregnant (Heberlein, Billings, Mattison-Faye, & Giese, 2016; Wilkinson et al., 2019). The imposition of any timing deadline deliberately creates a sense of urgency.

Studies of expulsion rates of IUDs inserted immediately postpartum consistently find that rates are significantly higher than when an IUD is inserted 4–6 weeks postpartum (Escobar & Shearin, 2019; Woo et al., 2015; Goldwaithe & Shaw 2015). Oregon's Medicaid guidance includes an analysis of expulsion rates and found general consensus that there is a slightly increased risk of expulsion if the insertion is performed within 10 min of placental delivery, and a significantly greater risk if the insertion is done between 10 min and 4 weeks of childbirth (Oregon Health Authority, 2016). Two policies (Georgia, Texas) specify a narrow time for eligible insertion, within 10–15 min of delivery. Most policies state that the insertion must happen sometime during the inpatient stay ($n = 25$), which may be more dangerous, considering that many doctors do not have special training in immediate postpartum insertion of IUDs (ASTHO, 2018). The remaining 19 policies will also cover LARC at a later outpatient appointment. However, the benefits of IPLARC are routinely described as worth the expulsion risk to prevent unintended pregnancy, reduce short-interval pregnancies, and save costs (Escobar & Shearin, 2019; Rodriguez et al., 2014).

Promotional materials emphasise that IPLARC insertion is 'medically and logistically favorable,' in an effort to ground the policy in a scientific logic (Heberlein et al., 2016). However, this discourse draws upon and reproduces long-standing racist, sexist, and classist logic that confines and restricts 'choice' temporally (Mann & Grzanka, 2018). This logic—based on ideas about patient 'noncompliance'—subtly creates ideas about how some patients are inherently irresponsible. The noncompliant Medicaid patient cannot be trusted to comply within a less restrictive window of voluntary postpartum contraceptive use. She cannot be trusted to take the oral contraceptive pill when needed or return to the doctor for a six-week check-up, at which time she could receive a LARC, so the sense of urgency is amplified.

Assumptions about the 'wily' nature of the patient (Bridges, 2011) are also produced by sites of silence in our data (Clarke, 2005), or what is *not* articulated in a given situation. The state Medicaid policies enumerate cost, time of insertion, and type of device; removal is rarely mentioned. Clarke (2000) called LARC 'imposable,' because of the focus on insertion, not the removal, which requires women to contracept for a period of time dependent upon the health care provider (i.e. the inserter and remover). If these policies compel a woman who already has limited access to health care to keep an IUD or implant in longer than she may prefer, these health policies may constitute reproductive oppression (Ross & Solinger, 2017). Importantly, no guidance specifies who is responsible for the cost of removal after the federally mandated 60 days of postpartum Medicaid coverage (ACOG, 2020). This critical absence in the policies cuts across all four axes. That these policies typically do not speak to the removal process is a troubling feature, especially considering the population they target and the justification for time of insertion (Isley, Brown, Rivlin, Keder, & Norris, 2019; Vela et al., 2018).

Alongside the push to increase access to IPLARC for women on Medicaid, there has been considerably less attention to unintended pregnancies covered by private insurance. Private insurance does not cover IPLARC. Most privately insured women who want LARC postpartum have it placed 4+ weeks after birth, when it is covered. IPLARC is extensively promoted amongst Medicaid recipients, but not available to women with private insurance, indicating there seems to be little concern for whether future pregnancies are planned for women who are not poor. That some unintended pregnancies require urgent intervention and others seemingly do not is a notable silence in LARC promotion more broadly.

Efficiency

The model South Carolina policy emphasises LARC *only* because of how efficient it is (e.g. an IUD is 98% effective at preventing pregnancy). There may be other means of preventing pregnancy, but LARC is principally efficient and safe (see, e.g. Hofler et al., 2017). When ACOG (2016) declares,

> The IUD and the implant are the most effective forms of reversible birth control available. During the first year of typical use, fewer than 1 in 100 women using an IUD or an implant will become pregnant. This rate is in the same range as that for sterilization,

the clear focus—and thus the main justification—is on the efficacy of the device. The rapid, near-universal uptake of the IPLARC Medicaid policies since 2012 underscores this point.

The IPLARC approach reflects an emphasis on efficiency above and beyond a more comprehensive approach to sexual and reproductive health. While the clinical literature references trade-offs or when the data shows a lower rate of continued usage at one year postpartum, most Medicaid guidance and clinical studies underline the pressing need to promote IPLARC to prevent pregnancy (e.g. Dole & Martin, 2017; Xing et al., 2019). For example, the State of Vermont (2016) argues, '[LARC] utilisation is being promoted as an efficient means to eliminate unplanned pregnancy. Women facing an unplanned pregnancy are at greater risk for a number of social, economic and health problems.' Likewise, Florida's Medicaid guidance explains: 'Research shows that LARCs are effective in reducing unintended pregnancies, premature and low birth weight births, and prenatal drug exposure.' The power of the devices to reduce or eliminate serious health consequences for women, children, and the state is presented as a matter of fact. In other words, IPLARC is an acutely expeditious means by which to accomplish the state's cost-saving costs by engendering responsible sexual citizenship.

Prioritising efficiency risks undermining patient-centered contraceptive counselling. In an analysis of the association between quality of postpartum contraceptive counselling and changes in contraceptive method preference between delivery and 3-months postpartum, Coleman-Minahan and Potter (2019) found that high-quality postpartum contraceptive counselling was 'relatively rare' and women of colour and of lower socioeconomic status received high quality counselling less often. Dehlendorf and colleagues (2014) found that younger women were more likely to receive 'foreclosed' counselling, in which providers direct patients toward particular methods. IPLARC Medicaid guidance exemplifies a 'foreclosed' approach, because the policies endemically limit contraceptive options. These policies and concordant clinical findings suggest that low income women of colour may be more likely to experience both subjective/interpersonal — and systems-level foreclosure of their contraceptive options, whereby IPLARC is framed as the obvious, reasonable, and most effective choice. Such hegemonic logic reinforces the idea that to choose to contracept (or not) with an approach other than LARC is irrational and irresponsible.

Cost-effectiveness

Changes to Medicaid policies are functionally motivated by political and financial variables. Accordingly, it is misleading to talk about Medicaid policies as exclusively or even primarily reflecting clinical judgments; they should also be understood as cost-saving strategies implemented by relatively autonomous state actors. State-level IPLARC policies are no exception. In their study of Medicaid officials' justifications for adopting or not implementing postpartum insertion policies, Moniz and colleagues (2016) found officials invoked two reasons to adopt or not adopt IPLARC guidance: health outcomes and costs. Officials from states who had adopted such policies cited overall cost savings and better maternal and child health outcomes. Officials from states who had not adopted such policies cited what Moniz and colleagues called misinformation about LARC's clinical effects and budgetary concerns related to the costs of training providers and purchasing LARC devices. These costs are not insignificant—and the difficulties associated with building a complex public health initiative, which IPLARC policies need, are well-documented (e.g. Cooper, Boydell, Heller, & Cameron, 2018; Harper, Loper, Louison, Morse, & Hill, 2019; Hofler et al., 2017). Moniz et al. conclude that the officials who have not yet embraced IPLARC policies should be lobbied with 'correct' information and convinced of IPLARC's cost-saving potentials.

Unintended pregnancies are often framed as a costly public health problem in which an unintended pregnancy is the cause, rather than effect, of structural inequalities (e.g. Peipert, Madden, Allsworth, & Secura, 2012). Indeed, IPLARC is actively promoted as a strategy for reducing poverty. Cost is a factor in three ways: (a) state expenditures related to unintended and short-interval pregnancies, (b) the state Medicaid budget for IPLARC and the associated training, and (c) a barrier for women who wish to obtain contraception. The ACOG LARC Program (2020) argues Medicaid programs remove barriers to using LARC, including education, time, and cost, and that IPLARC is the most cost-effective approach to reducing unintended pregnancies. When Georgia promoted its new Medicaid guidance, officials invoked this statistic: 'In 2010, the rate of unintended pregnancy was 60% of all pregnancies in Georgia and almost $917.5 million was spent on unintended pregnancy by the federal and state government' (Sonfield & Kost, 2015). The state emphasised women's lack of planning (an irresponsibility), implying those pregnancies are problematic *because* of the cost burden to the state. The Oregon Health Authority (2016) states, 'Effective contraception is cost-saving (not just cost-effective). Economic modelling predicts high levels of cost savings from immediate placement of LARC.' According to Washington and colleagues (2015), Oregon's economic forecasting found a cost savings of $282,540 and a gain of 10 quality of live years per every 1,000 women who desired a postpartum IUD. Overall, the key dependent variable in IPLARC policy analyses is cost savings. Oregon's enthusiasm for IPLARC comes despite their finding that 'there is insufficient data to show a reduced risk of unintended pregnancy from immediate placement.' Of the 44 Medicaid policies[3], three reference cost-savings for the state in the policy, 18 mention LARC's effectiveness, and 12 mention reducing rates of unintended pregnancy. That cost savings to the state are mentioned at all in a health care policy (which is functionally a reimbursement memo) is meaningful. The majority of the guidances have only one or two sentences explaining the policy change and then list the reimbursement codes. At least eight states and the Association for State and Territorial Health Care Providers have published detailed 'toolkits' that provide detailed justification for the policies, and all of them underscore substantial cost-savings.[4]

Outcomes

We observe axiomatic enthusiasm for these kinds of devices, and the data suggest an analytic anchor in what LARC does, not (a) how it is experienced, (b) when it does not work, or (c) patients' relationship to their own sexual and reproductive health and well-being. The effect of LARC is responsibility, so this goal supersedes other goals or even other outcomes, including device removal. In *Intrauterine Devices and Implants: A Guide to Reimbursement* (Armstrong et al., 2016), a section on removal reads:

> In spite of [federal Medicaid law that requires coverage], providers may encounter problematic coverage or reimbursement policies for removal of LARC methods. For example, some public or commercial plans may have payment policies that, in effect, deny separate reimbursement for removal in some contexts.

Hawaii's Medicaid guidance is one of the few that provides a code for removal, but it applies only if the woman is still receiving Medicaid. The Nevada guidance explicitly states, 'There is no process for Medicaid reimbursement [for removal] when the recipient is not Medicaid eligible.'

Where most articles cite cost, incomplete information, and concerns about safety as common roadblocks to LARC uptake (Glazer, Wolf, & Gorby, 2011; Paul et al., 2018), few studies probe the phenomenology of LARC use (e.g. pain or discomfort). In 2018, six years since South Carolina's initial IPLARC guidance, Carr and colleagues found low levels of pain and high rates of satisfaction. Conversely, Dole and Martin (2017) found that as IPLARC placements increased, so too did requests for early removal, primarily because of irregular bleeding patterns. However, their conclusion is that better education and counselling will improve rates of continued LARC usage. To return to work by Moniz et al. (2016), we find most telling their lack of attention to users' actual experiences. Beyond concerns about LARCs' effects on breastfeeding (e.g. Turok et al., 2017; Goldwaithe & Shaw, 2015), the physical or emotional experience of LARC remain under-investigated.

Clinical literature suggests a desire to gently but firmly make the case that LARC is the best choice notwithstanding the diverse desires, practices, and needs that might inform a choice to (not) contracept. Whereas medical professionals focus on efficacy, women choose contraception based on many factors, including side effects and non-contraceptive benefits. In an analysis of patient perceptions of IPLARC, women expressed a desire for autonomy in their contraceptive decision-making and described making internally motivated decisions based on their life goals and individual priorities (Sznajder, Carvajal, & Sufrin, 2020); however, the study showed that while some women were very satisfied with their LARC, some women felt pressured and coerced to choose LARC. These findings echo the argument by Gubrium and colleagues (2016) that 'No one form of contraception should be the first-line method for everyone' (p. e2). Mann and colleagues (2019) found that participants who accepted IPLARC on Medicaid but desired removal due to negative side effects encountered barriers ranging from cost to reluctant providers. In a study of providers' perceptions of LARC removal, Isley and colleagues (2019) found that providers expressed conflict, disappointment and irritation when patients asked for 'early' LARC removal. South Dakota's Medicaid policy notes 'providers must counsel the recipient about LARC side effect treatment options prior to removal of LARC [except in cases of medical emergency].' Despite calls for 'shared decision making' (Dehlendorf, Kimport, Levy, & Steinauer, 2014; Escobar & Shearin, 2019), LARC-first or LARC-*only* approaches that marginalise concerns about access to removal remain dominant in the clinical literature (Isley et al., 2019).

Notably, one outcome discussed in IPLARC promotion materials directly related to patients' experience of the devices is pain management. Across national policy documents and state-level materials (e.g. professional newsletters), IPLARC discourse sometimes invoke patient pain experiences as an unnecessary and avoidable side-effect of IUD insertion, in particular. If users' longer-term experiences with the devices were largely effaced in policy documents and clinical discourse, insertion-related pain was acknowledged as a serious deterrent to usage and, therefore, should be avoided through appropriate training.

The age of LARC

The rapid uptake of Medicaid policies across 43 states and the District of Columbia, the enthusiasm from national and international public health and medical organisations, and the growing clinical literature in support of LARC together construct a dominant narrative that positions one class of contraception as the *best* kind. These discursive practices represent hegemonic support for LARC, which we call 'The Age of LARC' to draw attention to a particular political consciousness that currently prevails in public health. We chose to signal 'the age' of LARC based on a number of theoretical concerns: we seek to critically name the cultural and historically contingent dynamics at play in LARC promotion discourse in the U.S. and to gesture toward a form of contraceptive ubiquity whereby LARC enthusiasm has exceeded the boundaries of the clinical encounter to inflect broader discourses of responsible sexual and reproductive health, well-being, and empowerment.

In the Age of LARC, LARC promotion discourse constructs sexual citizenship through explicit normative appeals to and silences around what makes a healthy, responsible subject and, conversely, an unhealthy, irresponsible subject. It is implicitly and explicitly racialized, classed, and gendered but should never be understood as nonsexual. In this sense, IPLARC is a nexus of intersectionality: systems of power co-constituted through a regulatory form of technoscience. Sexuality in LARC promotion discourse is (not just) about bodies, sex, and procreation, but also about relations of being. Importantly, these relations are always already national insomuch as IPLARC policies are justified by their effects on the state. Certain pregnant bodies are quantified in terms of their cost to the state; rather than fundamentally eliminate certain reproductive capacities, IPLARC policies leverage a logic of empowerment to compel sexual healthism. For example, IPLARC appeals to improving birth outcomes, while at the same time effacing the sexual dimensions of women's health. With rare exceptions (see Higgins et al., 2015), sexual health is not included in the conversation about LARC, and that particular silence is productive and regulating. We posit that a key feature of the Age of LARC is the obfuscation of sexuality even as LARC promotion techniques script normative sexual actors, i.e. ideal LARC users/uses. In the Age of LARC, these relations are indexed according to normative logics of responsible sexual citizenship that foreclose important questions about race, population control, and agency amid a discourse of health and empowerment.

The Medicaid guidances for IPLARC are not laws. Instead, these policies are liminal, interstitial bureaucratic techniques, though their material consequences are law-like. These laws are not health-driven but are normatively constituted by financial concerns that take sexual behaviour as their locus of control. Accordingly, mundane reimbursement policies have significant consequences for shaping sexual citizenship. The brevity of most of the Medicaid policies (i.e. most are between one paragraph and three pages) and the absence of attention to removal have significant consequences for providers, administrators, and patients. The impetus for the policies manufactures a preference for LARC above all other contraceptives, thereby promoting providers' power and control at the expense of patients' autonomy. Despite the recitation of patient 'choice' in the clinical literature, a LARC-first approach limits and constrains personal choices by situating LARC as the only responsible and appropriate choice. Further, a key element of the hegemonic status of LARC promotion is the consistent articulation of empowerment and choice rhetoric even as patients' options are circumscribed by Medicaid policies and other forms of subtle coercion, including foreclosed contraceptive counselling (Dehlendorf et al., 2014), public health messaging (Mann & Grzanka, 2018), and interactions among peers (Grzanka & Schuch, 2020).

We used Epstein and Mamo's (2017) examination of sexual healthism to explore the niche of sexual and reproductive health promotion as a site of disciplinary power enhanced by reproductive technoscience. But our argument also has clinical implications. While we are not suggesting these policies are intentionally nefarious, it is imperative that STS scholars, sociologists, and public health researchers continue to bridge disciplinary and epistemic divides with clinicians and policy-makers to better foreground reproductive justice concerns amid LARC promotion efforts. A reproductive justice framework, because it centres women of colour, social justice, and human rights (Ross & Solinger, 2017), potentially disrupts this hegemony by ushering more meaningful patient-centered, intersectionally-informed care (Gomez et al., 2014). Patient-centered care, in this context, means that all women have access to and information about the range of birth control methods, so they may make whatever choice best suits their goals. Reproductive justice perspectives can help unsettle the persistent policy link between unintended pregnancy and poverty, which buttresses the hegemonic status of LARC as a solution to social, economic, and health problems. The Age of LARC may have a contrary effect to what it names as priorities: health and empowerment. How do we actually engender well-being and agency—and even promote social justice—in clinical encounters beyond the responsibilizing discourse of LARC promotion?

Notes

1. We use 'woman' and 'women' throughout this paper; however, we recognize that these terms do not encompass the full range of people who use contraception and who may be impacted by particular public health initiatives.
2. A 2019 analysis in *JAMA* found no statistically significant change in trend in short-interval births for adults following the policy change (Steenland et al., 2019).
3. The ACOG LARC Program compiles all state Medicaid documents: https://www.acog.org/About-ACOG/ACOG-Departments/Long-Acting-Reversible-Contraception/Immediate-Postpartum-LARC-Medicaid-Reimbursement
4. The Association for State and Territorial Health Care Providers compiles the toolkits: https://www.astho.org/Programs/Maternal-and-Child-Health/Long-Acting-Reversible-Contraception-LARC/Toolkits-and-Guides/

Disclosure statement

No potential conflict of interest was reported by the author(s).

References

ACOG. (2016). Committee Opinion No. 670: Immediate postpartum long-acting reversible contraception. *Obstetrics & Gynecology, 128*(2), doi:10.1097/AOG.0000000000001587

ACOG. (2020). ACOG LARC Program. American College of Obstetricians and Gynecologists. Retrieved from https://www.acog.org/About-ACOG/ACOG-Departments/Long-Acting-Reversible-Contraception

Ahmed, S. (2006). The nonperformativity of antiracism. *Meridians, 7*(1), 104–126. Retrieved from https://www.jstor.org/stable/40338719.

Akrich, M. (1992). The de-scription of technical objects. In W. E. Bijker, & J. Law (Eds.), *Shaping technology/building society: Studies in sociotechnical change* (pp. 205–224). Cambridge, MA: MIT Press.

American Academy of Pediatrics. (2014). Policy statement: Contraception for adolescents. *Pediatrics, 134*(4), e1244–e1256. doi:10.1542/peds.2014-2299

Appareddy, S., Pryor, J., & Bailey, B. (2017). Inter-pregnancy interval and adverse outcomes: Evidence for an additional risk in health disparate populations. *The Journal of Maternal-Fetal & Neonatal Medicine, 30*(21), 2640–2644. doi:10.1080/14767058.2016.1260115

Armstrong, E., McKee, C., Gandal-Powers, M., Levin, S., Kelinson, A. K., Luchowski, A., & Thompson, K. (2016). *Intrauterine devices & implants: A guide to reimbursement.* San Francisco. Retrieved from https://larcprogram.ucsf.edu/

ASTHO. (2018). Guidance for Developing a Toolkit on Immediate Postpartum Long-Acting Reversible Contraception. Association of State and Territorial Health Official, Arlington. Retrieved from https://www.astho.org/Maternal-and-Child-Health/Increasing-Access-to-Contraception/Guidance-for-Developing-a-Toolkit-on-Immediate-Postpartum-LARC/

Bingham, D. (2017). *How South Carolina became a model for reproductive options.* The State, Dec 4. Retrieved from https://www.thestate.com/opinion/op-ed/article187968199.html

Bridges, K. M. (2011). *Reproducing race: An ethnography of pregnancy as a site of racialization.* Berkeley: University of California Press.

Carr, S. L., Singh, R. H., Sussman, A. L., Rogers, R. G., Pereda, B., & Espey, E. (2018). Women's experiences with immediate postpartum intrauterine device insertion: A mixed-methods study. *Contraception, 97*(3), 219–226. doi:10.1016/j.contraception.2017.10.008

Centers for Disease Control and Prevention. (2015). Preventing teen pregnancy: A key role for providers. Centers for Disease Control CDC Vitalsigns. Retrieved from http://www.cdc.gov/vitalsigns/larc/

Clarke, A. E. (2000). Maverick reproductive scientists and the production of contraceptives, 1915–2000 + . In A. R. Saetnan, N. Oudshoorn, & M. Kirejczyk (Eds.), *Bodies of technology: Women's involvement with reproductive medicine.* (pp. 368–383). Columbus: OSU Press.

Clarke, A. E. (2005). Situational analysis: Grounded theory after the postmodern turn. Thousand Oaks, CA: Sage.

Clarke, A. E., Shim, J. K., Mamo, L., Fosket, J. R., & Fishman, J. R. (2003). Biomedicalization: Technoscientific transformations of health, illness, and U.S. Biomedicine. *American Sociological Review, 68*(2), 161–194. doi:10.2307/1519765

Coleman-Minahan, K., & Potter, J. E. (2019). Quality of postpartum contraceptive counseling and changes in contraceptive method preferences. *Contraception, 100*(6), 492–497. doi:10.1016/j.contraception.2019.08.011

Conrad, P. (1992). Medicalization and social control. *Annual Review of Sociology, 18*, 209–232. doi:10.1146/annurev.so.18.080192.001233

Cooper, M., Boydell, N., Heller, R., & Cameron, S. (2018). Community sexual health providers' views on immediate postpartum provision of intrauterine contraception. *BMJ Sexual & Reproductive Health, 44*(2), 97. doi:10.1136/bmjsrh-2017-101905

Crawford, R. (1980). Healthism and the medicalization of everyday life. *International Journal of Health Services, 10*(3), 365–388. doi:10.2190/3H2H-3XJN-3KAY-G9NY

Dehlendorf, C., Kimport, K., Levy, K., & Steinauer, J. (2014). A qualitative analysis of approaches to contraceptive counseling. *Perspectives on Sexual and Reproductive Health, 46*(4), 233–240. doi:10.1363/46e2114

Dole, D. M., & Martin, J. (2017). What nurses need to know about immediate postpartum initiation of long-acting reversible contraception. *Nursing for Women's Health, 21*(3), 186–195. doi:10.1016/j.nwh.2017.04.003

Epstein, S., & Mamo, L. (2017). The proliferation of sexual health: Diverse social problems and the legitimation of sexuality. *Social Science & Medicine, 188*, 176–190. doi:10.1016/j.socscimed.2017.06.033

Escobar, M., & Shearin, S. (2019). Immediate postpartum contraception: Intrauterine device insertion. *Journal of Midwifery & Women's Health, 64*(4), 481–487. doi:10.1111/jmwh.12984

Ezer, P., Jones, T., Fisher, C., & Power, J. (2019). A critical discourse analysis of sexuality education in the Australian curriculum. *Sex Education, 19*(5), 551–567. doi:10.1080/14681811.2018.1553709

Geronimus, A. T. (2003). Damned if you do: Culture, identity, privilege, and teenage childbearing in the United States. *Social Science & Medicine, 57*(5), 881–893. doi:10.1016/S0277-9536(02)00456-2

Glazer, A. B., Wolf, A., & Gorby, N. (2011). Postpartum contraception: Needs vs. Reality. *Contraception, 83*(3), 238–241. doi:10.1016/j.contraception.2010.07.002

Goldthwaite, L. M., & Shaw, K. A. (2015). Immediate postpartum provision of long-acting reversible contraception. *Current opinion in obstetrics & gynecology*, 27(6), 460–464. https://doi.org/10.1097/GCO.0000000000000224

Gomez, A. M., Fuentes, L., & Allina, A. (2014). Women or LARC first? Reproductive autonomy and the promotion of long-acting reversible contraceptive methods. *Perspectives on Sexual and Reproductive Health, 46*(3), 171–175. doi:10.1363/46e1614

Gomez, A. M., & Wapman, M. (2017). Under (implicit) pressure: Young Black and Latina women's perceptions of contraceptive care. *Contraception, 96*, 221–226. doi:10.1016/j.contraception.2017.07.007

Grzanka, P. R., Mann, E. S., & Elliott, S. (2016). The neoliberalism wars, or notes on the persistence of neoliberalism. *Sexuality Research and Social Policy, 13*(4), 297–307. doi:10.1007/s13178-016-0255-8

Grzanka, P. R., & Schuch, E. (2020). Reproductive anxiety and conditional agency at the intersections of privilege: A focus group study of emerging adults' perception of long-acting reversible contraception. *Journal of Social Issues. Advance Online Publication*, doi:10.1111/josi.12363

Gubrium, A. C., Mann, E. S., Borrero, S., Dehlendorf, C., Fields, J., Geronimus, A. T., … Sisson, G. (2016). Realizing reproductive health equity needs more than long-acting reversible contraception (LARC). *American Journal of Public Health*, *106*(1), 18–19. doi:10.2105/AJPH.2015.302900

Harper, K. D., Loper, A. C., Louison, L. M., Morse, J. E., & Hill, N. (2019). Stage-based implementation of immediate postpartum long acting reversible contraception using a reproductive justice framework. *American Journal of Obstetrics and Gynecology*, doi:10.1016/j.ajog.2019.11.1273

Heberlein, E. C., Billings, D., Mattison-Faye, A., & Giese, B. Z. (2016). *The South Carolina Postpartum LARC Toolkit*. Choose Well Initiative and the South Carolina Birth Outcomes Initiative. Retrieved from https://www.choosewellsc.org/img/SC_Postpartum_LARC_Toolkit.pdf

Higgins, J. A. (2014). Celebration meets caution: LARC's boons, potential busts, and the benefits of a reproductive justice approach. *Contraception*, *89*(4), 237–241. doi:10.1016/j.contraception.2014.01.027

Higgins, J. A., Ryder, K., Skarda, G., Koepsel, E., & Bennett, E. A. (2015). The sexual acceptability of intrauterine contraception: A qualitative study of young adult women. *Perspectives on Sexual and Reproductive Health*, *47*(3), 115–122. doi:10.1363/47e4515

Hofler, L. G., Cordes, S., Cwiak, C. A., Goedken, P., Jamieson, D. J., & Kottke, M. (2017). Implementing immediate postpartum long-acting reversible contraception programs. *Obstetrics and Gynecology*, *129*(1), 3–9. doi:10.1097/AOG.0000000000001798

Isley, M. M., Brown, M., Rivlin, K., Keder, L. M., & Norris, A. (2019). Why do you want it out?: Provider perspectives on early LARC removal. *Obstetrics & Gynecology*, *133*, 204S.

Kavanaugh, M. L., & Jerman, J. (2018). Contraceptive method use in the United States: Trends and characteristics between 2008, 2012 and 2014. *Contraception*, *97*(1), 14–21. doi:10.1016/j.contraception.2017.10.003

Levitt, H. M., Motulsky, S. L., Wertz, F. J., Morrow, S. L., & Ponterotto, J. G. (2017a). Recommendations for designing and reviewing qualitative research in psychology. Promoting methodological integrity. *Qualitative Psychology*, *4*(1), 2–22. doi:10.1037/qup0000082

Madden, T., Mullersman, J. L., Omvig, K. J., Secura, G. M., & Peipert, J. F. (2013). Structured contraceptive counseling provided by the contraceptive CHOICE Project. *Contraception*, *88*(2), 243–249. doi:10.1016/j.contraception.2012.07.015

Mann, E. S. (2018). Sexual citizenship and everyday feelings. In S. Talburt (Ed.), *Youth Sexualities: Public Feelings and contemporary cultural Politics* (1st ed., Vol. 1, pp. 183–206). Santa Barbara: Praeger.

Mann, E. S., & Grzanka, P. R. (2018). Agency-without-choice: The visual rhetorics of long-acting reversible contraception promotion. *Symbolic Interaction*, *41*(3), 334–356. doi:10.1002/symb.349

Mann, E. S., White, A. L., Rogers, P. L., & Gomez, A. M. (2019). Patients' experiences with South Carolina's immediate postpartum long-acting reversible contraception Medicaid policy. *Contraception*, *100*(2), 165–171. doi:10.1016/j.contraception.2019.04.007

McNicholas, C., Madden, T., Secura, G., & Peipert, J. F. (2014). The contraceptive CHOICE project round up: What we did and what we learned. *Clinical Obstetrics and Gynecology*, *57*(4), 645–653. doi:10.1097/GRF.0000000000000070

Metzl, J., & Kirkland, A. R. (eds.). (2010). *Against health: How health became the new morality*. New York: NYU Press.

Moniz, M. H., Chang, T., Davis, M. M., Forman, J., Landgraf, J., & Dalton, V. K. (2016). Medicaid administrator experiences with the implementation of immediate postpartum long-acting reversible contraception. *Women's Health Issues*, *26*(3), 313–320.

National Women's Health Network and SisterSong. (2016). Joint statement of principles on LARC. National Women's Health Network. Retrieved from https://www.nwhn.org/nwhn-joins-statement-principles-larcs/

Oregon Health Authority. (2016). Health Evidence Review Commission (HERC): Coverage guidance: Timing of Long-Acting Reversible Contraceptive (LARC) Placement. Retrieved from https://www.oregon.gov/oha/HPA/DSI-HERC/EvidenceBasedReports/LARC-CG.pdf

Paul, R., Bayer, C., Braun, E., Mullen, M., Frisse, A., & Robbins, C. C. (2018). Immediate postpartum LARC reimbursement increases uptake of effective contraception after pregnancy [22G].

Obstetrics & Gynecology, 131, https://journals.lww.com/greenjournal/Fulltext/2018/05001/Immediate_Postpartum_LARC_Reimbursement_Increases.279.aspx.

Peipert, J. F., Madden, T., Allsworth, J. E., & Secura, G. M. (2012). Preventing unintended pregnancies by providing no-cost contraception. *Obstetrics and Gynecology, 120*(6), 1291–1297. doi:10.1097/aog.0b013e318273eb56

Puri, J. (2016). *Sexual states: Governance and the struggle over the antisodomy law in India*. Durham: Duke University Press.

Ricketts, S., Klingler, G., & Schwalberg, R. (2014). Game change in Colorado: Widespread use of long-acting reversible contraceptives and rapid decline in births among young, low-income women. *Perspectives on Sexual and Reproductive Health, 46*(3), 125–132. doi:10.1363/46e1714

Roberts, D. E. (1997). *Killing the black body: Race, reproduction and the meaning of liberty*. New York: Vintage Books.

Rodriguez, M. I., Evans, M., & Espey, E. (2014). Advocating for immediate postpartum LARC: Increasing access, improving outcomes, and decreasing cost. *Contraception, 90*(5), 468–471. doi:10.1016/j.contraception.2014.07.001

Ross, L. J., & Solinger, R. (2017). *Reproductive justice: An introduction*. Oakland: University of California Press.

Secura, G. M., Allsworth, J. E., Madden, T., Mullersman, J. L., & Peipert, J. F. (2010). The contraceptive CHOICE Project: Reducing barriers to long-acting reversible contraception. *American Journal of Obstetrics and Gynecology, 203*(2), 115.e1–115.e7. doi:10.1016/j.ajog.2010.04.017

Sonfield, A., & Kost, K. (2015). Public costs from unintended pregnancies and the role of public insurance programs in paying for pregnancy-related care: National and state estimates for 2010. New York: Guttmacher Institute. http://www.guttmacher.org/pubs/public-costs-of-UP-2010.pdf.

Steenland, M. W., Pace, L. E., Sinaiko, A. D., & Cohen, J. L. (2019). Association between South Carolina Medicaid's change in payment for immediate postpartum long-acting reversible contraception and birth intervals association between changes in Medicaid payment and immediate postpartum LARC use and birth intervals in South Carolina. *JAMA, 322*(1), 76–78. doi:10.1001/jama.2019.6854

Sznajder, K., Carvajal, D. N., & Sufrin, C. (2020). Patient perceptions of immediate postpartum long-acting reversible contraception: A qualitative study. *Contraception, 101*(1), 21–25. doi:10.1016/j.contraception.2019.09.007

Takeshita, C. (2011). *Global biopolitics of the IUD: How science constructs contraceptive users and women's bodies*. Cambridge, MA: MIT Press.

Tavernise, S. (2016). Medicaid finds opportune time to offer birth control: Right after birth. *New York Times* (Oct 28). Retrieved from https://www.nytimes.com/2016/10/29/health/birth-control-medicaid.html

Thomas, A., & Karpilow, Q. C. (2018). Long-acting reversible contraception: A silver bullet solution for unintended pregnancy? *American Journal of Public Health, 108*(8), 1007–1008. doi:10.2105/AJPH.2018.304523

Turok, D. K., Leeman, L., Sanders, J. N., Thaxton, L., Eggebroten, J. L., Yonke, N., ... Espey, E. (2017). Immediate postpartum levonorgestrel intrauterine device insertion and breast-feeding outcomes: A noninferiority randomized controlled trial. *American Journal of Obstetrics and Gynecology, 217*(6), 665.e1–665.e8. doi:10.1016/j.ajog.2017.08.003

Tyler, C. P., Whiteman, M. K., Zapata, L. B., Curtis, K. M., Hillis, S. D., & Marchbanks, P. A. (2012). Health care provider attitudes and practices related to intrauterine devices for nulliparous women. *Obstetrics & Gynecology, 119*(4), 762–771. doi:10.1097/AOG.0b013e31824aca39

Vela, V. X., Patton, E. W., Sanghavi, D., Wood, S. F., Shin, P., & Rosenbaum, S. (2018). Rethinking Medicaid coverage and payment policy to promote high value care: The case of long-acting reversible contraception. *Women's Health Issues, 28*(2), 137–143. doi:10.1016/j.whi.2017.10.013

Waggoner, M. R. (2017). *The zero trimester: Pre-pregnancy care and the politics of reproductive risk*. Oakland: University of California Press.

Walls, J., Gifford, K., Ranji, U., Salganicoff, A., & Gomez, I. (2016). *Medicaid Coverage of Family Planning Benefits.* Kaiser Family Foundation, San Francisco, CA. Retrieved from http://files.kff.org/attachment/Report-Medicaid-Coverage-of-Family-Planning-Benefits-Results-from-a-State-Survey

Washington, C. I., Jamshidi, R., Thung, S. F., Nayeri, U. A., Caughey, A. B., & Werner, E. F. (2015). Timing of postpartum intrauterine device placement: A cost-effectiveness analysis. *Fertility and Sterility, 103*(1), 131–137.

Wilkinson, B., Ascha, M., Verbus, E., Montague, M., Morris, J., Mercer, B., & Arora, K. S. (2019). Medicaid and receipt of interval postpartum long-acting reversible contraception. *Contraception, 99*(1), 32–35. doi:10.1016/j.contraception.2018.08.017

Winters, D. J., & McLaughlin, A. R. (2019). Soft sterilization: Long-acting reversible contraceptives and the carceral state. *Affilia.* doi:10.1177/0886109919882320

Woo, I., Seifert, S., Hendricks, D., Jamshidi, R. M., Burke, A. E., & Fox, M. C. (2015). Six-month and 1-year continuation rates following postpartum insertion of implants and intrauterine devices. *Contraception, 92*(6), 532–535. doi:10.1016/j.contraception.2015.09.007

World Health Organization. (2012). From evidence to policy: Expanding access to family planning: Strategies to increase use of long-acting and permanent contraception. Department of Reproductive Health and Research, World Health Organization, Geneva, Switzerland. https://www.astho.org/Maternal-and-Child-Health/Long-Acting-Reversible-Contraception/Policy-Brief-Increasing-LARC-Use-WHO/

Xing, J., Lyons, D., Fan, Z. J., Glenn, A., & Felver, B. (2019). *Improving Women's Access to Long-Acting Reversible Contraception: Role of Medicaid Reimbursement Policy Change.* Washington State Health Care Authority and Department of Social and Health Services Research and Data Analysis Division, Olympia, WA. Retrieved from https://www.dshs.wa.gov/ffa/rda/research-reports/improving-women%E2%80%99s-access-long-acting-reversible-contraception-role-medicaid-reimbursement-policy-change

Producing bodies at risk in sexual health: an ethnographic comparative analysis between the combined oral contraceptive pill and pre-exposure prophylaxis in Switzerland

Marlyse Debergh

ABSTRACT
This article demonstrates that 'bodies at risk' in sexual health are socially constructed. It does so via a heuristic comparison between two molecular technologies that are central to the promotion of sexual health: the combined oral contraceptive pill (COCP) and pre-exposure prophylaxis (PrEP). Drawing on ethnographic research conducted in two sexual health institutions in the western part of Switzerland, the article presents two main findings. First, it argues that bodies are constructed as being at low or high risk by sexual health professionals (based on health and lifestyle criteria). Second, it shows that access to either the COCP or PrEP is largely based on this former classification. The article also demonstrates that there are ambivalent situations in which sexual health professionals seek compromises between different risks, and pragmatically adapt their medical protocols.

Introduction

Drawing on ethnographic research conducted in two sexual health institutions in the western part of Switzerland, this article seeks to demonstrate that 'bodies at risk' in sexual health are socially constructed. It does so via a comparative analysis of two molecular technologies. The first is the combined oral contraceptive pill (COCP). Most commonly known as 'the birth control pill', or simply as 'the pill', the COCP is a hormonal treatment to avoid pregnancy, which is composed of two types of molecules: oestrogen and progestogen. The COCP is distributed in one of the two sexual health institutions where I conducted my fieldwork: a sexual health centre for the general public. The second molecular technology is pre-exposure prophylaxis (PrEP). PrEP is taken by seronegative persons to prevent getting infected by the Human Immunodeficiency Virus, better known as HIV (AIDS, n.d.). PrEP is composed of two molecules, tenofovir and emtricitabine, which are also present in triple therapies involving seropositive patients. PrEP is distributed in the second sexual health institution I visited for my fieldwork: a sexual health centre for men who have sexual relations with other men (MSM).

Although the COCP and PrEP are currently considered central technologies in the promotion of sexual health, scholarly research has paid little attention to their convergence. Yet, they are both taken at a preventive stage by bodies risking sexual health, who are 'neither sick, nor healthy' (Jeangros & Bourrier, 2014).[1] Issues of individual autonomy, the right to make decisions about one's own body, sexual pleasure and independence underpin both molecular technologies, echoing a central dimension of the definition of sexual health: '[T]he possibility of having pleasurable and safe sexual experiences [...]' (WHO, 2002). According to Paul B. Preciado (2019), the COCP and PrEP represent 'chemical condoms' that produce '[n]ew forms of relation, desire and affect' (pp. 103–104). Together they shape the constitution of a new form of sexuality characterised by 'biomolecular' technologies, which are marketed by pharmaceutical industries (Preciado, 2019, p. 103). But what is it that puts a body at risk in sexual health? How do sexual health professionals deal with risk, and with bodies at risk, in sexual health consultations?

Drawing on the governmentality perspective of risk (Aradau & Van Munster, 2007; Ewald, 1991; Gouilhers-Hertig, 2017; Lupton, 1999, 2013; Maffi & Gouilhers, 2019; Rich, Evans, & De Pian, 2011), in this article I argue that the category of bodies at risk in sexual health is the result of constitutive practices conducted by sexual health professionals, as they assess individuals according to a profile that determines their access to either the COCP or PrEP. More precisely, through ethnographic descriptions of both observations and in-depth interviews, this article demonstrates that sexual health professionals hierarchise bodies at risk in sexual health through a complex assessment of two levels of risk: (1) an individual risk, namely that of the individual whose health condition and lifestyle might pose a risk for her/himself; (2) a risk induced by molecular technologies, as they interact with the individual's body (i.e. side effects). Moreover, this classification determines the individual's access to molecular technologies. Finally, some situations are ambivalent, as they lead sexual health professionals to seek compromises between different risks and to pragmatically adapt their medical protocols.

The article is divided into four sections. First, I briefly discuss literature on bodies at risk, offering some examples from existing research on the topic. The second section is devoted to the theoretical framework: the governmentality perspective of risk. Next, I present my methodology and the context of the research. In the last part, I present my ethnographic findings, divided into two sub-sections.

Bodies at risk

In the field of the sociology of health, various studies have examined the links between bodies and risk. A first strand of research focuses on the relations between pregnant women's bodies and risk. Lupton, for example, explains that '["t]he pregnant woman is surrounded by a complex network of discourses and practices directed at the surveillance and regulation of her body" and that risk is a central discourse' (cited in McDonald, Amir, & Davey, 2011, p. 2). In another study, Karalyn McDonald et al. (2011) show that women who are pregnant or breast-feeding manage the risk not only of their own body, but also of the foetus' body: '[The] weighing of risks and benefits becomes immensely more complex because they are considering the effect on two bodies rather than one' (p. 1).

A second body of research has considered other bodies at risk. On the topic of the human papillomavirus (HPV), Geneviève Rail et al. (2018) speak of '[t]he discursive constructions of girls' and women's embodiment as both vulnerable (i.e. "at risk" of HPVs) and dangerous (i.e. as a threat of contagion)' (p. 626). A second interesting study is Maria Caiata-Zufferey's research on asymptomatic women living with the genetic risk of breast/ovarian cancer. Caiata-Zufferey (2015) demonstrates that '[t]he genetically at-risk status conveys an invitation to transform health into a project, i.e. into a set of planned activities realized in collaboration with the medical system in order to reduce the risk of developing cancer' (p. 141).

A study on policies favouring male plasma donors to female donors in the United Kingdom by Julie Kent and Anne-Maree Farrell (2015) shows that this policy reflects gender discrimination by presenting women as 'risky' (p. 49). As they explain, 'it constructs all women as risky plasma donors regardless of their age, reproductive history or antibody status' (Kent & Farrell, 2015, p. 49). The gender dimension of bodies at risk is also at the forefront of a comparative study on risk assessment practices regarding contraceptives for women and men by Jessika Van Kammen and Nelly E. J. Oudshoorn (2002). As they explain, '[t]he dominance of the individual-risk model and the low acceptance of risks in the male contraceptive community, industry, and in the culture at large, particularly if it concerns men, has culminated in a quest for zero risk' (p. 449).

While these studies offer relevant insights into the topic of bodies at risk, there is a lack of information on how, in practice, bodies at risk in sexual health are socially constructed. The aim of this article is therefore to unveil the process-based, constitutive nature of risk profiling in sexual health institutions. In doing so, it will draw on Elizabeth Wheatley's definition of bodies at risk. In her study on how 'bodies at risk' of heart disease are encouraged to do fitness in order to reduce this risk, Wheatley (2005) explains that '[p]eople are discursively constituted as bodies at risk, subjected to medical scrutiny, and objects of medical discipline, surveillance, and control' (p. 202). In this article, we see how this definition can be applied to the case of bodies at risk in sexual health.

The governmentality of risk

We are all surrounded by countless risks: environmental, lifestyle, medical, interpersonal, economic, criminal, and so on (Lupton, 2013, p. 22). As Lupton (2013) explains, '[r]isk is seen as something that can be managed through human intervention; and risk is associated with notions of choice, responsibility and blame' (p. 37). Furthermore, 'risk is considered as objective, as well as predictable and controlled by science' (Gouilhers-Hertig, 2017, p. 42). Yet, risk does not exist in itself, but is the product of social relations (Gouilhers-Hertig, 2017, p. 4). In other words, what societies consider to be 'risky' depends on socio-cultural contexts (Lupton, 2013, p. 21).

Drawing on Michel Foucault's definition of governmentality, in this article I adopt the 'governmentality of risk' perspective, as it can offer a heuristic account of the construction of risks (Aradau & Van Munster, 2007; Ewald, 1991; Gouilhers-Hertig, 2017; Lupton, 1999, 2013; Maffi & Gouilhers, 2019; Rich et al., 2011). This perspective is characterised by the situatedness of risk: '[It] is only through these discourses, strategies, practices and institutions that we come to know "risk"' (Lupton, 2013, p. 114).

Furthermore, the governementality of risk establishes a relation between risk, power and technologies of surveillance (Lupton, 1999, 2013; Maffi & Gouilhers, 2019, p. 2).

This is a top-down relation, in which experts are key actors. Among other actors, they formulate imperative statements '[on] individuals' behaviours and subjectivities in relation to health, risk and embodiment' (Lupton, 2011, pp. 637–638). For example, in addition to lay advice, pregnant women are surrounded by expert advice: '[t]old to avoid smoking, drinking alcohol and coffee and taking other drugs, to eat a nutritious diet and engage in regular exercise' (Lupton, 2013, p. 120).

However, the governmentality of risk approach does not imply that power relations are merely top-down (Gouilhers-Hertig, 2017, p. 38); rather, power can also be (re)produced by individuals themselves (Gouilhers-Hertig, 2017, p. 37). Following Foucault's (2004) definition of power, I argue that power is 'the conduct of the conduct' (pp. 3, 191, 327). In this perspective,

> Rather than mainly being externally policed by agents of the state, individuals police themselves, they exercise power upon themselves as normalized subjects who are in pursuit of their own best interest and freedom, who are interested in self-improvement, seeking happiness and healthiness. (Lupton, 2013, p. 119)

According to this approach, certain groups of individuals are, then, labelled as being 'at risk' and '[r]equiring particular forms of knowledges and interventions' (Lupton, 2013, p. 117). For instance, in her research on childbirth in Switzerland, Solène Gouilhers-Hertig (2017) shows that women who are labelled 'psycho-social cases' are under the surveillance of midwives (p. 280). Further, individuals considered to be at risk are expected to be 'responsible' (Maffi & Gouilhers, 2019, p. 2), and to regulate themselves according to social norms (Lupton, 2013, p. 37). Thus,

> [i]f a certain population group is identified through statistical calculations as being at 'high risk' of developing heart disease, based on such attributes as gender, age and diet, then members of that group are then encouraged to deal with the risk factors themselves. (Lupton, 2013, p. 130)

As Lupton explains, these labelling processes are linked to a dimension of otherness, based on gender, class, race and ableism dynamics: '[W]omen, the working class, non-whites, the disabled and gay men are set apart as the Other' (Lupton, 2013, p. 181). As she explains, 'such bodies are culturally represented as subject to the will of the flesh rather than that of reason, prone to emotionality, excessive desire, violence or disarray' (Lupton, 2013, p. 181). Further, labelling certain individuals as being 'at risk' has social consequences: '[It] often serves to reinforce the marginalized or powerless status of individuals' (Lupton, 2013, p. 155). By contrast, dominant bodies are not perceived as being 'at risk', as in the case of '[t]he white able-bodied, bourgeois, heterosexual masculine body' (Lupton, 2013, p. 181). Risk thus reveals the existence of power relations based on gender, class, race and ableism.

The governmentality of risk approach is particularly useful to my research mainly for two reasons. First, this theory represents a unique tool to analyse how risk in sexual health is (re)produced throughout social interactions. Secondly, by putting an emphasis on experts, we can better understand both the role of sexual health professionals and the power relations between them and the individuals who consult them on a voluntary basis.

In the case of my ethnographic research sexual health professionals represent key actors in the prescription and promotion of molecular technologies. As I will explain more in detail, they are 'the gatekeepers of molecular technologies'.

Methodology and context of the research

As explained previously, this article is based on ethnographic fieldwork, conducted in two sexual health institutions in 2018: a sexual health centre for the general public, and a sexual health centre for MSM. I used two qualitative methods: ethnographic observation and in-depth interviewing. During seven months of fieldwork, I attended the two institutions as an observer, surveying their staff members' daily routines. Following the workflow of the two centres, I was present four half-days per week and I observed 91 sexual health consultations in the sexual health centre for the general public. At the sexual health centre for MSM, I attended between two to three half-days per week and I observed 73 sexual health consultations. During the consultations, I took notes in a field notebook, without intervening. All descriptions were transcribed to a computer file that same evening or the following day.

In addition, I conducted in-depth interviews with all sexual health professionals working in the two institutions. In this article, I focus on six in-depth interviews with three sexual health counsellors and three physicians, all of them women.[2] The interviews lasted between one to three hours, and were audio-recorded with the agreement of the participants, and transcribed verbatim. I used the qualitative software Atlas.TI to code and inductively analyse the gathered data (Holton, 2007, p. 265). Both participant observations and in-depth interviews are examined in this article. The language of the ethnography was French, and I translated the excerpts presented here into English myself.

My research project was evaluated by the research ethics committee located in one canton where part of the fieldwork was conducted. As it judged that my research did not fall under the scope of the 'Federal Act on Research Involving Human Being' (Admin.ch, 2011), the committee decided that the ethical guidelines were to be set up independently. Hence, permissions to conduct the observations and interviews were first obtained from the hierarchy of the two institutions. Next, permissions were obtained from sexual health professionals, as well as from individuals who were consulting the professionals at the time. In the case of the in-depth interviews, I obtained written permissions before starting the discussion. Participants were given enough time to read the informed consent form and ask questions, and were given a copy. Participants were also given the right to ask me to leave their consultation, or to interrupt the interview at any time. Finally, both the organisations and the participants' identity have been anonymised.

The COCP and the sexual health centre for the general public

In the Western world, women gained access to the COCP in the 1960s (Mottier, 2008, p. 54), and this event was part of what Caroline Rusterholz (2015) describes as a 'contraceptive revolution' (p. 41). It introduced a new social norm of sexuality, by separating 'erotic sexual activity' from 'procreation' (Giami, 2016, p. 5). Moreover, according to Claire Grino (2014), the COCP was part of a process of 'biologisation of contraception' with three main tendencies: '[a]n investment in physiological processes within women's bodies to prevent pregnancies, a prescription of a medication to individuals who are not sick, and a treatment presenting no therapeutic purposes' (p. 2).

In Switzerland, the COCP became available in 1961 (Rusterholz, 2015, p. 44). It is currently delivered under a medical prescription. In 2017, it was one of the most common methods of contraception in Switzerland (27%), following the male condom (33.9%) (OFS, 2019). A quarter of women aged 15–49 years old are taking the COCP (Obsan, 2017, p. 1). One blister pack (one-month dosage) costs between 9 and 24 Swiss Francs (CIAO.ch, 2003). The Swiss Compulsory Health Care does not reimburse the COCP.

The COCP is prescribed in the sexual health centre for the general public that was one of the sites for my ethnographic research. Most commonly known as a 'family planning clinic', as they were previously called, these centres were created in the 1970s (Praz, 2017). They are public institutions, or private institutions recognised by the State. Their services include the following main areas: contraceptive methods, Sexually Transmitted Infection (STI) tests, 'pregnancy ambivalences' (described by medical science as 'the conflict of wanting or not wanting to have a child' (Holmgren & Uddenberg, 1993, p. 15)), and abortion. Sexual health consultations are free. STI tests, pregnancy tests and contraceptive methods (mainly external condoms and the COCP) are sold at a reduced price. In some institutions sexual health counsellors collaborate with gynaecologists; in others, sexual health professionals work independently.

The sexual health centre in this research is located in a small town servicing a mostly rural area. The centre employs three female sexual health counsellors, who work part-time, and there are no gynaecologists. In this article, I use the term 'client' – widely used by sexual health counsellors – to indicate individuals who consult counsellors on a voluntary basis. According to the centre's 2018 annual report, most clients are women (71%) and under the age of 20. During my fieldwork, I noticed that, although I met some individuals with a relatively high socio-economic background, such as university students, most women were white, and many had a relatively low socio-economic background.

PrEP and the sexual health centre for MSM

In 2016, the Swiss Federal Commission for Sexual Health (an extra-parliamentary commission providing strategic and political advice to Government in the fight against HIV/AIDS and other sexually transmitted infections, FCSH, n.d.) published a list of medical recommendations for the use of PrEP (FCSH, 2016). Most notably, it ruled that PrEP can only be prescribed by a physician and requires medical supervision every three months (AIDS, n.d.). In Switzerland, '[PrEP] is available under the name Truvada® for CHF 900 per month (packs containing 30 tablets)' (FCSH, 2016). It is therefore a rather expensive treatment, however, as sexual health professionals explained to me, some generic drugs are imported online by individuals. Since PrEP is a preventive medication, the Swiss Compulsory Health Care does not reimburse it. There are currently between 1200 and 1700 users of PrEP in this country (PrEPWatch, 2020), almost exclusively MSM (OFSP, 2019, p. 10). According to the Federal Office of Public Health, this can be explained in two ways: First, MSM are particularly at risk of getting infected by HIV because of the prevalence of HIV among MSM; and second, there is a 'density of

MSM sexual networks', meaning that it is assumed that MSM have numerous partners (OFSP, 2019, p. 10).

PrEP is prescribed in the sexual health centre for MSM that was my second fieldwork site. This type of institution is dedicated to gay men, bisexual men, MSM, trans* persons and male sex workers. They were established in the 2000s to provide HIV testing to the gay community. Initially, it was a peer-to-peer service, provided by members of the gay community. Subsequently, the centre became progressively 'medicalised', although it remained a community service. Today, sexual health professionals working in this type of institution are physicians, nurses and sexual health counsellors. The mandate of these institutions is focused on testing, diagnosis and treatment of STIs, vaccinations for hepatitis and HPV, and PrEP and post-exposure prophylaxis (PEP), (a medication taken in case of potential exposure to HIV (NHS.UK, n.d.)).

The sexual health centre for MSM in this fieldwork is located in a large city. Three female physicians, two male nurses and one male sexual health counsellor are employed part-time. The nurses and the sexual health counsellor define themselves as part of the gay community. Sexual health professionals in this institution refer to the term 'users' to indicate individuals who consult them on a voluntary basis. According to my observations, users are mainly white men. The institution's 2018 annual report states that the average age of users is 34 years. During my fieldwork, I also noted that it is not uncommon to meet men with a middle or high socio-economic status. Yet, there were also users who struggle to pay for their tests or their treatments. Finally, I found that when users define their sexual orientation during the sexual health consultations, they usually define themselves as gay men.

Findings

The findings of my ethnographic fieldwork are divided into two sections. First, I show how sexual health professionals classify bodies at risk by doing a risk assessment of individuals based on their health condition, as well as their lifestyle. As other sociological studies of health have demonstrated, risk is classified along a continuum, running from low to high risk (Maffi & Gouilhers, 2019, p. 2). The result of this assessment determines if individuals will get access to the molecular technology. If this is the case, sexual health professionals accept the risk induced by the molecules, namely the side effects, which are considered 'trivial' or 'small' risks. These trivial or small risks were evident in my observations. Regarding the COCP, these 'trivial' risks mainly consist of a feeling of tension during menstruation, bleeding between menstruation cycles, decrease of libido, mood changes, weight gain and water retention. In the case of PrEP, 'small' side effects mainly regard digestive issues, allergies and insomnia, as well as potential damage to the liver, kidneys, and bones.

By contrast, the second section demonstrates that bodies considered to be at high risk might not get a prescription of molecular technology, or may have their treatment interrupted. In other words, sexual health professionals estimate that the interactions between individual risk and risk induced by molecular technologies are too important in those cases. This section also shows that sexual health professionals encounter borderline situations that lead them to make compromises between different risks and they adapt medical protocols accordingly.

Hierarchising bodies at risk

In the sexual health centre for general public, I found that a large number of women use the COCP, or wish to start using this method of contraception. Even though they are not physicians, the centre's sexual health counsellors are allowed to prescribe the COCP for three months. The first COCP blister pack (one-month dosage) is usually prescribed during a consultation lasting approximately one hour, when the sexual health counsellors estimate the client's individual risk by asking questions about their health condition and lifestyle. For example, the following fieldnotes describe a counsellor estimating the risk for two twin sisters:

> During the medical investigation, the sexual health counsellor asks the two women if they feel pain during menstruation. Then, she asks them if they smoke, if any of their family members has medical antecedents regarding specific health issues, such as cardiovascular illness, diabetes, thrombosis, hypertension and cancer. Then, the sexual health counsellor asks them if they have any allergies and if they have got acne.

This excerpt shows that, in order to get a COCP prescription, individuals must be healthy and have no medical antecedents among their blood relatives. Lifestyle, especially a smoking habit, is also an important element when classifying profiles of risk factors. In other words, women who would like to get a COCP prescription should preferably be young non-smokers, without medical issues, and without medical antecedents in their blood relatives' health history. This low-risk profile must be completed in order to avoid one main risk induced by molecules, which the sexual health counsellors labelled as a 'non-trivial risk': thrombosis. According to them, the risk of thrombosis increases by five to six times for women who are taking the COCP.

If women corresponded to a low risk profile, the sexual health counsellors accepted a series of risks, labelling them as 'trivial side effects' (feeling of tension during menstruation, bleeding between menstruation cycles, decrease of libido, mood changes, weight gain and water retention). They also said that these 'trivial side effects' usually only occur between the first and third months after starting the medication.

If a counsellor decided to prescribe the COCP, the three blister packs (three-months dosage) were not instantly delivered to women. They only received the first blister pack, and had to come back two more times for the other two blister packs. The COCP thus clearly implies a medical surveillance (Lupton, 2013, p. 156). After three consultations and the prescription of three COCP blister packs, the sexual health counsellors were not allowed to prescribe a fourth one. If women want to keep using this method of contraception, they have to make an appointment with a gynaecologist or a general practitioner (GP). Hence, there is a hierarchical work division between the different gatekeepers of molecular technologies. Not surprisingly, in the case of the COCP, gynaecologists represent the highest-level experts, followed by sexual health professionals, and in most cases, I observed that sexual health counsellors advise women to make an appointment with a gynaecologist, rather than with a GP.

In the sexual health centre dedicated to MSM, PrEP is a central molecular technology used for the promotion of sexual health. If users wish to start this treatment, they must first go through a medical consultation of approximately 30 minutes, with one of the three physicians. As in the case of the COCP prescription, the sexual health professionals assess a risk profile of MSM by evaluating their health condition and lifestyle. Based on a medical protocol, this assessment is necessary to decide if PrEP can be prescribed. Similarly to the women who want to use the COCP, users must correspond to a low-risk profile in order to be eligible for PrEP treatment. More precisely, they must have a negative HIV serology at least six weeks after the most recent risk situation; they must present a 'normal' renal function; they should not suffer from hepatitis infection; and they must have undergone additional laboratory investigations for hepatitis A, B and C, and for syphilis (FCSH, 2016). If users prove not to be immune to hepatitis A and B, they must get a vaccination (FCSH, 2016). Users also have to get anal, oral and urethral smears for two bacterial STIs: Gonorrhoea and Chlamydia (FCSH, 2016). Additionally, users might need to get an optimisation of vitamin D (FCSH, 2016). The sexual health professionals also ask users if they are under medical treatment, if they have been hospitalised and if they have any allergies (FCSH, 2016). As with the COCP prescription, their lifestyle is also evaluated. Notably, the sexual health professionals check if users are taking any illicit drugs, as is illustrated in the following extract:

> She [the physician] asks him if he takes illicit drugs. The man replies that he smokes cannabis and takes poppers, on average once per month. He also adds that he smokes. The physician exclaims: 'And you smoke! OUCH!!! This is almost the worst!' She suggests he tries to quit smoking. The man then says that he already took GHB [gamma-Hydroxybutric acid] twice. The physician tells him to be careful with this drug.

As in the case of the COCP, certain risks induced by the molecular technology – such as digestive side effects, allergies and insomnia – are accepted if the individual presents a low-risk profile. For example, during one consultation that I attended, the user received negative laboratory results, and told the physician that he has been completely abstinent for the past five months. Regarding this low-risk profile, the extract below shows the physician's choice to take these side effects risks and the man's willingness to run these risks himself:

> The physician prescribes the treatment [PrEP] for one month. She says: 'It may affect your digestion a little'. She adds that he may also have allergies and insomnia. The man replies: 'If we read the side effects of medications, we would not take any of them!' The physician says: 'I agree with you!'

In addition to digestive symptoms, allergies and insomnia, PrEP may provoke other undesirable effects that medical practitioners are willing to accept if users present a low-risk profile. These risks concern potential damage to the liver, the kidneys and the bones. With regard to the latter, these effects can be explained by the fact that PrEP may interrupt the attachment of calcium, consequently leading to osteoporosis in the long run. Hence, physicians need to check the user's vitamin D level before prescribing PrEP, as it plays a key role in the absorption of nutrients by the body. For instance, in the following consultation with one of the three physicians, a man expresses his willingness to start PrEP. The physician discusses the side effects of PrEP with the user:

> The physician explains to the man that studies have shown that PrEP has allowed for an incidental decrease of HIV infections in London. She explains what the side effects of PrEP are. She says: 'This drug, it has some small side effects!' She explains that these effects are rare, but that PrEP may have effects on the kidney, on bones. Therefore, it is necessary to check the D vitamin level before starting the treatment. She explains that concerning bones, the effects of PrEP are completely reversible as soon as the treatment is stopped.

If users start taking PrEP, they have to undergo medical supervision in the sexual health centre for MSM every three months, as encapsulated by this comment made by a physician to a man who came to the centre for information on the treatment: 'PrEP is accompanied by medical monitoring!'.

During medical supervisions, the sexual health professionals re-evaluate users' risk profiles via an HIV test, a syphilis test, and anal, oral and urethral smears for Gonorrhoea and Chlamydia (FCSH, 2016). This medical check-up also represents an 'evaluation and promotion of drug treatment adherence' and an 'evaluation of adverse effects and potential interactions' (FCSH, 2016). Hence, as for the COCP, PrEP implies continued surveillance (Lupton, 2013, p. 156) of MSM under PrEP treatment, even if they present a low-risk profile.

High risk bodies and borderline cases

Regarding both the COCP and PrEP, sexual health professionals will not accept risks associated with molecular technologies if the individuals do not present a low-risk profile. In other words, certain bodies are too risky. Even though I rarely encountered these situations, they offer relevant insights into the issue under examination here. In the case of COCP, following the rules of the medical protocol, if risks are perceived as cumulative, or if individuals present a 'non-trivial' risk, the sexual health professionals may not prescribe it. In this case, they will send the female client to a gynaecologist. As one counsellor explained during an interview,

> […] for me … as soon as the blood pressure is too high, or if their mothers had breast cancer, if there is hypertension and if the girl smokes a lot of cigarettes … for me, it is difficult. I send them to the gynaecologist.

I encountered some of these situations during my fieldwork. For example, one woman who came to the sexual health centre to start the COCP eventually did not receive it. During the consultation, she said that she occasionally smokes, and that she is allergic to aspirin. She explained that her brother has cardiac insufficiency, because he was born prematurely. Also, her mother had gestational diabetes and her grandmother had a thrombosis. Finally, she noted that several women in her family have had breast cancer. The sexual health counsellor decided to send this woman to a gynaecologist, because she concluded that the client had a high-risk profile. In this situation, the woman's profile was judged too risky, both in terms of health condition and lifestyle, and she therefore did not get a COCP prescription. Moreover, this situation once again shows that there is a hierarchy in the expertise of risk assessment, with gynaecologists being located at its top.

Similarly, physicians may refuse to prescribe PrEP if they find that users do not correspond to a low-risk profile. Contrary to the sexual health centre for the general public, though, physicians in the sexual centre for MSM stand at the top of the hierarchy of expertise. Thus, during an in-depth interview, one of the physicians explained to me that she almost refused to prescribe PrEP to one user, because he did not present a low-risk profile:

> [Me]: *Could you describe situations where you would not have recommended PrEP?*
>
> [Physician]: So, there was a person with whom I hesitated because of the anamnesis. He started to explain that he has got renal disease. And this is indeed a counter-indication. One of the components of the Truvada®, the tenofovir can, in some rare cases, have an impact on the renal function. So, with someone who already has a damaged renal function, we do not recommend prophylaxis medication that may risk worsening his renal function. I once had to face this situation. In the end, the renal function was not ... it was not a big issue, so the person could still use it [the PrEP], but that, that would have been a reason to say 'no' if there was a real issue with his renal function.

Nevertheless, there are situations where things run less smoothly, as shown by the following borderline case. A woman comes to the sexual health centre to get a prescription for the COCP. She smokes 10 cigarettes per day, which sexual health professionals consider as a risk factor.

> The sexual health counsellor asks the woman: 'Do you smoke?' The woman says 'yes'. The sexual health counsellor grimaces and tells her: 'Cigarette increases the risk of thrombosis, so I am currently I little bit embarrassed ... ' [the counsellor sighs, and pouts]. She adds, with a slightly ironic smile: 'Don't you have any intention to quit smoking?' The woman seems a bit confused, she puts her hands together and replies: 'Yes, I do!'

As this woman does not present any other risk, the sexual health counsellor eventually decides to prescribe the COCP. According to my fieldnotes, she tells the woman the following:

> 'So, okay, I do agree to prescribe the COCP. IF (!), there is an IF! [she stops speaking for a few seconds, to place emphasis on her words] IF you do not increase your tobacco consumption, or IF you decrease it!' The woman replies that she will not increase her consumption. She adds that, during the week, she only smokes three to four cigarettes a day.

This excerpt shows that sexual health professionals make compromises between different risks if individuals do not present a clear low-risk profile. In between two sexual health consultations, I asked one counsellor to explain how she evaluates the risk of associating the COCP with tobacco, as the medical protocol does not give any quantitative indication of a maximum threshold of cigarettes:

> Regarding cigarettes, she tells me that she estimates that women should not smoke more than ten cigarettes per day. She also explains that arterial problems are considered an eliminatory factor. She adds that she adapts the risk assessment to different criteria: sometimes certain risks are 'stronger', sometimes it is 'the combination, the cumulation of small risks' that is determining.

In their study on classifications, Geoffrey C. Bowker and Susan Leigh Star (1999) state that 'people do not really follow formal rules; they make up their own' (p. 71). As the previous excerpt shows, sexual health professionals tend to adapt protocols in borderline situations.

Regarding PrEP, sexual health professionals face specific ethical dilemmas in borderline cases, which again lead them to seek compromises between risks. Since some users take PrEP without the required risk assessment and without medical prescription, physicians fear its misuse. Sexual health professionals have labelled this phenomenon as 'wild PrEP'. According to them, misuse by non-experts is particularly worrying, because it could lead to resistance to triple therapies. Thus, one physician explained to me that the risk implied by PrEP should be managed exclusively in a medical context, with regular medical supervision (every three months):

> I tell myself, I prefer to prescribe PrEP, even though I tell myself that 'it is maybe not completely indicated', but the person is absolutely willing to take it, so rather than for him to take a random Truvada®, without any control [*sic*]. Because there are a lot of people who do that! [People who] certainly buy anywhere online, or people who trade stuff, wrong stuff, [...], because they have bad knowledge of it [the PrEP].

As this example shows, physicians make compromises between different risks, on a case-by-case basis, in order to avoid misuse of PrEP that could lead to resistance to triple therapies.

According to Gouilhers-Hertig (2017), medical protocols are mainly 'manufactured' by physicians, following the principles of evidence-based medicine (p. 139). In her research on childbirth, she shows that health practitioners, however, renegotiate the protocols through 'informal practices' (p. 160). The excerpts taken from my ethnographic research show that an assessment of the various risks in sexual health is an ongoing process that can lead to an adaptation of the protocols via these 'informal practices' (Gouilhers-Hertig, 2017, p. 160).

Conclusion

Through a heuristic comparison between the COCP and PrEP, distributed in two Swiss sexual health institutions, I have made an empirical contribution to the literature on bodies at risk. By putting an emphasis on the process-based risk profiling in two sexual health institutions, I have argued that the category of the body at risk in sexual health is a complex social construction, which determines access to molecular technologies. As gatekeepers of molecular technologies, sexual health professionals play a key role, since they represent experts with the power to grant or deny access to these technologies.

I have demonstrated two main empirical results. First, bodies are constructed as being at high or low risk by sexual health professionals (based on the individuals' health condition and lifestyle). Second, access to molecular technology is based on the former classification. On the one hand, bodies with a low-risk profile get access to molecular technologies, and certain risks (side effects) thereof as they interact with the individual's body are accepted. On the other hand, if bodies are classified as high risk, they may not get access to molecular technology. Furthermore, sexual health professionals encounter borderline cases. This leads them to make compromises between different risks, notably by pragmatically adapting medical protocols.

The implications of these results are significant. First, they reveal that risk, in sexual health, is not limited to sexual practices or safe sex. Rather, risk in sexual health is about whether a person's body is considered healthy enough to accept molecular technologies. Therefore, the process described in this study medicalises not only sexuality, but it also medicalises bodies. In other words, sexual and reproductive bodies become medical risks themselves, through the process of the sexual health consultations. Secondly, ethnographic studies like this one can deepen our knowledge on the dynamics of risk construction, at a micro-level. The findings highlight the complexity of social interactions that take place and interlink risk, bodies, sexuality, and health. By focusing on the relations between sexual health professionals and individuals who consult on a voluntary basis, our understanding of this nexus, and of the power relations at play is enhanced.

In a nutshell, by putting the emphasis on constitutive practices of risk profiling, this ethnographic research has shown that gatekeeping, expertise and risk assessments have concrete effects on bodies seeking molecular technologies. A person's access to molecular technologies is fully determined based on sexual health professionals' classification of risky bodies. Moreover, as molecular technologies become more central to the management of sexual health risk, the risk assessment procedure by sexual health professionals becomes more routinised for certain individuals. Further studies would benefit from a more focused examination of this routinisation on individuals' sexual health, and particularly that of precarious, racialised, and *trans individuals' sexual health. Finally, in line with what Bowker and Star (1999) have stated, this research proves that 'whatever appears as universal or indeed standard, is the result of negotiations, organizational processes, and conflict' (p. 61).

Notes

1. All translations of French citations are mine.
2. In this article, the notions of 'woman' and 'man' refer to cisgender persons, meaning that their gender identity matches the one they were assigned at birth.

Acknowledgements

I would like to thank Claudine Burton-Jeangros, Armelle Weil, Camille Bajeux, Carolina Topini, and the researchers of the Reproductive Sociology Research Group (ReproSoc) for their precious suggestions. Thanks to the editors and the anonymous peer reviewers for their insightful comments. I would also like to thank the participants who took part of this research. Finally, thanks to Andrea Hajek, and Anouk Severin for their language editing.

Disclosure statement

No potential conflict of interest was reported by the author(s).

References

Admin.ch. (2011). *Federal Act on Research Involving Human Being*. https://web.archive.org/web/20200527081839/https://www.admin.ch/opc/en/classified-compilation/20061313/

Aide Suisse contre le SIDA (AIDS). (n.d.). *PrEP*. https://www.aids.ch/en/faq/protection-and-risk/prep/

Aradau, C., & Van Munster, R. (2007). Governing terrorism through risk: Taking precautions, (un)knowing the future. *European Journal of International Relations*, *13*(1), 89–115.

Bowker, G. C., & Star, S. L. (1999). *Sorting things out: Classification and its consequences.* Cambridge, MA: MIT Press.

Caiata-Zufferey, M. (2015). Genetically at-risk status and individual agency. A qualitative study on asymptomatic women living with genetic risk of breast/ovarian cancer. *Social Science & Medicine, 132*, 141–148.

CIAO.ch. (2003). *Combien coûte la pilule ?* https://www.ciao.ch/questions/379580-combien-coute-la-pilule/

Ewald, F. (1991). Insurance and risk. In P. M. Miller, G. Burchell, & C. Gordon (Eds.), *The Foucault effect: Studies in governmentality: With two lectures by and an interview with Michael Foucault / edited by Graham Burchell, Colin Gordon, Peter Miller* (pp. 197–210). Chicago: The University of Chicago Press.

FCSH. (2016). *Recommendations of the Swiss Federal Commission for Sexual Health (FCSH) on pre-exposure prophylaxis (PrEP) for HIV prevention.* https://www.bag.admin.ch/bag/en/home/das-bag/organisation/ausserparlamentarische-kommissionen/eidgenoessische-kommission-fuer-sexuelle-gesundheit-eksg.html

FCSH. (n.d.). *Swiss Federal Commission for Sexual Health.* https://www.bag.admin.ch/bag/en/home/das-bag/organisation/ausserparlamentarische-kommissionen/eidgenoessische-kommission-fuer-sexuelle-gesundheit-eksg.html

Foucault, M. (2004). *Naissance de la biopolitique: Cours au Collège de France (1978-1979)* (M. Senellart, F. Ewald, & A. Fontana, Eds.). Paris: Gallimard/Seuil.

Giami, A. (2016). De l'émancipation à l'institutionnalisation: Santé sexuelle et droits sexuels. *Genre, Sexualité & Société, 15*, 1–14.

Gouilhers-Hertig, S. (2017). *Gouverner par le risque: Une ethnographie comparée des lieux d'accouchement en Suisse romande.* [Unpublished doctoral dissertation]. Geneva: University of Geneva.

Grino, C. (2014). La pilule: Biologisation de la contraception et régulation sociale. *Genre, Sexualité et Société, 12*, 1–24.

Holmgren, K., & Uddenberg, N. (1993). Ambivalence during Early pregnancy among Expectant mothers. *Gynecologic and Obstetric Investigation, 36*(1), 15–20.

Holton, J. A. (2007). The coding process and its challenges. In A. Bryant & K. Charmaz (Eds.), *The SAGE handbook of grounded theory* (pp. 265–289). Los Angeles: SAGE.

Jeangros, C., & Bourrier, M. (2014). *Ni malades, ni en bonne santé.* Paris: Publications de la Sorbonne.

Kent, J., & Farrell, A.-M. (2015). Risky bodies in the plasma bioeconomy: A feminist analysis. *Body & Society, 21*(1), 29–57.

Lupton, D. (1999). *Risk.* London: Routledge.

Lupton, D. (2011). 'The best thing for the baby': Mothers' concepts and experiences related to promoting their infants' health and development. *Health, Risk & Society, 13*(7/8), 637–651.

Lupton, D. (2013). *Risk* (2nd ed.). Abingdon: Routledge.

Maffi, I., & Gouilhers, S. (2019). Conceiving of risk in childbirth: Obstetric discourses, medical management and cultural expectations in Switzerland and Jordan. *Health, Risk & Society, 21* (3–4), 185–206.

McDonald, K., Amir, L. H., & Davey, M.-A. (2011). Maternal bodies and medicines: A commentary on risk and decision-making of pregnant and breastfeeding women and health professionals. *BMC Public Health, 11*(5), 1–8.

Mottier, V. (2008). *Sexuality a very short introduction.* Oxford: Oxford University Press.

NHS.UK. (n.d.). *Can post-exposure prophylaxis (PEP) stop me getting HIV?* https://www.nhs.uk/common-health-questions/medicines/can-post-exposure-prophylaxis-pep-stop-me-getting-hiv/

Observatoire suisse de la santé (Obsan). (2017). *Communiqué de presse. En Suisse, quatre personnes sur cinq recourent à la contraception.* https://www.bfs.admin.ch/bfs/fr/home/statistiques/catalogues-banques-donnees/communiques-presse.assetdetail.2905775.html

Office fédéral de la santé publique (OFSP). (2019). *VIH, syphilis, gonorrhée et chlamydiose en Suisse en 2018: Survol épidémiologique* (pp. 10–36). https://www.bag.admin.ch/bag/fr/home/krankheiten/krankheiten-im-ueberblick/hiv.html

Office fédéral de la statistique (OFS). (2019). *Santé reproductive.* https://web.archive.org/web/20191115201521/https://www.bfs.admin.ch/bfs/fr/home/statistiques/sante/etat-sante/reproductive.html

Praz, A.-F. (2017). Pionnières et pionniers du planning familial en Valais. Annales Valaisannes. *Numéro spécial consacré à l'histoire des femmes*, 199–219.

Preciado, P. B. (2019). *Un appartement sur Uranus: Chroniques de la traversée.* Paris: Bernard Grasset.

PrEPWatch. (2020). *Switzerland.* https://www.prepwatch.org/country/switzerland/

Rail, G., Molino, L., Fusco, C., Norman, M. E., Petherick, L., Polzer, J., … Bryson, M. (2018). HPV vaccination discourses and the construction of "at-risk" girls. *Canadian Journal of Public Health = Revue Canadienne de Santé Publique, 109*(5–6), 622–632.

Rich, E., Evans, J., & De Pian, L. (2011). Children's bodies, surveillance and the obesity crisis. In E. Rich, L. F. Monaghan, & L. Aphramor (Eds.), *Debating obesity: Critical perspectives* (pp. 139–163). Basingstoke: Palgrave Macmillan.

Rusterholz, C. (2015). Reproductive behavior and contraceptive practices in comparative perspective, Switzerland (1955–1970). *The History of the Family, 20*(1), 41–68.

Van Kammen, J., & Oudshoorn, N. E. J. (2002). Gender and risk assessment in contraceptive technologies. *Sociology of Health & Illness, 24*(4), 436–461.

Wheatley, E. E. (2005). Disciplining bodies at risk: Cardiac rehabilitation and the medicalization of fitness. *Journal of Sport and Social Issues, 29*(2), 198–221.

World Health Organization (WHO). (2002). *Sexual health.* https://www.who.int/topics/sexual_health/en/

Index

Page numbers in **bold** refer to tables and those in *italic* refer to figures.

Taylor & Francis Group
an **informa** business

Taylor & Francis eBooks

www.taylorfrancis.com

A single destination for eBooks from Taylor & Francis with increased functionality and an improved user experience to meet the needs of our customers.

90,000+ eBooks of award-winning academic content in Humanities, Social Science, Science, Technology, Engineering, and Medical written by a global network of editors and authors.

TAYLOR & FRANCIS EBOOKS OFFERS:

- A streamlined experience for our library customers
- A single point of discovery for all of our eBook content
- Improved search and discovery of content at both book and chapter level

REQUEST A FREE TRIAL

support@taylorfrancis.com

Routledge
Taylor & Francis Group

CRC Press
Taylor & Francis Group